Vectors of Death

Vectors of Death

The Archaeology of European Contact

Ann F. Ramenofsky

University of New Mexico Press

Albuquerque

Library of Congress Cataloging-in-Publication Data

Ramenofsky, Ann F. (Ann Felice), 1942–
Vectors of death.

Bibliography: p.
Includes index.
1. Indians of North America—Population.
2. Indians of North America—Diseases.
3. Epidemics—North America—History.
4. Diseases and history—North America.
I. Title.
E98.P76R36 1987 304.6′08997 87-19232
ISBN 0-8263-0997-6

First edition.

Contents

Figures

Tables

Preface

This project began when I was a graduate student at University of Washington. In a casual conversation with Bob Dunnell, I mentioned that I was interested in doing some research on the contact period of North America. In his off-handed way, Bob suggested that I look into the "disease business." I began reading, and the more I read, the more confusing the topic became. There was no consensus beyond the common recognition that European contact had forever changed the nature of Native American cultures. Major questions remained, including the timing of disease introduction, temporal onset of fundamental changes in relation to disease contact, and the placement of historical documents in the sequence of events of the contact period. Emotionally charged differences on these issues were so fundamental that acceptance of one stance meant the rejection of others.

It seemed to me that resolution of these basic problems were significant for two different but related reasons. Beginning with Boasian Anthropology, we have accepted, and even cherished, the assumption that historical documents or ethnographic descriptions were relevant analogues for reconstructing prehistoric systems. Yet, at the core of the debates on European contact sat the question of the nature of even the earliest descriptions. If these problems could be resolved in a preliminary way, we could contribute to a more objective rendering of the postcontact experience of Native Americans. Resulting descriptions could serve both scientific and humanistic ends.

In the end I decided that rather than accept anyone else's definitions and assumptions of European contact, I would focus my attention on the sixteenth century and attempt to resolve some of the key issues of contact period studies. Of major importance in my approach was the independent treatment of regional archaeological and historical records. This decoupling made the analysis far more difficult than I had anticipated. It meant, for instance, that I could not use existing archaeological chronologies, since they, by in large, were based on documents which were as biased and incomplete as the archaeological records and were themselves under investigation. New chronological work had to be undertaken in order to create archaeological sequences that were as free as possible of historically derived assumptions. Changes derived from archaeological analyses could then be compared with changes described in historical documents.

The results of this approach appear in the text and appendices of this book. I hope that I have clarified some of the basic issues in contact period studies, have provided new perspectives on some of these issues, and have suggested fruitful avenues of research that can be investigated for sometime to come.

Acknowledgments

I could not have completed this book without the assistance and support of numerous individuals. Bob Dunnell, Don Grayson, Robert Rausch, and Peter Nute were excellent guides and teachers and are now valued friends. Hank Dobyns encouraged me to seek publication even before my dissertation was completed. Bruce Trigger carefully read the Iroquois analysis and provided numerous comments and insights. I am also grateful to Jim Griffin for his meticulous and critical reading of the Lower Mississippi Valley sequence.

The collection of data was carried out at several institutions. Ray Wood opened his office and library (including Don Lehmer's notes) to me. Michael Trimble, then a graduate student working on the nineteenth-century smallpox record from the Middle Missouri, gave me access to microfilms from the Office of Indian Affairs. Jeff Brain provided copies of unpublished manuscripts on sites and sequences in the lower valley.

I would also like to thank colleagues and friends for helping me through the numerous drafts. Linda Cordell made several important suggestions on the organization of the text. My editor, Claire Sanderson, has been patient, supportive, and thorough. Ann Whitmer, Linda McQueen and Kathy Joiner read and reread the manuscript. Diane LeNoir handled all the revisions on the word processor. Mary Lee Eggart and Clifford Duplechin drafted my figures.

I owe a special thanks to my husband, Tom Wood, for his continuing support of this project and for suggesting an excellent title for the book. I thank our children, Ben and Kate, who, although too young to understand what I was doing, helped maintain my humor and perspective. I dedicate this work to all three.

This research was supported by several grants, including one from the American Association of University Women and an award from the Louisiana State University Council on Research.

One

The Population Debate in Perspective

For nearly a century, ethnologists, ethnohistorians, and demographic historians have carried on a lively debate that centers on the size of Native American population immediately prior to European contact. Three issues are at the heart of the debate: (1) precontact population size and magnitude of postcontact decline; (2) timing of the decline relative to the earliest census counts; (3) role of infectious disease in that decline.

Ethnologists of the American Historical School (Helm 1965, 1980; Kroeber 1934, 1939; Steward 1949) generally take a conservative position on these issues. They do not accord disease a major role in the early postcontact period, but date the recognized onset of aboriginal decline subsequent to historical documentation and sustained European settlement. Because the earliest census counts do not necessarily represent grossly reduced populations, they can provide indices for estimating population size during the late precontact period. Employing such counts typically results in a small aboriginal population base for A.D. 1492.

Ethnohistorians, typified by Dobyns (1966, 1981, 1983) and Krech (1978, 1983) and historical demographers, such as S. F. Cook (1976) and W. Borah (1976), envision an entirely different sequence of events during the contact period. They assume infectious diseases, a major cause in the destruction of aboriginal populations, reached regional groups decades, if not centuries, prior to historical documentation. Consequently, even the earliest census counts may describe populations as much as 95% reduced from precontact maxima; precontact estimates must then be orders of magnitude larger than postcontact counts. Given contrasts between positions, it is no wonder that for A.D. 1492, suggested totals for aboriginal North America range from 0.9 million (Kroeber 1939) to 18 million (Dobyns 1983).

Differences between estimates are, in part, explained by a series of historical factors. Ethnologists of the American Historical School focused on reconstructing native cultures prior to the arrival of Europeans. This focus initially grew out of a strong commitment to salvage the past and the belief that, although not racially inferior, native populations had not changed greatly throughout their development (Stocking 1976; Trigger 1981a, 1984). This school of thought believed that major changes including the introduction of disease occurred following European documentation and settlement and were of less concern. As Kroeber states:

> After some hesitation I have omitted . . . accounts of the relations of the natives with the Whites and events befalling them after such contact was established. It is not that this subject is unimportant, or uninteresting, but that I am not in a position to treat it adequately. It also is a matter that has comparatively slight relation to the original condition. . . . I might better contribute to the future writing of such a history by concentrating effort in the field to which my training and predilection has led me. . . . I have, therefore, considered contact only in special cases; as when necessary to form an estimate of an ancient vanished culture through the medium of its modern and modified representative (1925:VI).

Ethnologists employed informant memory, individual traits, and historical documents to recreate the past from the modified present. The static reconstruction set at the beginning of regional contact with Europeans became known as the ethnographic present.

The development of regional archaeological chronologies, acculturation studies, Native American land claim cases, and ethnohistory began to change the perspective on the American Indian. Chronological work on the archaeological record of North America began in earnest in the 1930s (Trigger 1984; Willey and Sabloff 1980). As studies accumulated, it became apparent that change, rather than stability, dominated the record. Acculturation studies that began during or shortly after World War II (Herskovits 1958; Malinowski 1945; Tax 1952) focused on gradual accommodations of Native American societies to European culture. Like archaeological investigations, these studies demonstrated that native populations and systems experienced considerable disruption. (See for example, Spicer 1961, 1962.) The study of ethnohistory developed with American Indian land claims and reinforced the impression of change.

The consequence of all this research resulted in a reevaluation of the ethnographic present. In 1955, Steward argued that ethnographic descriptions of Native Americans were not "primary data" and should not be construed to represent pristine populations or systems. More recently still, Dobyns writes that the ethnographic present

> may be termed "divorced from reality." No such cultural phase existed; ethnographies written in the ethnographic present are like paintings of extinct birds based on hearsay and on the artist's imagination. The methods and techniques traditionally employed by ethnographers are not capable of recovering from a very small handful of survivors an accurate portrait of societies that have not functioned for decades—and in many instances centuries—prior to the arrival of the ethnographer (1983:26).

Despite the growing recognition of discontinuity in aboriginal populations and systems through the contact period, the position advanced primarily by Kroeber continues into the present (see for example, Fenton 1985; Helm 1965, 1980). Consequently, ethnologists and ethnohistorians continue to debate problems of timing, magnitude, and cause(s) of aboriginal population change during the early contact period. Moreover, because scholars are using the same type of data to reach contradictory conclusions, the debate cannot be resolved solely within the field of ethnology.

As Borah (1976) and others (Dobyns 1983; Heizer 1941; Trigger 1985) have noted, archaeologists could make significant contributions to the question of population change during the contact period. The record is temporal and incorporates data on population size or density. Nonetheless, archaeologists, with few exceptions (Heizer 1941; Perttula 1984; Ramenofsky 1982; Smith 1984; Snow and Starna 1984; Trigger 1985; Upham 1982), have not entered this field of research. The reason for this oversight seems to lie in the current goals and methods of demographic archaeology.

Even though the archaeological record of population is not comparable to historic period census counts, a major goal of demographic archaeology is to develop absolute counts of people (Hassan 1981). To derive such estimates archaeologically requires the use of some sort of modern standard or analogue. More often than not, these analogues, taken from historical or ethnographic counts of population, are drawn from the low end of the population scale. Low estimates fail to consider questions of early disease introduction and resulting decline of population. Consequently, archaeologists who employ these estimates as analogues are accepting the position of demographic continuity throughout the period of European contact.

Thus, while ethnologists and ethnohistorians are debating an issue to which archaeologists could make genuine contributions, the archaeological goal of developing absolute estimates of population has limited that contribution. This situation is all the more ironic since, as noted by several archaeologists (Dunnell 1980; Leone 1972), American archaeologists have always been consumers of ethnological ideas and models. In the field of Native American demography, archaeologists have largely accepted the conservative stance and have not considered the alternative approach.

This work approaches the population debate from an archaeological perspective. Because the archaeological record is not isomorphic with the historical record, the scope of the study does not include many of the fine points of the ethnological debate. Nonetheless, it does address the following key questions: whether the decline postdated A.D. 1492 (but predated sustained European settlement and documentation at a regional scale), whether the decline was catastrophic in nature, and whether disease was causal in that decline.

This investigation necessitates that the archaeological record of population change be evaluated independently of historical or ethnographic records. Consequently, although archaeological and historical records are considered, they are treated as independent sets of data. While this approach precludes providing absolute estimates of people, it does not prevent an assessment of the validity of each side of the debate. Positions are so fundamentally different that relative or ordinal estimates of population change are sufficient for resolving these questions.

The pattern of archaeological change in population is developed through analysis of settlement, the archaeological variable most closely tied to population (Hassan 1981; Schacht 1981, 1984). If Kroeber's position is correct, then analyses of settlements should suggest a pattern of stability until the period of historic documentation. If, on the other hand, Dobyns's position is correct, patterns of settlement should show drastic changes commensurate with population loss prior to the beginning of written records.

Since the primary goal of this work is to build a pattern of population change through the contact period, settlement analyses must be regional in scope. Although it would be convenient to identify and trace changes in population size or density at a single site, such an approach is not appropriate. As suggested by twentieth-century census counts of native populations, some individuals have survived in almost all situations; thus, a local archaeological record could be at variance with the larger pattern. While learning something about continuity in population, this approach would not systematically consider the question of discontinuity.

Although this work addresses the role of disease, evidence for or against an early introduction is, at best, indirect. With very few exceptions (Jackes 1983), disease-causing micro-organisms are not preserved in the archaeological record. Thus, arguments for disease as causal in the decline hinge on the nature, rapidity, and timing of the loss. Under virgin soil conditions and in the absence of medical assistance, initial introductions of infectious parasites typically result in large-scale epidemics with mortality ranging from 30 to 100%. Catastrophes of this magnitude can completely alter the structure of population within one or two generations. If the loss is registered in the archaeological contact record and predates sustained European presence in the region, then disease is the only reasonable explanation of the event. If loss follows sustained colonization, then other variables could be responsible.

The organization of this book follows from the archaeological questions. First, it presents the necessary background for understanding the population debate. Historical and archaeological goals and methods of estimating population are specifically emphasized. A description of the archaeological methods employed in this analysis follows. Because the timing and pattern of population change has implications for the causes of such change, documentation of three regional test cases precedes consideration of the cause of population change. In Chapter 4, archaeological patterns are built and compared. The following chapter is devoted to the question of acute infectious disease. In Chapter 6, the results of this study are summarized and the implications discussed.

Two

Estimates of Aboriginal North America

THE ETHNOLOGICAL DEBATE

In recent decades the debate continues, if anything with greater participation and, one suspects, with no diminution of emotion (Borah 1976:13).

Numerous scholars have considered the North American population question; but, in recent years, Kroeber and Dobyns have been the major protagonists in the debate. Kroeber's landmark study *Cultural and Natural Areas of Native North America* (1939) established the modern precedent for low population estimates. Dobyns's recent book, *Their Number Become Thinned* (1983) challenges all Kroeber's conceptions. As seen in Table 1 differences in their estimates are so great that any single figure is rendered meaningless.

Since Kroeber and Dobyns are at opposite ends of the population question, and since both men have had major impacts on the field of aboriginal American demography, this discussion examines their positions in some detail. Other ethnologists, ethnohistorians, and demographers will be considered in light of the intellectual differences between these protagonists.

The most crucial distinction between Kroeber and Dobyns hinges on the role accorded disease during the period of European contact. Intellectual differences on this issue have ramifications regarding the evaluation of historic census counts and the methods used to reconstruct precontact population size.

The American Historical School excludes acute infectious disease as a major cause of population decline in the early postcontact period (Helm 1965, 1980;

Table 1 Comparison of Kroeber's and Dobyns's Estimates of Aboriginal North American Population

Area	*Kroeber (1939)* Size	Density[a]	*Dobyns (1983)* Size	Density[a]
Arctic and Subarctic	146,430	4.02–1.35	3,443,007	34
California	125,000[b]	5.0–70.0	336,060	77–120
Northwest Coast	129,000	28.30	1,204,723	116–120
N. Great Lakes	37,300	7.18	907,893	43
Plateau/Great Basin	74,350	2.47–7.15	3,722,323	43
Southwest	60,500	2.26–75.7	600,000	85
S. Great Lakes	42,500	9.61	3,800,000	386
East	426,400	6.95	4,008,000	253–572
TOTAL	1,041,480		18,022,006	

[a]Density per 100 km²
[b]Kroeber 1925

Helm et al. 1978; Kroeber 1934, 1939; Rosenblat 1976; Steward 1949; Thornton and Marsh-Thornton 1981). Consequently, native populations decline slowly if at all, justifying an assumption of continuity in population across the contact border. Precontact population size can be estimated from the earliest historical census counts through "dead reckoning or simple additive procedure" (Kroeber 1939:180).

If, because of disease, there was a substantial and rapid drop in population (Borah 1976), continuity in population size or density cannot be assumed. The earliest census counts must then be considered in light of catastrophic death from disease. The chasm between the earliest census counts and estimates of precontact population is filled by mathematically determined depopulation ratios (see for example, W. Borah and S. Cook 1963; N. Cook 1981; S. Cook 1973a; S. Cook and L. Simpson 1948; H. Dobyns 1966, 1983).

Dead Reckoning

Although Schoolcraft (1853–1857) made continental wide population estimates, Mooney (1910, 1928) is credited with the earliest systematic assessment of Native American population size. Drawing on all available historical documents, Mooney made a head count of Native Americans on a tribe-by-tribe basis. He filled in gaps in knowledge by projecting spatially from documented to unknown population units. Subsequently, tribes were divided into geographic areas, and estimates were presented for two different times (Table 2). The earlier dates correspond to Mooney's assessment for the beginning of European contact; the later date marks the beginning of his study.

According to Swanton, who edited *Aboriginal Population* after Mooney's

Table 2 Mooney's Aboriginal Population Estimates by Geographic Area

Area	*Date*	*Contact Population Size*	*1907 Population Size*	*Percentage Loss*
North Atlantic States	1600	45,600	21,900	61.0
South Atlantic States	1600	52,200	2,170	96.0
Gulf States	1650	114,400	62,700	45.0
Central States	1650	75,300	46,126	39.0
Plains	1780	141,800	55,338	62.0
Columbia Plateau	1780	89,300	15,431	82.7
California	1769	260,000	18,797	93.0
Central Mountains	1845	19,300	11,544	40.0
New Mexico/Arizona	1680	72,000	53,837	25.0
Other Areas (Canada, Alaska, Greenland)	Variable	273,100	176,000	Variable
TOTAL		1,153,000	406,000	

death, Mooney's estimates were lowered from his earlier investigations, but were "still somewhat high" (1928:2). Despite the high numbers, however, Mooney did recognize attrition of aboriginal population from alcohol and disease. Comparison of population size at the two intervals is evidence of this recognition. Decreases from the beginning of contact to 1907 range from 25 to 96%.

Mooney's estimates became the point of departure in Kroeber's demographic studies (1925, 1934, 1939). Like Mooney, Kroeber used a simple additive method and spatial projection. He also considered all available information: explorer accounts; missionary records; house and village counts; federal census counts; and informant memory.

While recognizing Mooney's contribution to the field of aboriginal demography, Kroeber went beyond simply enumerating people. Although not an environmental determinist, he viewed environment as setting broad limits for population density. "We infer a denser population from a rich ecology, or among agriculturalists, from a larger area of more fertile soil" (1939:180). As seen in Table 1, a rich ecological setting such as the Northwest Coast could support hunters and gatherers at densities greater than that of eastern agriculturalists.

Kroeber, more conservative than Mooney, believed that the latter's estimates for the beginning of European contact were "mostly too high rather than too low" (1939:132). Several assumptions lay behind this belief. Contemporary estimates were derived from figures taken from explorers' journals and mission records. Because both missionaries and explorers inflated their figures for political reasons, "the vast majority of figures made by contemporaries are too large" (1939:180). "Competent ethnologists with interest in concrete facts" (1939:180) could correct these errors by reducing counts.

In California, the state Kroeber knew best, Mooney's estimates were unrealistically high. Mooney derived his estimates for Californian populations from Merriam (1905). Merriam, in turn, estimated native Californians by projecting spatially from mission to nonmission areas and projecting backward temporally. He also considered population decline following European contact. Since Kroeber distrusted missionary records, he lowered Merriam's and Mooney's population estimates for California from .26 million to .125 million (Kroeber 1925). Ultimately, Kroeber thought his North American population total of 1.043 million would shrink to around .9 million.

Largely as a result of his California experience, Kroeber recognized that Indians had disappeared by the early twentieth century; but unlike Mooney, he did not consider aboriginal depopulation from disease (1925, 1939). "There is one Indian in California today for every eight that lived in the same area before the white man came" (1925:887). Kroeber, saddened by the attrition, refused to admit disease was a factor in the decline because he feared it would lead to overestimation of predisease populations. "Excessive exaggerations need also to be guarded against, such as the statement sometimes cited that 70,000 California Indians died of epidemic disease in a few years following 1830" (1925:881).

Nonetheless, Kroeber had to account for the obvious decline. In California, he attributed the loss to the intensity of European-native interaction: the more intense the interaction, the greater the aboriginal depopulation (1925). He used a different argument for the mound-building areas of the East (1939). Like numerous earlier investigators (Barton 1799; Harris 1835; Haven 1856; Thomas 1894), Kroeber acknowledged the discontinuity between the density of mounds and the thinly scattered historical populations. Also, like others, he assumed that the mound builders had been an agricultural society, which supported a greater population than the historically recorded tribes. Kroeber attributed the decline in population to persistent and unrelenting warfare and lack of political organization.

The most recent debate regarding depopulation from disease concerns band-level societies of the Arctic drainage lowlands of Canada and eastern Alaska. Helm (1965, 1968, 1980) and Krech (1978, 1983) are the key protagonists, and the principal question concerns the stability of the social structure of subarctic bands through the period of European contact. Population change enters into this conflict as the reason behind change or stability in their social forms.

Helm holds the conservative position. Although she does not make continental- or regional-scale estimates of precontact population, she uses many of Kroeber's assumptions to draw inferences about the structure of subarctic bands.

Helm's position (1965, 1968, 1980) is a reaction to the position of Service (1962) and Krech (1978, 1983). Both Service and Krech argue that because of epidemic mortality from infectious disease, the band structure of the Arctic drainage lowland Dene changed from a unilineal to a bilateral form. Because Helm can find no convincing evidence of epidemic mortality in the Hudson Bay records (1980), she argues that disease is not a factor in the initial period of European contact.

Several important consequences follow from Helm's position: First, population loss does not occur during the first several hundred years of European contact. Occasional losses due to disease or starvation are offset by a cessation of the practice of female infanticide. Because population is stable, band structure is also stable. Accordingly, bilaterality, in the Mackenzie Region, does not evolve following European contact; it predates the arrival of Europeans and persists until 1945. All major changes among these groups postdate 1945. The stability in population and social structure is reflected in Helm's chronological divisions of the contact period: Early contact, 1780–1821; contact traditional, 1821–1945; modern 1945–present (Helm et al. 1978).

In summary, Kroeber is primarily responsible for the argument that disease does not have catastrophic consequences on native populations either before or after sustained European settlement. As a consequence, large estimates of native populations taken from documents must be reduced or rejected; smaller estimates are accepted and projected back to 1492. The empirical result is a low population base for the beginning of contact; the theoretical result is the creation of Kroeber's "demographic present" fully comparable to the ethnographic present. Helm's position on disease and catastrophic decline demonstrates the continued popularity of the Kroeberian argument.

Depopulation Ratios

Although the argument that introduced disease caused a demographic catastrophe among Native Americans has intellectual roots in the sixteenth century, S. F. Cook and his associates (Borah and Cook 1963; Cook 1937, 1940, 1943, 1955, 1973a, 1973b, 1976; Cook and Borah 1960; Cook and Simpson 1948) are responsible for systematically defining this position. In a long series of studies, Cook attempted to document the magnitude of population loss and use that data as a baseline for projecting population back to the precontact period. Like Kroeber, California was a research area for Cook, but because his assumptions were different than Kroeber's, his estimates of population were much higher.

Cook was a historical demographer, not an ethnologist; consequently, he drew data from all the relevant historical records. Kroeber's ethnological knowledge related to the present and could not be extrapolated across a temporal gap that spanned some 400 years. When describing the epidemic environment of California some years after European contact began, Cook states:

> It is necessary to emphasize this demographic catastrophe of 1833–1845 in order to justify the statement that none of the twentieth century ethnographers is to be trusted with respect to estimates of population. The reason is simple. Barrett, Kroeber, Merriam and others used informants of no more than 70 years of age. These persons could not remember events prior to 1850 or 1860. They could name and locate former villages, but they had no knowledge of the number of inhabitants (1976:12).

Equally important was Cook's recognition of the effects of Old World diseases on aboriginal populations. Instances of local or epidemic disease outbreaks were recorded in historical documents; from available data, mortality rates could be calculated.

Cook's demographic methods differed from those of Kroeber. He took population estimates from all available records. Employing a larger battery of information allowed Cook to cross-check estimates and to control mathematically for the problem of over- or under-representation. He averaged estimates with the same calendrical date, and established ratios of population change between successive temporal units. Cook and his colleagues (Cook 1973a; Cook and Borah 1971) then determined a series of ratios for a single region. These, in turn, allowed the calculation of an average rate of change through the entire interval. In most instances, because aboriginal population was declining, the rate described depopulation trends. Finally, the rate of decline was used to estimate the original population size.

The results of such a different approach appear in Table 3. In 1943, Cook estimated the aboriginal population of California, exclusive of desert groups (for example, Madoc, Paiute, Washo, eastern Mono, Colorado tribes, and Mojave), and his final figure showed a 7% increase over Kroeber's figure for the same area. New data and the completed analysis of the coastal zone and Sacramento Valley raised Cook's later estimate (1976, 1978) for aboriginal California, exclusive of desert groups, to 300,000. The final precontact figure is more than 100% higher than that of Kroeber for the same area.

Table 4 summarizes several precontact estimates for Mexico. Borah and Cook (1963) limit their precontact estimates to central Mexico, the region for which

Table 3 Estimates of Aboriginal Californian Populations

Merriam (1905)	*Kroeber (1925)*	*Cook (1943)*	*Cook (1976, 1978)*
260,000[a]	125,000[b]	133,500[b]	300,000[b]

[a]All of California.
[b]Exclusive of native populations in desert areas.

Table 4 Comparison of Some Population Estimates for Mexico (in Millions of People)

Area	*Kroeber (1939)*	*Steward (1949)*	*Borah and Cook (1963)*
Mexico	3.2	4.5	not estimated
Central Mexico	not estimated	not estimated	25.2

they had documentary evidence of population change. Kroeber and Steward, however, estimate precontact populations for all of Mexico. There is considerable disparity between estimates that does not correlate with spatial differences. Borah and Cook's estimate for a smaller area is 87.3% higher than Kroeber's estimate for all of Mexico.

Dobyns, following the tradition established by Cook, has added new and forceful dimensions to Native American demographic studies (1963a, 1963b, 1966, 1976, 1981, 1983). First, he is the clearest spokesperson for the recognition that microbial contact and depopulation are independent of, and may have occurred prior to, the arrival of Europeans in particular locations. Based on his analysis of Andean epidemic history and aboriginal decline, Dobyns suggests a new definition of contact:

> Most analysts have confused the concept of 'aboriginal times' with 'pre-conquest' in the Andean area without realizing that aboriginal times terminated prior to conquest, at least in biological terms. The Inca Empire conquered by Pizarro's few hundred adventurers probably numbered less than half as many subjects than it had a decade earlier (1963b: 494).

In 1983 Dobyns carries the distinction between aboriginal and pre-conquest to its logical conclusion. He argues that the documented smallpox epidemic in Mexico in 1520 is, in fact, a pandemic, spreading through native channels as far south as Chile and as far north as Canada. Because of catastrophic depopulation from the microbe, aboriginal conditions in the Americas end in 1520. Dobyns defines the temporal unit between 1520 and the onset of face-to-face interactions as the protohistoric.

If Dobyns is correct in proposing that the spread of Old World diseases precedes other European introductions, then even the earliest historical descriptions are a record of populations adjusting to new conditions. Dobyns pursues this line of thought by arguing that fusion and fission of populations and the abandonment of entire regions are responses to catastrophic death (1963a, 1983). Using the Seneca as a test case (1983), he establishes an epidemic chronology that links relocation of villages to particular epidemic events.

A second and equally important implication of this position is that all figures for precontact populations of native North America, exclusive of those by Cook, are unrealistically low. Dobyns sets about changing this biased perspective by developing new precontact estimates.

In 1966, Dobyns's starting point is Borah and Cook's (1963) depopulation ratio of 16:1 for Central Mexico. Because, according to Dobyns, Borah and Cook had been too cautious in estimating native deaths from disease; he raises precontact population of Central Mexico from 25 to 30 million. Consequently the depopulation ratio over the first 130 year period becomes 20:1. In the end, the depopulation ratio for North America becomes 20 or 25:1. When these ratios are multiplied by selected nadir populations, the total ranges from 9 to 12 million. In 1983 Dobyns reestimates the total North American population to be 18 million. (See Table 1.)

Much of the 1983 work is devoted to establishing precontact estimates for the Timucua of northern Florida and southeastern Georgia. As seen in Table 5, Dobyns's figure for these chiefdoms is orders of magnitude larger than that of any other twentieth-century scholar.

To reach this astronomically high figure, Dobyns employs a series of independent demographic methods. The logic of this approach is to achieve comparable results from variable and frequently conflicting data sets. Estimating procedures include: carrying capacities of wild and domesticated plants and meat protein; historical documents; settlement variables; and general mortality rates derived from a temporal series of recorded or presumed epidemics. Because results of these methods are consistent, Dobyns is convinced that the estimates

> lie within the correct order of magnitude. The mutual consistency is also great enough to indicate that previously published estimates of the number of aboriginal native Americans in Florida have definitely not been of the correct order of magnitude (1983:294).

Dobyns's position on disease and Native American depopulation contrasts strongly to that of Kroeber. Yet it is difficult to accept his estimates of precontact aboriginal populations because of his biases and methods of reconstruction that derive from incomplete data.

Unlike Kroeber, Dobyns is never conservative in estimating aboriginal popu-

Table 5 Twentieth-Century Estimates of Precontact Timucua[a]

Mooney (1928)	*Swanton (1946)*	*Goggin (1952)*	*Tebeau (1971)*	*Deagan*[b] *(1978)*	*Dobyns (1983)*
13,000	13,000	5–8,000	15,300	15–20,000	722,000

[a]After Dobyns 1983 [b]Eastern Timucua only

lation. He assumes there were millions of Indians in North America prior to European arrival; his goal is to prove this assumption. By his own admission, however, because disease contact precedes census counts, the latter are biased by some factor in a data base that necessarily excludes the requisite information. To overcome this methodological problem, Dobyns employs a nested set of assumptions and analogies that may or may not be appropriate.

For instance, to derive a precontact estimate for the Timucua, Dobyns first establishes an estimate for the historical baseline at 1560 by using the size of warrior population or a type of analogical reasoning termed the principle of military parity (1983:179). Both methods are problematical. There are gaps in the documentary evidence on the number of warriors in Timucua chiefdoms, and the principle of military parity is based on the reasonable but untested assumption that enemy polities must be able to field standing armies of equal size. To convert warriors to total population, Dobyns uses Borah and Cook's conversion ratio (1963) from their study of Aztec populations in the Valley of Mexico. Like Aztec warriors, Timucuan warriors were 35% of total population. Unfortunately, there is no way of assessing the accuracy of the conversion ratio for Timucuan chiefdoms.

To recapitulate, the Cook and Dobyns school, in contrast to the Kroeberians, argues that native populations were far from stable during the early centuries of European contact. Because of introduced disease, populations precipitously decline; in the wake of that decline, settlement, subsistence, and political forms change. To estimate the magnitude of loss requires the use of depopulation ratios. Because of the nature and magnitude of change that begins before and continues after documention, both the ethnographic and demographic present do not reflect reality.

Even with an excellent historic record (for example, N. D. Cook 1981) the problem of estimating precontact population is difficult. When assumptions of stability or change are added to this already difficult task, the outcomes are extreme. In the end, scholars must solve the problem through the use of analogues. If populations are assumed to be stable, the historic or ethnographic record can become an adequate guide to the past. If scholars assume that populations were precipitously declining, however, they must reinterpret the historical record or employ other analogues for the past. Cook and Dobyns use both approaches. Unfortunately, until contrasting assumptions of stability or change in population are tested against an independent body of data, it will not be possible to determine which position is correct.

ARCHAEOLOGICAL ESTIMATES OF POPULATION

Two major aspects of the archaeological record make it particularly appropriate for investigating the question of population continuity or discontinuity through the contact period. Because the archaeological record is a record of people, signatures of population are certainly present in all archaeological deposits. Secondly, because the record is time-transgressive (Plog 1973; Trigger 1978), it begins before and continues after documentation and sustained European settlement. Consequently, evidence for or against demographic stability ought to be easily tested.

Despite these advantages, the difficulties in estimating population archaeologically are easily comparable to, and perhaps greater than, problems arising from estimates based on historical records. The difficulties explain, in part, why no archaeologist has developed a continental scale estimate of precontact population. Most demographic archaeologists want to develop an absolute estimate of people. (See Hassan 1981; Schacht 1981, 1984 and associated references.) Although some part of the archaeological record is employed in deriving the estimate, the archaeological reconstruction is based on analogy. More often than not, the analogue is ethnographic in origin but does not consider the ethnological debate. Because of the debate, serious doubt is cast on the reliability of any ethnographic estimate for reconstructing precontact population size. Consequently, potentially fallacious analogues are obscuring evidence of population change incorporated in the archaeological record.

Some archaeologists (for example, Heizer 1941; Perttula 1984; Ramenofsky 1982, 1984, 1985; Smith 1984; Snow 1980; Starna 1980; Upham 1982, 1984a) are aware of the controversy regarding precontact population size, and do not use analogues in deriving population estimates. Consequently, these studies of population are sounder methodologically than many others previously conducted. With few exceptions (Heizer 1941; Ramenofsky 1982; Starna 1980), however, archaeologists do not consider the population evidence present in the archaeological record in developing estimates. Instead, they limit their analyses of population to the period of regional documentation, and interpret historical estimates in light of the Cook-Dobyns disease hypothesis.

The Use of Analogy

This study limits the use of analogy in reconstructing population size to the discussion of settlement parameters. Archaeologists and historical demographers agree that settlement variables, such as house size or site size, have the closest ties with population.

In outline, the use of analogy in archaeological estimates of population is deceptively simple. First, some archaeological variable such as settlement area or house area is quantified. If the settlement has a "long" occupational history, decisions regarding spatial extent per unit time must be made. Then, the variable is multiplied by some constant, such as family size or number of people per unit area, creating an archaeological estimate of population.

In North America, archaeological estimates of population size or density from settlement parameters are an outgrowth of similar work conducted with settlements and populations from the historical period. In California, Cook and Treganza (1950) used a sample of sixteen ethnographically documented societies and four prehistoric settlements to determine the relationship between population size, settlement area and house counts. In a log-log regression they demonstrated a linear relationship between population size and settlement area. When houses were multiplied by a factor of six, the number assumed to best represent historic Californian Indian family size, Cook and Treganza (1950) established a figure they considered reasonably accurate. Cook and Heizer (1965, 1968) carried these experiments farther, estimating Californian population from a whole series of settlement relationships. Concluding that the relationship between population and settlement data was allometric, or nonlinear, they suggested that in estimating population, 13.92 m^2 should be allowed for the first six persons; and 9.29 m^2 for each additional person.

Naroll (1962) pioneered a slightly different approach to the relationship between population and settlement area. Naroll was interested in whether there was a universal mathematical relationship between population size and domestic floor area within a settlement. He employed a cross-cultural sample of eighteen ethnographic societies and demonstrated an allometric relationship between population and total roofed area of settlement. As population was added to a settlement, domestic floor area measured in square meters decreased. The formula for the relationship was:

$$A = 21.7\ p^{.84195}$$

Where:
A = area;
p = population.

At the end of the article, Naroll simplified his equation to one of constant density, suggesting that 10 m^2 is required for every person. As correctly pointed out by Schacht (1981:127), the simplification was unfortunate because "it obscures the central point of Naroll's article that the ratio of people per area is not a constant. . . ,[and] Naroll's rule of thumb seems not to be a very good approximation of his own results."

Naroll's formula has been reexamined and modified by several authors (B. Brown 1985; Casselberry 1974; LeBlanc 1971). Using a sample of three ethnographic societies, LeBlanc (1971) found that consideration of total roofed area was insufficient to account for variability in the standard deviations between samples. He suggested two modifications of Naroll's formula: a separation of rooms by function; and restricting inferences to roofed or walled space only. Casselberry's interests (1974) focused on population size of multifamily dwellings. For eight ethnographic societies, Casselberry discovered that 6 m^2 was required for each person. B. Brown's mathematical result (1985) agreed with Casselberry's requirement. He was interested in a constant, not an allometric, growth model. From reanalysis of Naroll's samples and an analysis of sixteen other ethnographic samples, Brown showed that 6 m^2 was required to accommodate a single person.

This brief review emphasizes several points. Ethnographic estimates of population begin with people. Defining the relationship between people and their habitually utilized space is based on records and observations made during the late nineteenth or twentieth centuries. Even when information is reasonably accurate, the relationship appears to be variable.

Archaeological estimates begin with space. If archaeologists are going to use one or another of the spatial conversions as analogues, they must address the central question of whether the analogue developed from recent observations can be applied to the past. Two conditions must prevail before an analogue can be applied: Time must be precisely controlled, and twentieth-century population size or density must be shown to be analogous to the precontact period. Rarely, if ever, are both of these conditions met.

It is no accident that the use of spatial analogues to develop archaeological estimates of population has been most popular in the Southwest (for example, Hill 1970; Longacre 1975; Plog 1975; Watson et al. 1980) or Mesoamerica (for example, Blanton 1972; Parsons 1971; Sanders 1965, 1970). In both regions, the survival of some aboriginal groups into the twentieth century permits an assumption of spatial continuity between prehistoric and historic populations.

Hill (1970) attempted a synchronic reconstruction of population size at Broken K Pueblo by limiting the reconstruction to the period of time when the pueblo was prosperous. After separating room types functionally, he estimated population only for habitational rooms. He used Kroeber's and Stubbs's twentieth-century data on population size from Hopi and Zuni as analogues for estimating percentage of rooms inhabited, number of people per room, and household size. Estimates so derived were then compared with those based on Naroll's formula, and on Cook and Heizer's formula. Archaeological estimates of total population ranged from 55 to 193 people. In the absence of independent evidence by which the adequacy of various estimates of population size could be judged, Hill employed subjective criteria.

Although Longacre (1975) attempted a trend analysis of population at Grasshopper Pueblo, he was less cautious than Hill. In estimating the population there, Longacre (1975) simply assumed that Hill's assessments of the number of people per room and percentage of rooms occupied were correct.

Recently, Watson, Redman and LeBlanc (1980) have offered a series of estimates for total population of El Morro Valley during the El Morro phase, which dates to the thirteenth century. They derived room counts from tracing room outlines and from excavation. Based on demographic data from Hill, Kroeber, and Stubbs, they assumed 80% occupancy of rooms at any one time. If population to room ratio is 1:1, total population is 2500. If population to room ratio is 2:1, the estimate doubles. Using Casselberry's conversion they obtained a figure for El Morro Valley of 3125 people.

Plog's study in the Upper Little Colorado drainage (1975) departed from those previously described. First, he did not present an absolute estimate of people. He was interested in the pattern of growth in regional population and employed several formulas to estimate population change from settlement parameters. Because of incomplete excavation, Plog had to estimate room counts from rubble, and he relied on ethnographic information for this estimate. Room count was a function of the formula:

$$N = .1A \times 4.0$$

where:
N = number of rooms of the pueblo
A = area of rubble mound.

Because of long occupations in the Upper Little Colorado, Plog also had to control for number of rooms occupied through time. His formula for this determination was based on the assumption that the growth of settlement followed the growth of population at that settlement. Settlements were divided into 50–year occupational increments; and at the maximum, 78% of all rooms per pueblo were occupied. Before and after the maximum, "the number of occupied rooms is half that of the preceding period" (1975:96). Changes in settlement size and percent occupancy through the span of existence of individual pueblos were then used to suggest change in population.

In the Valley of Mexico, Sanders pioneered the use of ethnographic analogy to reconstruct population size (1965, 1970). The size of surface scatter and arbitrary samples of 50 to 100 temporally sensitive sherds constituted the primary archaeological data in these experiments. Sanders used the following assumptions to estimate people from these data: (1) that limits of particular sherd types marked the limits of the settlement during that time period; (2) that density of debris corresponded to population density; (3) that twentieth-century, rural, Mexican village types were analogous to those of precontact Mexico. These assumptions allowed Sanders to equate certain densities of sherds with certain densities of population. As in the Hill-Longacre case, subsequent investigators (Blanton 1972, Parsons 1971) accepted Sander's assumptions as appropriate for estimating population density.

In all these studies, researchers are aware that the control of time must precede estimates of population. Consequently, there is a minimal attempt to group excavated units or surface remains by some temporal interval. Because of the scale of archaeological time, the interval is never as precise as that used by ethnologists when estimating population.

With the exception of Plog, however, none of the archaeologists question the relevance or reliability of the analogues they employ. They simply assume that population structure or distribution is stable from the pre-European period through the twentieth century. Therefore, if the number of people inhabiting a dwelling in the twentieth century is seven, the assumption is that same number occupied a dwelling in the thirteenth century. The result is a static population size. This creation violates the diachronic nature of archaeological data and obscures the question of change. Although there are other problems with his approach (see Hassan 1981; Schacht 1984), Plog perceives the analogical difficulty and does not attempt to convert archaeological data into numbers of people.

As currently practiced, the reconstruction of archaeological population size or density from ethnographic estimates has serious shortcomings. Where ethnologists debate the question of Native American population decline in the historical period, archaeologists assume that population is stable through time, and that ethnographic estimates are accurate. Before employing ethnographic analogy for demographic purposes, archaeologists must address the disease-depopulation question. This work could be successfully accomplished by estimating demographic change archaeologically through the contact period and then comparing the pattern with census counts from the historical period.

Ethnohistory and Archaeology

Some archaeologists with an interest in ethnohistory have considered the question of precontact population size in light of the Kroeber-Dobyns debate. They have evaluated historical documents to determine whether catastrophic change in population did, indeed, occur. The general consensus is that Kroeber's failure to consider epidemic mortality made his precontact estimates unrealistically low. Upham's study (1982) of the Western Pueblo, Hopi, Zuni, and Acoma, is an excellent case in point.

As in the California case, some ethnologists have argued that large estimates of the western Pueblo are exaggerated by a factor of ten. Upham questions this position since it "presupposes that our current understanding of Western Pueblo culture satisfactorily accounts for all the changes and variation among the Pueblos in the prehistoric and modern periods" (1982:38).

Upham first graphs historic estimates of Western Pueblo population for the 400 years since the beginning of documentation, 1583. These graphs demonstrate a 75–80% attrition in population during the first hundred years of contact. Because comparable depopulation rates are found in the work of Cook and Dobyns, Upham suggests that for the beginning of Western Pueblo history, population counts, while lower than some historic figures, are orders of magnitude greater than traditional ethnological estimates. His 1982 total for the Western Pueblo in 1583 is 36,000.

In a more recent paper (1984a) Upham argues that because contact in the Southwest began with the Coronado *entrada* of A.D. 1540, and because disease contact precedes history, his initial estimate is too low. He raises that figure to 51,514 by multiplying the 1583 figure by a smallpox mortality rate of 30%. The 1984 total is six times larger than Kroeber's 1939 figure for these populations.

Snow (1980; Snow and Starna 1984) shares Upham's opinion that traditional ethnology has seriously biased archaeological perception of precontact population size. In one of his New England studies (1980), Snow discusses the Kroeber-Dobyns debate and provides new precontact population estimates for New England on a culture-by-culture-basis. His estimates are derived largely from early seventeenth-century documents that included village and warrior counts and postepidemic figures. Snow's precontact estimate of 21,900 for the Abnaki is seven times larger than Kroeber's.

While recognizing catastrophic decline from disease, Snow (1980; Snow and Starna 1984) does not think that disease contact precedes documentation in the Northeast. After evaluating Dobyns's epidemic arguments and regional historical documents, Snow concludes that disease contact begins in 1616. This date is more than 100 years after contact began in the St. Lawrence Basin. He states:

> The testimony of the Indians themselves and the horrible effects the epidemic had on the population all combine to strongly indicate that this was the first major epidemic to strike New England. This and subsequent epidemics in the Northeast reduced some Indian populations up to a total of 98% of their 1600 populations over the course of the seventeenth century. Thus, while the epidemic may have been delayed for several decades in the Northeast as compared to Mexico, their effects were similar (1984:17).

Because disease postdates documentation, Snow does not face the methodological dilemma that Dobyns is continually trying to overcome. Pre-epidemic population figures are employed to estimate precontact population size, while postepidemic figures indicate the magnitude of population loss.

Although the logic of Snow's argument is clear, the question remains whether the argument itself is correct. Whether disease contact in the Northeast truly postdated documentation can only be resolved by evaluating the sixteenth- and seventeenth-century archaeological records for the area. Snow's archaeological work in the Middle Mohawk Valley is certainly a step in that direction.

Although limiting his study to the seventeenth century, Starna (1980) employs both archaeological and historical records in estimating pre-epidemic Mohawk population. Historical documents of the seventeenth century provided estimates of Mohawk village and house counts. To determine the size of Iroquois long houses and number of hearths and compartments per house, Starna employs the known archaeological record from New York and Ontario. He estimates population on a per house basis by multiplying the number of compartments by a conservative family count of four and five. This figure is converted to total population by multiplying it by Iroquois house counts. Since Starna is aware of arguments involving population loss from disease, he assumes his initial figures are postepidemic. He derives pre-epidemic figures for the Mowawk by multiplying the postepidemic figures by disease mortalities that range from 50% to 70%. The resulting Mohawk estimates are higher than earlier precontact estimates for the entire New York Iroquois population. Starna does not consider whether the pre-epidemic figures are also precontact.

The ethnohistorical studies of population are superior to those based on analogues because they avoid the methodological pitfalls of analogical reasoning by extracting information from historical documents. These studies challenge the Kroeberian position on aboriginal population size and density by reestimating population in light of catastrophic decline from disease. At the same time, the exclusion of the archaeological record in estimating population limits the validity of this research. Because the archaeological record is the most appropriate and accessible independent test of this issue, it must be evaluated before either assumption can be accepted.

CONCLUSIONS

Although ethnologists, demographic historians, and archaeologists have investigated the issue of aboriginal population size and density, there is no consensus of opinion. The major conflict is between Kroeber and Cook-Dobyns. As shown, however, assumptions of contact period events have major implications for the numbers generated and the meaning of those numbers.

To date, archaeological estimates of population are of little use in deciding how many people lived in North America prior to European arrival. The coupling of the archaeological record with ethnographic analogy results in a small but static population size from prehistory through the twentieth century. When archaeologists become historians and evaluate records of the contact period, they conclude that population attrition ranges from 50% to 95%. Whether populations remain stable or decline catastrophically can only be established by the independent evaluation of archaeology and history.

Three

Methods and Definitions

To facilitate the archaeological investigation of the population debate, I shall frame divergent ethnological models into a single testable question: Did Native Americans experience a population collapse immediately following initial contact with Europeans but predating written records and sustained colonization?

Because the relevant change or lack of it takes place prior to written documents, the question places the problem within an archaeological realm. Although the archaeological record is appropriate for such a research question, it may not be empirically adequate. After all, infectious parasites do not preserve well in the archaeological record (see Jackes 1983 for a possible exception); and previous archaeological research has not been directed toward obtaining data on this issue. Nonetheless, the kind of change required by the Cook-Dobyns model is of such magnitude that it should be readily detected even by relatively primitive measures and with data of admittedly poor quality. Furthermore, once the general question has been answered, more specific questions, such as absolute rates of change or regional variability, can be pursued.

The term *collapse*, the key word of the research question, is defined as an *abrupt and catastrophic decline in population*. This type of decline meets the expectations of disease contact and is fundamentally different from a gradual attrition of the population base. If the record indicates that this type of population loss postdates initial contact, but predates sustained colonization, it can be concluded that introduced epidemic diseases were a major factor in the loss. If population loss is not catastrophic and/or occurs following sustained colonization, other mechanisms, such as those envisioned by Kroeber, must be responsible. Archaeological records and historical documents from pertinent periods must be systematically analyzed to determine whether the decline (1) was abrupt or gradual, (2) was extensive or minimal, and (3) predated or postdated sustained colonization.

MEASUREMENT AND DESCRIPTIVE REQUIREMENTS

To determine whether Native Americans experienced a demographic collapse, population units must be counted across space and through time. Direct archaeological measures of population are available either through grave counts or settlement data.

Grave Counts

Milner (1980) has argued that for the period following first contact, but prior to sustained colonization, analysis of mortuary populations is the most direct means for assessing the magnitude and nature of aboriginal decline from infectious diseases. Although Milner's point is valid and has been considered in certain burial contexts (Owsley and Bass 1979; Palkovich 1981), I am excluding this class of data for several reasons: Most importantly, I am not an osteologist with training in the analysis of death assemblages. Such training is however important for the temporal periods of concern in this study. In addition to the demographic biases typically present in burial samples (see Buikstra and Cook 1981), the possibility of catastrophic death from disease may introduce others. If large portions of population are dying from disease, then causes of death, and the representativeness of burial samples for living populations take on added significance. Do burial populations, for instance, represent those individuals who died from disease? Do cemeteries represent some proportion of unknown normal and abnormal attrition?

Furthermore, there are indications that some North American populations simply ceased interring their dead during the historical period. In 1701, Iberville named Dauphine Island on Mobile Bay, Massacre Island, because human skeletons were scattered along the southwest beach (McWilliams 1981:38). Although a single instance of this sort can be attributed to warfare, repetition of this phenomenon suggests that factors other than warfare were causative.

Vancouver recorded similar skeletal scatters when he first entered Puget Sound (Meany 1949). After the California and Oregon malarial epidemic of 1830, trappers reported finding unburied human bodies in aboriginal settlements in northern California (Cook 1955); Lewis and Clark recorded exposed human skulls and teeth in abandoned Mandan villages (Thwaites 1904,1).

Repetition of the breakdown of burial practices in different regions suggests that death from disease may have been causal. This suggestion is supported by documentary evidence on the Black Plague in Europe. Because so many people died so quickly, survivors were too few in number to accord the dead proper burial. Dead bodies were abandoned in streets or stacked one on top of another and burned (Tuchman 1978).

If the North American experience is at all comparable to the European experience, then information necessary for the question of population collapse is not contained in cemeteries. Before cemetery data can be employed, the problem of differential interment between and within regions during the historic period must be addressed.

Settlement Data

Settlement data constitute the second and archaeologically more reliable measure of population. Because of the nature of the problem addressed in this research and because of the impossibility of tracing particular communities over time archaeologically (that is, looking at community fission, fusion, variability in settlement location), regional population is the appropriate measure. Expressed in terms of settlement, regional population is the sum of population at individual settlements:

(1)
$$P_r = \sum_{i=1}^{n} S_p$$

where:
P_r = regional population
S_p = the population of individual settlements.

Although equation (1) correctly depicts the relation between settlement population and regional population, it is not sufficient empirically. The underlying assumption that it is possible to count the number of people at a single point in time is not applicable to archaeological data. Two modifications, therefore, are required: (1) The equation must include a temporal element; and (2) a substitute for settlement population count must be devised. Each modification is considered below.

Even when archaeologists seek a population estimate for a single area and for a single period, the results are not comparable to population counts developed from census data because of the problem of determining contemporaneity of settlement (Schacht 1984). When estimates are to be compared over time, the duration of the periods used to assemble settlement counts will exert a major influence on population estimates. Consequently, a temporal term is introduced to control for period duration such that the archaeological population of a region is the sum of populations at single settlements divided by a standardized temporal interval:

$$P_{ar} = \frac{\sum_{i=1}^{n} S_p}{(T/100)} \qquad (2)$$

where:

P_{ar} = the archaeological population of the region
S_p = the population of individual settlements
T = the duration in years of the period of time represented by settlement counts.

Since the means of assessing time available to archaeologists does not permit the use of periods of the same length in absolute years, T can be expected to vary from case to case. In order to be able to compare estimates derived for periods of different durations, T is adjusted to an interval of 100 years. The selection of 100 years is arbitrary representing a compromise between the usually finer archaeological periods that can be recognized at the end of a sequence and the longer periods that are characteristic of the prehistoric ones.

In spite of this modification for calculating regional population, time can still seriously influence derived estimates. Equation (2) will overestimate or underestimate regional population if the duration of settlements themselves relative to the duration of the counting periods is either not constant or is not normally distributed about the mean.

Although it might be convenient to assume that settlement duration is more or less constant over the period of time of this study, this assumption is clearly unwarranted. During the historical period, documentary sources indicate considerable population movement and relocation. (See for example, Bowers 1965; Brain 1980; I. Brown 1985; Chomko 1977; Dobyns 1983; Fairbanks 1978; Schroeder 1979; Wray 1983; Wray and Schoff 1953.) Suites of absolute dates sufficient to bracket settlement duration would be the most appropriate means for measuring the effects of settlement duration on regional estimates of population. Such data, however, do not exist for any region in the United States. Typically, a single date or small series of dates are obtained for components or strata, and then the dates are treated as if they represented the mean or median age of the unit. (See Finlayson and Pihl 1980 for a similar discussion.) Although investigators have occasionally suggested settlement duration, lack of a sound empirical basis for such assessments and the variability inherent in these less than rigorous statements precludes their use here.

For the periods of time involved in this study, however, general trends in settlement duration can be identified. As a consequence of population reduction and political or economic disturbance, I expect settlement duration to decrease following European contact. Thus, although there are no means available to measure the magnitude of bias introduced by this parameter, it is possible to assess its direction. Overestimation of regional population should occur as settlement duration decreases relative to archaeological periods of a longer duration. Although this expectation identifies a major source of error plaguing regional estimates of archaeological population, it does not solve the problem of settlement duration. The solution lies in the rigorous control of the time during which single settlements are occupied.

The next consideration is a suitable substitute for head counts that can be reliably measured in the archaeological record. Since counts of archaeologically known settlements are not equivalent to the total number of settlements actually occupied during a given period, a simple sum of head counts for each settlement is not possible. Consequently, Equation (2) must be modified to reflect this condition:

$$P_{ar} = \frac{S_c}{(T/100)} \times \overline{S_p} \qquad (3)$$

where:

P_{ar} = archaeological regional population

T = the duration in years of the period of time represented by the settlement count

S_c = number of settlements

$\overline{S_p}$ = mean population of settlements.

In Equation (3) the archaeological population of a region is the product of settlement counts divided by the standardized temporal interval and the population at each of those settlements expressed as a mean. Since the biases and problems affecting the measurement of the number of settlements (S_c) are different from those affecting the measurement of the populations (S_p) of those settlements, the two components must be separated. Using mean settlement population has further advantages given the kinds of information typically available for single settlements.

Since archaeological samples of settlements typically do not meet parametric assumptions, P_{ar} cannot be treated as an interval or ratio measure but must be accorded either nominal or ordinal significance. Of the two alternatives, an ordinal measure is more appropriate. Statements of greater precision than "people are present or absent" are certainly possible. To employ Equation (3) as an ordinal measure, however, requires that S_c represent approximately the same fraction of total settlements for each period and region being compared. Each of these points is discussed in turn.

While it is not possible to assign numbers to the magnitude of population change recorded in the archaeological record, the change can be generally ranked. Further, according to the Cook-Dobyns model, population is fundamentally different after contact than before it; to treat these two classes of population as equivalent and symmetrical violates the model being tested. Consequently, in all interpretations, P_{ar} is treated as an ordinal measure, even when specific analyses produce interval or ratio measures.

As noted above, the value of P_{ar} as an ordinal measure depends on the assumption that the same fraction of the record is tabulated for each estimate. While the nature of archaeological sampling has not been directed toward obtaining this type of information, every effort is made to identify and control biases affecting this assumption. Rarely, if ever, is this assumption correct. The fraction of the record actually known varies in terms of the visibility of settlements in the archaeological record, differential archaeological interest in settlements of different periods and regions, and how settlements, that is, archaeological sites, become known. (See for example, *ad hoc* reports of sites vs. systematic survey, etc.) Fortunately, these biases are minimized within regions where the following conditions prevail: historical factors are responsible for similar cultural remains; similar postdepositional processes have operated on the visibility and accessibility of the record; and the history of archaeological research is more or less similar. As a consequence, regional sequences are separated since there is no way to precisely quantify the effects of these biases from region to region. Even in comparing regional sequences, it must be remembered that differences in estimates may arise from these sources.

In terms of period to period comparisons within a region, differences that arise as a consequence of archaeological interest are the strongest, since the other kinds of biases are controlled to some extent by the selection of regions studied. American archaeologists have long used a general research strategy termed the "direct historical approach" (e.g., Bandelier 1890; Dixon 1913; Steward 1942; Strong 1935, 1940; Thomas 1894), in which documents guide the identification and location of historically occupied settlements. Before the development of probability-based sampling designs in archaeology there was no comparable method for discovering prehistoric sites. Consequently I expect that the effect of this differential sampling will result in an increase in historical period settlement counts relative to settlement counts of earlier periods. The exact magnitude of the bias cannot be calculated, but the direction is clear. It should lead, once again, to rejection of the Cook-Dobyns model.

Variability in human settlement strategies is the last problem that can seriously influence estimates of population. Here, the relevant contrast is between mobility and sedentism. Although these didactic terms represent two ends of a continuum with considerable variability between (for example, Binford 1980, 1982; Cordell and Upham 1984; Jochim 1976, 1981; Upham 1984b), the simple dichotomy is sufficient for this study.

In a mobile organization, population relocates periodically, and this, in turn, results in a number of residental locations during an annual cycle. From an archaeological perspective, these loci could represent either different populations or the same population at different seasons. To estimate population from the residues of a mobile organization requires documenting the annual cycle of moves and determining whether the residues represent special activity, logistical, or residental locations. Although archaeologists have considered these problems, they have not resolved them. Without resolution, tabulating residental locations of a mobile strategy can overestimate population.

Given the state of the art, sedentism is a more reliable organization to use for estimating population. Because units of population tend to remain in the same location through an annual cycle, problems of duplicate counting occur less frequently. Furthermore, since settlement duration within regions and temporal units tends to be comparable, settlement counts can be employed as a substitute for census counts in the absence of other types of settlement data.

Biases that derive from restricting analysis of population to regions characterized by sedentary strategies relate to the concept and consequence of permanence. A common assumption of sedentism is that the entire population unit remains in the same location throughout the year. This is not the case, since one consequence of a sedentary strategy is an increase in logistical moves (Cordell and Upham 1984). Fortunately, differentiating between logistical stations and residental locations is easier within a sedentary organization.

Because a sedentary settlement strategy implies clustering of people, the risk of infection from communicable diseases is higher than among populations who practice a mobile strategy (Bartlett 1960; Black 1966). Analysis of sedentary settlements are more likely to include data pertinent to answering the question of population collapse. At the same time, because mobile strategies are a dominant part of the North American record, descriptions based on sedentary settlements cannot be assumed to represent the total pattern of demographic change during European contact. A whole pattern, in fact, depends on the integration of data from mobile and sedentary settlements; but the integration must await the development of rigorous methods of population analysis of mobile settlements.

A surrogate for S_p is still required. Two archaeological measures, settlement area and roofed area, are consistently used (see Chapter 2). Each describes a different spatial aspect of population, and each is subject to particular biases.

Where areal measurements of sedentary settlements are known, P_{ar} can be described by mean settlement area of a region:

(4) $$P_{ar} = \frac{S_c}{(T/100)} \times \overline{S_a}$$

where:
P_{ar} = archaeological population of the region
S_c = sedentary settlement counts
$\overline{S_a}$ = mean area of sedentary settlements
T = duration in years of the period of time represented by settlement counts.

Several considerations dictate that S_a be measured as a mean. Knowledge of $\overline{S_a}$ presumes knowledge of settlements. The number of settlements for which S_a is known, however, is always empirically less than S_c. If areal data were available for all settlements uniformly, a simple sum could be used:

$$P_{ar} = \frac{S_a}{(T/100)}$$

In using a mean, it is recognized that S_a is normally a sample of S_c, and I assume that there are no systematic biases involved in reporting settlement area (for example, that the value of settlement area does not correlate with the decision to report settlement area). This must remain an assumption as the data necessary to evaluate it are not available. Were such data known, the simple sum could be used, but again, the sum presumes knowledge of the area of all settlements.

Other, more fundamental problems intrinsic to the meaning of S_a limit the utility of Equation (4). Although S_a is typically defined as the daily-use area of a population, in the absence of structural features such as palisade lines or ditches, there is no archaeological agreement on how to establish boundaries. Furthermore, postdepositional processes or multiple occupations may obscure the precision with which site boundaries are identified (Finlayson 1985). Consequently, estimates for even single sedentary settlements may vary widely because of subjective archaeological opinion involved, or because of the time when the estimate was made, rather than because of the type of habitual use.

Even if biases in the definition of $\overline{S_a}$ are controlled for, there remains the problem of how settlement area relates to population size. A common assumption is that settlement area is a function of population size (for example, Blanton 1972; Johnson 1972; Parsons 1971), but settlement area is actually a complex function of population size, settlement structure, and cultural geography. A large settlement area need not correlate with a large population; nor a small settlement area with a small population. The small area may be filled by a few, large, multifamily houses; and the large area may include a few single family houses, work areas, and garden plots. In the absence of information on settlement structure, estimates of settlement area are not very meaningful in population studies.

There may be contexts, however, where Equation (4) could be reliably employed. If variability in settlement structure is known or is constant, changes in regional settlement area may reasonably reflect changing population size.

Roofed area is the second measure of settlement population size. Like S_a, roofed area of settlement (S_{ra}) varies according to S_p but, in contrast to S_a, roofed area is less variable and largely free of measurement and definitional problems. These advantages partially explain archaeological attempts to convert roofed area into a ratio measure of population (for example, B. Brown 1985; Casselberry 1974; LeBlanc 1971; Naroll 1962; Schacht 1984.) Unfortunately, the relation between population and roofed area is a complex allometric function yet to be understood mathematically.

In spite of the imprecision as a ratio measure, S_{ra} is the most reliable ordinal measure of archaeological settlement population. As opposed to the definition of S_a, archaeologists tend to agree that a certain complex of traits, wall features, storage pits, sleeping areas, and hearths, constitute a habitational structure. This agreement facilitates consistent field definitions of house versus non-house areas of settlements.

Where measurements of some houses of known settlements are available, population is described as the mean roofed area of known sedentary settlements:

(5) $$P_{ar} = \frac{S_c}{(T/100)} \times \overline{S_{ra}}$$

where:

P_{ar} = archaeological population of the region
S_c = sedentary settlement counts
$\overline{S_{ra}}$ = mean roofed area of sedentary settlements
T = duration in years of the period of time represented by settlement counts.

For the reasons discussed in conjunction with equation (4), the appropriate measure of S_{ra} is a mean. Although a more reliable estimator of population size, the information necessary to calculate $\overline{S_{ra}}$ is less frequently reported. If a settlement has been excavated in its entirety, then a simple sum of the area of the houses could be used; but such information is rarely available. Consequently, the calculation of $\overline{S_{ra}}$ must assume that the number of houses in a settlement can be accurately counted or estimated (using symmetry or spacing) and that the sample of houses for the area reported is not systematically biased in terms of house dimensions.

Because $\overline{S_{ra}}$ ultimately rests on house measurements, a kind of information only meagerly represented in archaeological descriptions, sampling errors, most of which are probably substantial and unknown, are involved in many estimates. There are no reasons to suppose that these errors are affecting archaeological knowledge unevenly. They should act only to increase the "noise" of the comparisons.

In summary, data derived from sedentary settlements will be employed for estimating regional population. Among the variety of settlement data, settlement counts, settlement area, and roofed area are most accessible in, and least subject to difficulties of, the archaeological record. These parameters are employed to develop archaeological equations (For example, see Equations (4) and (5)) that, under appropriate circumstances, can monitor population change. Each of the equations is subject to temporal and/or sampling biases; but since the direction of biases is generally known, reliability of estimates can be judged.

Nature and descriptive accuracy of regional data sets determine which equation is appropriate for particular test cases. Where possible, I will employ multiple equations to create a description of population that is as reliable and accurate as is possible within the confines of the data base.

By taking this explicit approach to estimating population, even in a relative sense, I have revealed the general weakness of most archaeological data for making any statements about regional population. If population issues are to be dealt with in archaeology in anything more than an impressionistic fashion, we must improve the general quality of data available. Because of the quality of data used in this research, a rigorous solution is simply not possible; in fact, research is feasible only because the test involves a catastrophic collapse. Research that entails the documentation of more subtle, gradual changes in population, often implied by ecological and evolutionary models, simply cannot be attempted with this quality data.

Chronology

Time is an important variable in this study because I want to determine when aboriginal decline began relative to other European introductions. Since most archaeological chronologies that incorporate contact define its origin by documentation or trade, they are inappropriate for my purposes. Consequently, I define existing temporal units that include the historical period, but these units do not entail the assumption that contact begins with European trade goods, sustained European presence, or historical documentation. Rather, I compare the timing of these introductions with the population evidence for or against collapse to determine whether disease contact and population collapse are prior to other types of European introductions. If collapse postdates colonization, then it is legitimate to define European contact by European products or people, whichever is earlier.

In building regional sequences, I will employ relative and absolute methods. To create the most accurate sequence from existing data, I will use multiple ordering methods, making it possible to verify the temporal placement of settlements. Once the most accurate regional sequence is created, changes in style and/or function will mark the beginnings and ends of periods.

Presence/absence and frequency seriations are well established in archeology. (See for example, Cowgill 1972; Dunnell 1970; Marquardt 1978.) I will employ both types of seriation to order stylistic classes of aboriginal ceramics. Although I will try to use traditionally defined classes in the seriations, this may not always be possible. If ceramic classes are not truly stylistic, it will not be possible to develop an order that I can infer is chronological (Dunnell 1970). Should this situation occur, it will be necessary to create new stylistic classes before building a temporal order.

In his research in the Lower Mississippi Valley, I. Brown (1979) has employed cumulative frequency curves of European trade material to create temporal orders of historically occupied aboriginal settlements. Brown, however, is unique in this regard. Except for the temporal treatment of trade beads (for example, Ahler and Swenson 1985; Brain 1980; Hayes 1983; Kidd and Kidd 1970), archaeologists typically do not expend much effort on the analysis of aboriginal assemblages from the postcontact period. This gap in archaeological method is explained by the fact that the presence of European items moves prehistoric archaeology into the realm of historic archaeology in the New World; historic archaeology tends to be treated as the archaeology of Europeans (South 1977; Trigger 1985).

In this study, I adopt I. Brown's approach. First, I will develop a classification of European function modified from South (1977). Although the classification is functional, no assumption regarding native function is implied. The classification is strictly a method for monitoring the appearance of European material in aboriginal contexts. Component frequencies are calculated for each class and are converted into component cumulative frequency curves. Class frequencies determine the shape of the curve. Since sampling biases preclude the use of parametric statistics to correlate curves, relative temporal orders are developed by visually comparing the shape of component frequency curves.

In building temporal orders, I will also employ absolute dates from radiocarbon determinations and from historical documents. Radiocarbon is of less utility than documents not only because of archaeological practices but because of changes in the ^{14}C reservoir curve during the recent period (Klein et al. 1982), and because of statistical problems that result when radiocarbon years are calibrated to bristlecone pine chronologies (see Browman 1981 for a recent review of radiocarbon research). As already noted, archaeologists typically date a component by a single radiometric determination; and there are always more undated than dated components. This shortcoming is particularly serious for late prehistoric and historic periods where contamination of the carbon reservoir can seriously bias determination of true radiocarbon age (Browman 1981).

Furthermore, calibrating radiocarbon years magnifies ambiguities by calibration. Not only are there numerous calibration curves (for example, Clark 1975; Damon et al. 1974; Klein et al. 1982; Ralph et al. 1974), but a single date may be associated with two or more calendrical dates (Renfrew and Clark 1974) (See Figure 1). To compensate for this problem, researchers suggest a 95% confidence interval to bracket the date. The resulting calendrical range may be as great as 400 years (Ralph et al. 1974).

Thus for the period of time of this study, radiocarbon dates are not reliable temporal indicators. To overcome some of the identified biases, I will present absolute dates as minimum, mean, and maximum temporal estimates. Besides demonstrating the imprecision in the temporal dimension, this approach provides three separate estimates of period duration against which changes in S_c can be judged. Where appropriate, multiple dates for single components are averaged according to Long and Rippeteau (1974) and, although admittedly inaccurate, all dates are calibrated to the bristlecone pine chronologies developed by Damon et al. (1974).

Dates taken from historical documents may prove more useful than those from radiocarbon assays. Documentary dates may confirm the placement of a settlement ordered by a relative method, may indicate inaccuracies in the order, or may suggest the possiblity that some settlements had multiple occupations.

In summary, since archaeologists traditionally define European contact by the presence of Europeans, written documentation or trade goods rather than by any type of population change, existing chronologies are clearly inappropriate for addressing the problem of population collapse. Consequently, new regionally based, chronological units defined independently of traditional markers are developed through seriations, cumulative frequencies, documentary and radiocarbon dates. Once I have established these units, I can estimate

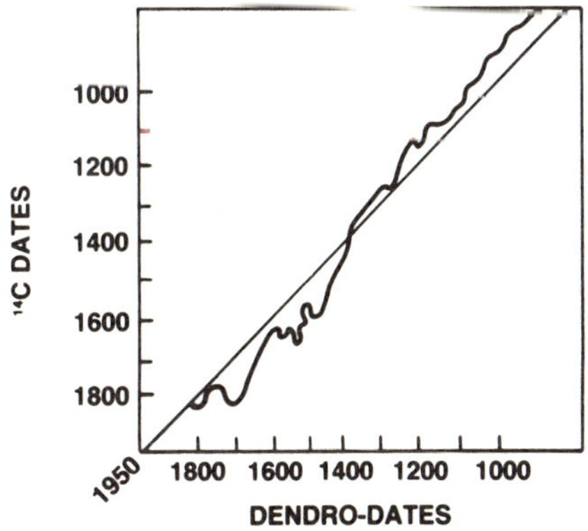

Figure 1. Radiocarbon Time Scale

the timing of population reduction relative to other introductions. One important result of this approach will be that the empirical record rather than assumptions will define the onset of aboriginal change that occurred because of European arrival in North America.

TEST CASES

Multi-regional samples are necessary in this study to establish a reasonably accurate pattern of population change despite data of admittedly poor quality. Several criteria, in addition to sedentism, governed the selection of test cases:

To minimize the effect of bias that occurs when data collected for one purpose are used for another, regions must have witnessed comparable archaeological treatment. This requirement did not necessarily mean that one person or institution had done all the field work, but it did imply a standard archaeological methodology.

Selected regions had to have a large sample of at least one settlement characteristic such as house size, settlement area, or settlement location. Initially, I had hoped for large samples of all settlement characteristics, but this desire turned out to be unrealistic. Typically, one aspect of settlement is better known than others, and the reliability of this measure had to be weighed against total sample size. A large sample of house measurements in a small number of villages might produce a more reliable ordinal estimate of population than a large number of village locations with few house measurements.

Determining the timing of population loss relative to traditional markers of European contact required the persistence of aboriginal settlement records through the appearance of trade goods, written records, and colonization. This requirement excluded obviously important data bases where the record abruptly terminated at the contact boundary. Examples of such data bases include Ohio (Graybill 1981; Griffin 1946b), Upper Great Lakes (Brose 1976; Green 1984; Mason 1976). Although the exclusion of these sequences introduced another source of bias that could lead to rejection of the Cook-Dobyns model, I preferred this alternative. Without persistence, I could not judge the accuracy of either model.

Regional archaeological samples must have different contact histories. Different contact histories facilitated comparison of native responses to Europeans and their products including disease.

In the end, I chose three regions: Lower Mississippi Valley, central New York, and the Middle Missouri Valley. (See Figure 2.) Although I had hoped to add part of the data base from the middle or upper Rio Grande, a series of unforeseen problems necessitated exclusion of that region.

Although each region met the criteria, they were still problematical. Since these problems have influenced archaeological knowledge, they need to be

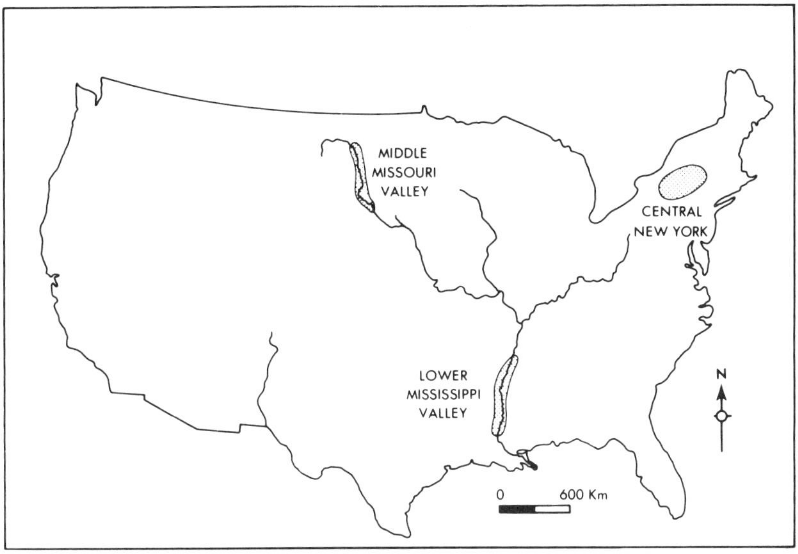

Figure 2. Location of Test Cases

considered before presenting relevant data. The discussion is not, however, directed toward blind criticism (Haag 1985: 278 for a similar point). Without previous large-scale syntheses, this study could not be attempted.

Sampling Biases

Regional data bases are a product of judgmental sampling. The problem with this strategy for this study is that the spatial pattern of settlements may not be representative of either total population size or the spatial distribution of that population. Although this difficulty can be partially controlled by large sample sizes, such samples are not available in all cases.

The surveys of Phillips, Ford, and Griffin (1951) and Phillips (1970) constitute the primary data of the sample from the Lower Mississippi Valley. Although Figure 3 gives the appearance of even spatial coverage, this is not the case (Table 6). Dense vegetation within the alluvial valley makes locating and identifying settlements difficult. Traditionally, archaeologists have employed two approaches for the discovery of settlements: the direct historical approach (Brain et al. 1974; I. Brown 1985; Ford 1936, 1961; Giardino 1984; Swanton 1939), and topographic changes (mounds and large trash heaps) readily detectable above the generally low elevation of the floodplain. As a result, the historical record is better known than the prehistoric record, and the latter is biased in favor of the large and the obvious.

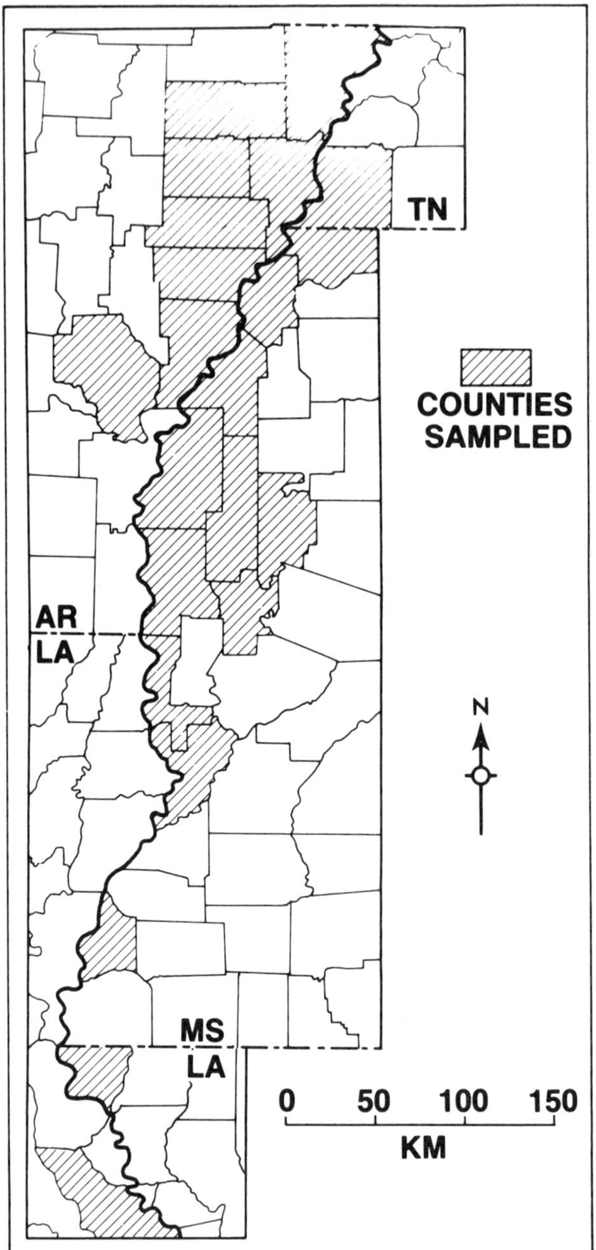

Figure 3. Spatial Distribution of the Lower Mississippi Valley Sample

Table 6 Lower Mississippi Valley Settlement Count by County or Parish

State	*County or Parish*	*Unique Location*
Tennessee	Shelby	1
Arkansas	Mississippi	3
	Cross	5
	Poinsett	1
	Crittendon	3
	St. Francis	3
	Lee	3
	Phillips	2
	Arkansas	2
Mississippi	De Soto	1
	Tunica	2
	Coahoma	4
	Bolivar	2
	Sunflower	7
	Le Flore	2
	Washington	6
	Humphreys	1
	Yazoo	2
	Issaquena	1
	Warren	3
	Adams	5
Louisiana	West Feliciana	1
	Iberville	1
TOTAL		61

The second major problem of the known record from the Lower Mississippi Valley is the absence of quantitative data on house or settlement size. Major surveys, focusing on surface collections, have produced relatively large ceramic samples that are useful in developing relative temporal orders. Unfortunately ceramic samples are not helpful for developing descriptions of house patterns or settlement size. Thus, while archaeologists know something about the spatial distribution of population from the Lower Mississippi Valley, they know very little about intra-settlement distribution of population. (See I. Brown [1985]; Klinger [1975–1977]; and Morse [1981] for exceptions.)

The central New York region is approximately 37,000 km^2, but within that general area, the sample is not spatially continuous. Of the twenty counties within the study area (Figure 4), only ten have archaeological data useful in this research (Table 7). In addition, settlements with areal measures of size from central New York is small, representing only a fraction of all late prehistoric and historic settlements that could be reliably fixed in time. Restriction of settlement samples to units that could be given a temporal assignment does not imply comparable excavation techniques.

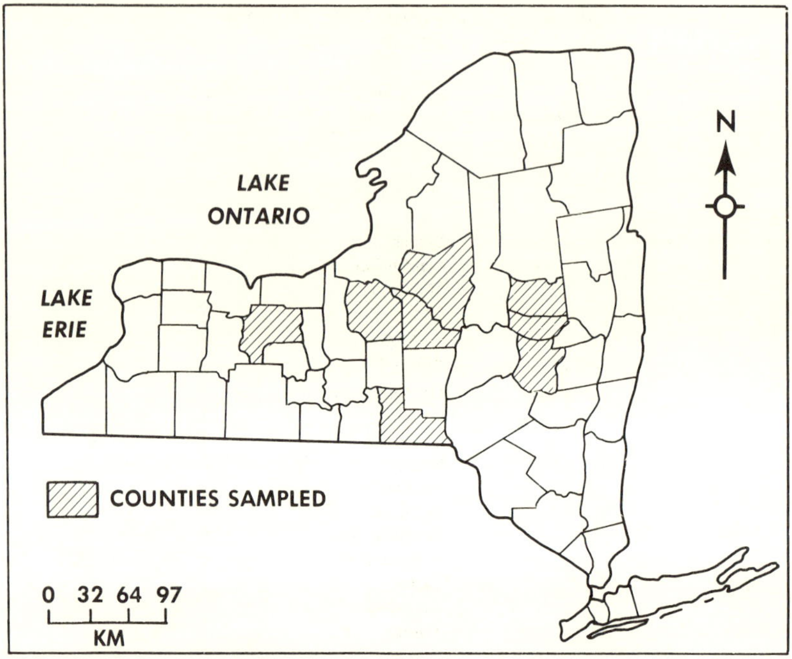

Figure 4. Spatial Distribution of the Central New York Sample

Table 7 Central New York Settlement Count by County

County	*Unique Location*
Ontario	1
Onondaga	9
Onondaga/Madison	2
Oneida/Madison	1
Oneida	1
Madison	9
Montgomery	1
Broome	1
Schoharie	1
Fulton	1
TOTAL	27

Caughnawaga (Grassman 1969) is the only settlement from the region in which all structures have been excavated and reported. In the other 24 settlements, houses are less consistently excavated; in fact, only sixteen (62%) of all settlements have roofed area data. When excavation focuses on settlement, surfaces are typically stripped to expose postmold patterns suggestive of palisade lines or houses. Some houses may be excavated, areas between houses are frequently ignored. At best, recovered assemblages from central New York represent house samples rather than component samples. (See Finlayson 1985 for an excellent discussion of settlement excavation.)

The sample from the Middle Missouri is a product of the River Basin Surveys (J. Jennings 1985; Lehmer 1971). The involvement of the federal government had both positive and negative effects on resulting descriptions. Expenditure of federal moneys meant the exploration of more archaeological resources than could ever have been done on an individual basis. In the Middle Missouri trench, a minimum of eighty sites were excavated or surveyed. Furthermore, although reporting lagged behind field work, the use of federal moneys and personnel guaranteed a publication outlet and standardization of descriptions. At the same time, archaeology was clearly secondary to hydroelectric construction; and this meant that archaeological projects operated within major temporal and spatial constraints.

Figure 5 and Table 8 summarize that fraction of the Middle Missouri site record that I have been able to use. The sample is weighted toward the west side of the river and has a strong southern orientation. Since hydroelectric constructions, not probability, determined where archaeologists worked, it is not possible to know whether the spatial distribution reflects sampling bias, actual distribution of population, or both.

The southern orientation appears to reflect both aboriginal land use and sampling. River terraces are lower in the south than in the north part of the region, permitting more space for construction of settlements and garden plots. At the same time, 50% of all sites used in these analyses are drawn from Stanley, Lyman, and Hughes counties; and three hydroelectric plants are located in this stretch of the river.

Temporal constraints and inadequate archaeological procedures have adversely affected excavation and recovery of samples within the Missouri trench. No site in this sample has been completely excavated. Since houses are essentially pit features, their surface visibility has created a ready focus for excavation. Some of these features are trenched to define boundaries, center posts, and fire pits. As in central New York, areas between houses are typically unexplored. Further, since settlement boundaries are not consistently marked by structural features, settlement dimensions tend to be unreliable. Consequently, samples recovered from excavation are biased not only to house areas, but to floor or near floor contexts.

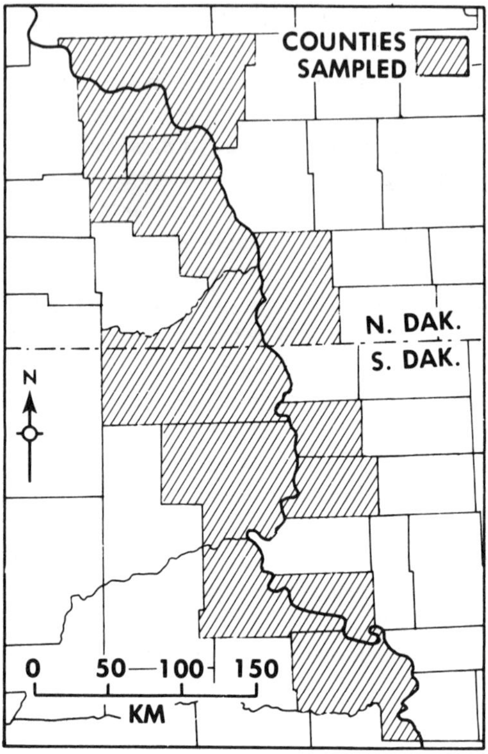

Figure 5. Spatial Distribution of the Middle Missouri Sample

Archaeological treatment of multiple occupations within the Middle Missouri is the last sampling bias to be considered. Residential locations are confined to terraces where space is limited. This, in turn, means that many locations along the trench witnessed multiple occupations. Because previous archaeological treatment was not directed toward obtaining representative samples from all cultural strata, I have found it difficult and frequently impossible to unravel the complex histories. Consequently, although some twenty locations are known to have multiple occupations, my final sample includes only ten.

In summary, I shall employ archaeological and historical records from the Lower Mississippi Valley, central New York, and the Middle Missouri Valley to test for the timing and nature of aboriginal population decline. One of the strengths of this analysis is the multi-regional approach. Because biases are present in each data base, the analysis of a single region could produce ambig-

Table 8 Middle Missouri Settlement Count by County

Side of River	*County*		*Settlement Count (n)*
West	Mercer		6
	Oliver		2
	Morton		1
	Sioux		2
	Corson		1
	Dewey		2
	Armstrong		0
	Stanley		11
	Lyman		4
		Subtotal	29
East	McLean		2
	Burleigh		0
	Emmons		1
	Campbell		0
	Walworth		2
	Potter		0
	Sully		0
	Hughes		3
	Buffalo		0
		Subtotal	8
TOTAL			37

uous results. This problem is less likely with a multi-regional sample. Repetition of results can only improve knowledge of contact period events and contribute to a more complete resolution of the problem. If, despite biases, I observe comparable patterns of change in spatially segregated regions with differing contact histories, conclusions will be strengthened.

Four

Archaeological Test Cases

We have become so accustomed to rely upon the testimony of word-written records that we lose sight of the fact that words are but thought symbols, ideaphones, *and ideagraphs, and that written records may be erroneous and incomplete while material objects may convey clearer meanings by which a much more accurate knowledge may be gained (Parker 1907:467).*

LOWER MISSISSIPPI VALLEY

The archaeological sample used in this analysis is a linear area, approximately 600 km long, that extends from Memphis, Tennessee south to Iberville Parish, Louisiana (Figure 6). Besides Quaternary-Age surfaces of the Natchez Bluffs the sample is restricted to Holocene floodplain surfaces and near surfaces of the St. Francis Lowlands, Yazoo Basin, and Taensa Basin. In addition to the Mississippi River, a number of major drainages flow through the area in a general north-south direction.

The area is one of low elevation, characterized by older ridges, swales, abandoned meander belts, oxbow lakes, active natural levees, and backwater swamps (Fisk 1944; Saucier 1974). Levee developments are extensive along drainages, channeling the direction of normal tributary flow parallel to the main channel of the Mississippi. Because flooding has always been a persistent problem in this section of the valley, most of the human habitation throughout the Holocene has occurred along the levees, which are topographic high areas of the landscape.

Historical Aboriginal Population

Documentation of aboriginal populations within the study area began with the

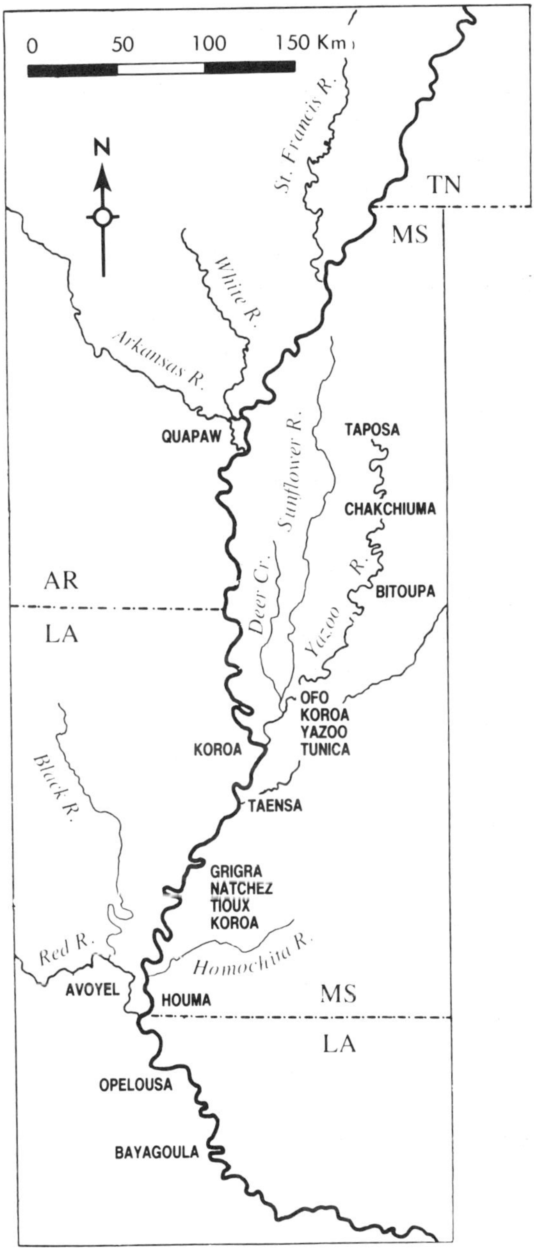

Figure 6. Study Area, Lower Mississippi Valley

De Soto *entrada* in the spring of 1541, when he spent approximately six weeks in the valley before moving west into Texas (Swanton 1939). The French period in the Lower Mississippi Valley began in 1673 with the explorations of Marquette and Jolliet (Shea 1903). The explorations of La Salle and Tonti in 1682 (Kellogg 1917) marked the beginning of consistent documentation of aboriginal groups. Although French settlement along the coast dated to 1699 (Biloxi Bay), permanent French settlements in the Valley occurred roughly a decade later (Swanton 1911).

Aboriginal populations did not persist long after the beginning of European colonization and settlement. Some groups disappeared completely, and even those who survived seemed to have been quite unstable (I. Brown 1985; Davis 1984; Giardino 1984; Swanton 1911). Abandoment, relocation, or amalgamation were frequent descriptions. As a consequence of their early disappearance, anthropologists have based their knowledge of aboriginal groups largely on Spanish and French documents. Swanton (1911, 1928) was responsible for synthesizing and analyzing the major French sources.

For the lower valley, Swanton places the ethnographic present in 1699, the date coincident with the Biloxi colony. According to his map (1911), in 1699 at least eighteen tribal groups were located along the Mississippi between the Yazoo Basin and New Orleans (Figure 6). North of the Yazoo, the valley was largely unoccupied except for the Chickasaw, who lived inland, and north of the study area, on the east side of the river. Although total tribal count could easily give the impression of a sizable population in the valley, this is not the case. Some groups identified in Figure 6 have passed into history only as a name; and the largest population, the Natchez, had no more than 1500 warriors (Swanton 1911). The Natchez War in 1730 marked the terminus of aboriginal systems and the final dispersion of Natchez, as well as other groups.

Significance of the Test Case

The archaeological analysis from the Lower Mississippi Valley is the first systematic test of Dobyns's sixteenth-century disease hypothesis. Since Dobyns (1983) bases his arguments on historical analyses from Florida, a study from the Southeast is crucial for confirming or disconfirming his position. If the lower valley record supports Dobyns's position, the case in favor of the general hypothesis is greatly strengthened. Although evidence for a seventeenth-century collapse does not necessarily exclude disease as causal, the case is simply not as strong. Since sustained European presence began in the late seventeenth century, other variables, including warfare and stress, could be contributing to trends in population; thus, regardless of outcome, the lower valley test is crucial to the general issue.

In addition, the test may help clarify archaeological treatment of the contact period in the lower valley. Although archaeologists interested in this region have entertained discussions of disease and population collapse, there are logical contradictions that make it difficult to determine the timing and nature of demographic change. Before presenting specific hypotheses to be tested, traditional approaches must be discussed.

Lower valley archaeologists have defined De Soto's arrival in 1541 (Bourne 1904) as the beginning of history, but these contacts were irregular and short-lived. As a consequence they were

> a false dawn. . . . These were not enduring affairs, and contact was soon broken, so that the area again receded into the realm of the unknown until European contact was reestablished and the historic period truly begun at the conclusion of the seventeenth century (Williams and Brain 1983:381).

Several cascading consequences have followed from this perspective. The 132 years that separate Spanish from French contact are a vague and largely undifferentiated interim, defined as the protohistoric (Morse and Morse 1983). Significant aboriginal change from Europeans was a late seventeenth-century process that began with French colonization, settlement, and documentation (Brain 1980; Brown 1985; Morse and Morse 1983; Phillips 1970; Williams 1980; Williams and Brain 1983).

Beginning with Collins (1927) and Ford (1936, 1961), the direct historical approach has guided the location and identification of archaeological sites (Brain 1975a, 1980; Hudson et al. 1985; Klinger 1975–77; Morse 1981). Ian Brown's recent work (1985) in the Natchez area is a good example. Although he tested and analyzed a number of deposits from later time periods, the final sample was weighted in favor of the protohistoric. "Sites were chosen on the basis of having protohistoric/historic materials"(1985:188). While it is reasonably certain that most of the sites from the French period are known (Brain 1970, 1973, 1975b, 1980; Brown 1975, 1979, 1985; Ford 1936, 1961; Neitzel 1965), the same statement cannot be made for prehistoric sites or even those occupied in 1541.

Furthermore, the use of the direct historical approach has led to a reliance on documents to reconstruct historic and prehistoric systems (Davis 1984; Ford and Willey 1941; Morse and Morse 1983). According to Griffin:

> The Mississippi Period was in full bloom at the time of the De Soto *entrada* into the Southeast, and at the time of other intermittent Spanish and French contacts in this area. We can, therefore, utilize with considerable confidence the information obtained from these chronicles and from the late seventeenth and eighteenth century European explorers . . . for the reconstruction of the social structure as it existed in the Mississippi Period in the Southeast (1952:362).

The Natchez are most significant in this regard. Because the Natchez persisted longer than many other, perhaps smaller, groups, there are a number of quite good eighteenth-century descriptions of their culture (Le Page du Pratz 1975; Swanton 1911). In addition, because the Natchez social system was seemingly based on ranks, it has become incorporated into the chiefdom model (Service 1962). This model has been used to describe ranked societies in the Southeast in both prehistoric and historical periods. (Davis 1984; Gibson 1973, 1980; Steponaitis 1978). The question of whether the Natchez system is a relevant analogue depends on whether the system was stable when first described. There has been some debate on this issue.

Among the Natchez, the primary class division was between nobility and Stinkards or commoners. Nobility, in turn, was comprised of three hierarchical classes: Suns, Nobles and Honored (Swanton 1911). While Suns provided the political and religious leaders—Tatooed Serpent and Great Sun—Stinkards made tribute payments to the nobility. A form of redistribution was accomplished through feasts, which occurred at regular intervals.

Although classes were permanent, marriage patterns were exogamous, creating an asymetrical structure in favor of nobility. Descriptions of the structure point to a progressive loss of commoners, which would have completely undermined the structure of the chiefdom.

Swanton (1911) thought the asymetrical structure was a social curiosity. When Hart reanalyzed the structure, he found it to be a "biological impossibility" (1943:374), headed toward a crisis if not a total collapse. Quimby (1946) was more generous in his analysis. He suggested that the Natchez practice of absorbing other native people into the social system at the rank of Stinkard compensated for loss of Stinkards through marriage. Given this practice, he concluded that the structure could persist for seven generations. Brain rooted Natchez classes in the prehistory of the Lower Mississippi Valley but suggested that exogamous marriages and the asymetrical structure were "adjustments to a new situation" (1971:221) that postdated De Soto. A grossly reduced population forced Natchez to absorb outsiders into their system with exogamous marriages providing the integrating mechanism. Despite differences in interpretation, it is clear that eighteenth-century Natchez social structure was in a state of flux quite possibly due to earlier population loss.

While assuming continuity, there are extensive discussions of discontinuity. Brain (1978:358) has suggested that during the French period "the great aboriginal climax witnessed by De Soto had passed, and the cultural inventory of the indigenous tribes was a poor reflection." Phillips's archaeological and historical research is primarily responsible for this perspective. (Phillips, Ford, and Griffin 1951). After comparing Spanish and French documents, Phillips concludes that aboriginal populations and cultural adaptations of the French period

> . . . are almost revolutionary in their nature and extent. They are not only in excess of the normal development; changes that might take place in a century and a half, but they are in the wrong direction, regressive rather than developmental (Phillips, Ford, and Griffin 1951:419).

According to Phillips, attrition of population was the most dramatic aboriginal change. Sometime between 1541 and 1682, Phillips estimated a population loss "amounting to at least eighty percent" (Phillips, Ford, and Griffin 1951:419). As population fell precipitously, settlement structure and political institutions also changed. By the late seventeenth century, there were not only fewer settlements, but those that persisted were infrequently associated with mounds. Simultaneously, complex political structures (chiefdoms) described in the De Soto chronicles gave way to decentralization and political equality of cultural units.

Since Phillips's convincing interpretations, other archaeologists (for example, Brain 1978, 1980; Ford 1961; Morse and Morse 1983) have adopted a perspective that recognizes significant disruptions of aboriginal population. There is no consensus, however, regarding either the timing or cause of the disruption. While some researchers (for example, Brain 1978; Williams and Brain 1983) think that the population decline began prior to De Soto, Ford (1961), like Phillips, placed its onset sometime between the Spanish and French periods.

The vagueness in terms of time is also expressed in terms of causes of the loss. As early as 1911, Swanton argued that the Natchez decline was due to both warfare and disease:

> What actually did destroy, or very nearly decimate the Natchez nation was the attrition of numberless encounters with other Indians, losses in the swamp from sickness and exposure, and epidemics which would have reduced them in any event, with or without warfare (1911:248).

Phillips's perspective is somewhat different (Phillips, Ford, and Griffin 1951) from Swanton's. He placed the origin of disease contact, especially that of smallpox, as a phenomenon of the French period. If disease was a late introduction, then warfare caused the massive loss of population. Since, during the eighteenth century, the Chickasaw were relatively intact and were frequently described as the "Iroquois of the South, the villains responsible for every calamity" (Phillips, Ford, and Griffin 1951:420). Phillips, therefore, suggests that the Chickasaw caused the catastrophic decline.

Milner (1980) and Brain (1980) disagree with Phillips. Milner suggests that disease played a significant role in the decline of southeastern aboriginal populations prior to the French period. Brain (1980) makes an even stronger point, stating that disease was the earliest European introduction and was responsible for massive depopulation episodes prior to sustained European presence:

> The European had many advantages over native aborigines of North America. One advantage, unknown to the participants at the time, was a biological constitution that withstood the new environment with relatively little stress and at the same time contributed diseases which were virulent, epidemic, and all too often fatal to the Indian. Thus, during the protohistoric period, before most Indians had even seen a white man, vast populations were wiped out, and any social, political, or other developments (and these were considerable as De Soto found at great expense) that might have withstood some of the European threat were lost with them. The European then, found only "inferior" cultures when he finally came to exploit and colonize North America (1980:270).

To recapitulate, the test case is significant for two specific reasons: It considers Dobyns's hypothesis in a region where the hypothesis was developed initially, and it may help resolve some of the ambiguities that pervade archaeological treatment of the record of European contact in the lower valley. While archaeologists recognize that the De Soto *entrada* ushered in history in the Lower Mississippi Valley, they equate European contact and its attendant changes with sustained European presence which began with French exploration in the late seventeenth century. This perspective allows archaeologists to make extensive use of documentary evidence. The question is whether such evidence describes populations essentially unaltered by Europeans or in the process of adjusting to catastrophic decline from disease. Only by separating archaeology and history and assessing the archaeological record of population collapse can this question be answered.

If the De Soto *entrada* was, indeed, a "false dawn," archaeological analyses should demonstrate stability of population until French colonization and settlement. If, on the other hand, the De Soto *entrada* marks the terminus of aboriginal population size and distribution, then significant changes in the nature and distribution of settlements ought to precede the late seventeenth century. Moreover, the timing of the collapse has implications for its cause. If the collapse predates sustained European presence in the valley, then Dobyns's idea about infectious disease is most likely correct. If the collapse occurs during the French period, then a combination of factors including both warfare and disease are probably responsible.

I frame alternative views into two hypotheses for testing against archaeological and historical records:

Hypothesis 1 (H1) states: Although European contact begins with De Soto in the lower valley, aboriginal collapse dates to the late seventeenth century and thus coincides with French colonization and settlement. The cause of the decline is a combination of factors including warfare and disease.

Hypothesis 2 (H2) states: Aboriginal collapse is a sixteenth-century event that occurs simultaneously with the earliest documentation in the lower valley. By the time of French colonization, aboriginal populations are drastically reduced. The timing of the event implicates infectious disease as causal in the collapse.

Late Mississippi Period Chronologies

As employed in this work, *Mississippi* refers to the period, and *Mississippian* refers to one cultural tradition of the Lower Mississippi Valley during that period. There are several integrative schemes for the Late Mississippi period in the Lower Mississippi Valley (Table 9), largely developed from analysis of ceramics. Because ceramics have been the primary basis for ordering the record, different theories of classification (Hill and Evans 1972) have affected final outcomes. The works of Ford and Phillips offer major contrasts. Ford was the primary temporal architect of the first Lower Valley Survey (Phillips, Ford and Griffin 1951); all other integrative schemes (Phillips 1970; Willey and Phillips 1958) basically modified Ford's early work.

Ford's interest was primarily chronological, extracting time from space and form. He defined ceramic types accordingly, and ordered archaeological units

Table 9 Late Mississippi Period Chronologies, Lower Mississippi Valley

TIME (A.D.)	PHILLIPS, FORD & GRIFFIN (1951) PERIODS	PHILLIPS (1970) YAZOO BASIN PHASES	WILLIAMS & BRAIN (1983) YAZOO BASIN PHASES	MORSE & MORSE (1983) MIDDLE MISSISSIPPI PHASES	BROWN (1985) NATCHEZ BLUFFS PHASES	RAMENOFSKY PERIODS
1800						
						III
1700						
		RUSSELL	RUSSELL	QUAPAW	NATCHEZ	
1600						
	A		WASP LAKE		EMERALD	II
1500				NODENA/PARKIN KENT/WALLS		
1400		DEER CREEK/ LAKE GEORGE/ WASP LAKE	LAKE GEORGE		FOSTER	I
	B		WINTERVILLE			
1300						
					ANNA	
1200						
1100						
1000						

through seriations (Ford 1954, 1962; Phillips, Ford and Griffin 1951). Phillips (1958, 1970), on the other hand, had both cultural and temporal interests. Although his pottery types were basically a reworking of Ford's types, his search for a finer resolution of the record led to the use of types and varieties. Temporocultural units, phases, were established through cumulative frequency curves of ceramics, spatial discontinuities and radiocarbon dates.

Differences are readily apparent. In Ford's order, the Late Mississippi period, A-B, crosses the historic baseline and continues until French settlement. During the Late Mississippi period, the Morses suggest there are a number of phases in the St. Francis Lowlands. At least two of these phases, Kent (House 1984) and Parkin (Morse 1981), cross the De Soto border. In the most recent chronology for the Yazoo Basin, Williams and Brain (1983) separate the Wasp Lake phase as part of the protohistoric or Spanish Period phase. I. Brown's Emerald phase (1985) occupies a similar temporal position in the Natchez Bluffs area.

Although specific sequences may be correct for each area, there is no way to determine which sequence is correct for the whole region. Chronologies of Phillips, Ford, and Griffin and of the Morses, though derived from different epistomologies, do not segregate the sixteenth century. To employ their units would mean that I could not investigate the hypothesis of a sixteenth-century collapse. While Williams, Brain, and Brown separate out the sixteenth century, it cannot be assumed *a priori* that their orders apply to the entire study area. Further, since their orders treat the protohistoric temporal unit as a continuation of earlier prehistoric traditions, they are assuming some degree of continuity through the sixteenth century. Such an assumption is not possible in this work. The creation of another chronology for the entire region that has no assumptions about stability or change is a reasonable alternative.

Although disputing the temporal divisions of the latest period, archaeologists generally agree that during the Late Mississippi period the Mississippian and Plaquemine traditions were present in the lower valley. Vicksburg, Mississippi is a convenient boundary between these two: the Mississippian tradition extended north from the upper part of the Yazoo Basin, while the Plaquemine tradition extended from the southern part of the Yazoo Basin to the coast.

The Mississippian tradition of the Late Mississippi period is composed of numerous and areally distinct phases (Brain 1978; Morse and Morse 1983; Phillips 1970; Williams and Brain 1983). Subsistence was based on maize agriculture, and sedentary settlements were associated with large platform mounds. In some areas, population lived in large, fortified settlements, such as those at Nodena (Morse 1973) and Powers (Price 1978). In other areas, such as Natchez, population was more dispersed (I. Brown 1985; House 1984).

Ceramics, one of the hallmarks of the Late Mississippi period, showed a variety of forms and styles. Subglobular jars with straight or slightly outcurved rims and lug handles, and simple bowls with round bases and curved sides continued from the Early Mississippi period. New forms, including bottles, and effigy bowls or jars, miniature vessels, ladles, discs, discoidals, and rattles were added. Decorative techniques included engraving, incising, and punctating, as well as monochrome or polychrome painting. Motifs occurred on the body, rim, and lip of vessels and included types such as Parkin Punctated, Barton Incised, Leland Incised, Rhodes Incised, Kent Incised, Ranch Incised, Avenue Polychrome and Bell Plain (Phillips 1970; Phillips, Ford, and Griffin 1951).

Mississippi period traits, not specifically limited to the Late Mississippi period, included shell tempered ceramics, willow leaf or half willow leaf projectile points with flat bases, thumbnail scrapers, and square button style beads (Morse and Morse 1983; Phillips, Ford, and Griffin 1951; Williams 1980).

The settlement pattern of some phases may have been hierarchically organized, but this was not a consistent feature of all phases. In the St. Francis Lowlands, Klinger (1975–1977) and Morse (1981) have suggested two different types of settlement hierarchies to account for settlement distribution during the Late Mississippi period. Klinger's model included five settlement types that ranged from specialized ceremonial centers (Parkin) to farmsteads of less than half a hectare. Morse's model, similar to that proposed by Flannery for the Formative in Mesoamerica, included four settlement types. The Parkin site was the major ceremonial center and occupied a strategic location during the Parkin phase. Small centers were removed from Parkin at regular intervals, and in between these centers were villages of two hectares or less. Based on a survey of the area, Morse suggested that there were no isolated farmsteads during the phase. In contrast to both Morse and Klinger, House (1984) suggested that the settlement pattern of the Kent phase was not hierarchically organized. If House is correct, then the variability between adjacent areas was, indeed, impressive.

In addition to a variable settlement pattern, archaeologists (Brain 1978; Brown and Brain 1983; Morse and Morse 1983; Phillips, Ford and Griffin 1951) have suggested that the distribution of population may have changed during the latest prehistoric period. Populations were relocating into fewer but larger settlements away from the main channel of the Mississippi.

Although Quimby (1951) was the first to define traits of the Plaquemine tradition, it had been known for some time in the archaeology of the Lower Mississippi Valley (Griffin 1946a). Like Mississippian, Plaquemine was associated with platform mounds; and settlements may have been organized into some sort of hierarchy. Also, like Mississippian, ceramics were one of best documented features of the tradition. Plaquemine ceramics were clay- or grog-tempered, and included such types as Addis Plain (Baytown Plain var. Addis), Evansville Punctated, Plaquemine Brushed, L'eau Noire Incised, Medora Incised, Fatherland Incised (Leland Incised var. Fatherland), Coles Creek Incised, Manchac Incised (Mazique Incised var. Manchac) (Phillips 1970;

Quimby 1951). Incision was a very common decorative technique in Plaquemine ceramics, and motifs included whorls, swastikas, and geometric designs applied to the body, lip, and rim of a wide variety of vessel shapes. Dominant vessel forms were carinated bowls, beakers, and jars with slightly constricted necks and outflaring rims.

Archaeologists have viewed the Plaquemine tradition as an indigenous lower valley culture that developed out of Coles Creek with the addition of Mississippian traits. Brain (1978), in fact, defined Plaquemine as a "Mississippianized Coles Creek." Beck (1981) has recently challenged this opinion, suggesting that Plaquemine was not a stylistically separate tradition, but a generalized subsistence strategy associated with sedentary settlements. Based on significant statistical correlations between site location and soil types, she contended that the change from a generalized to specialized, or maize-based, subsistence, did not occur until sometime after 1400.

In summary, although there is no consistently applied chronology of the Late Mississippi period for the entire study area, archaeologists generally agree that from roughly A.D. 1400 to 1700, Mississippian and Plaquemine traditions were present in the lower alluvial valley. They defined Mississippian by its stylistic motifs of shell tempered ceramics. Population distribution was variable, ranging from large, fortified and nucleated settlements to dispersed farmsteads. Many settlements were associated with platform mounds. Plaquemine, also defined by sedentary settlements and platform mounds, was distinct from Mississippian tradition because of clay- or grog-tempered ceramics.

Alternative Chronology

I have developed a new chronology (Table 9) that crosses into historical periods but does not prejudge the nature of changes that occur in those periods. Instead, I shall compare demographic indicators of population between temporal units to define whether or not populations catastrophically declined in the sixteenth century.

I employed radiocarbon assays, occurrence seriations of pottery and analysis of European trade goods, to assign sixty-six components to one of my three chronological periods. (See Appendix A for detailed discussion of orders). Radiocarbon dates were of limited utility in developing the chronology. Since only three of sixty-six components had absolute dates (Appendix A, Table 57), I placed greatest weight on the two relative methods.

Forty-nine components were ordered in one of the occurrence seriations; these were largely a reanalysis of Ford's seriations (Phillips, Ford, and Griffin 1951). After subdividing the region into five areas defined by Ford—St. Francis Lowlands, Memphis, Lower Arkansas, Upper Sunflower, and Yazoo Basin (Appendix A, Figure 18)—I employed Mississippi period types defined by Phillips, Ford, and Griffin.

Seventeen components had European material, but I had to limit my temporal analysis to sixteen, because the specific composition of the European assemblage from Haynes Bluff has not been reported. Of the seventeen components, five were also ordered by one of the seriations. Based on a new classification of European material, I analyzed European assemblages qualitatively because counts of individual European items were inconsistently reported in the literature. Finally, I employed dates from documents to determine whether archaeological assignments of components were consistent with the designations from the historical record.

To counteract the imprecision in the temporal dimension, I created minimum, mean, and maximum estimates of each period (Table 10) to bracket period durations. This control afforded three different temporal measures against which changes in settlement counts could be judged. Since settlement counts were the only demographic indicator available in this part of the valley, the control was of some importance.

Table 10 Length of Archaeological Periods in the Lower Mississippi Valley

	Period Length (A.D.)			*Period Duration (Years)*		
Period	*Minimum*	*Mean*	*Maximum*	*Minimum*	*Mean*	*Maximum*
III	1700–1730	1700–1750	1700–1764	30	50	64
II	1541–1673	1541–1682	1541–1699	132	141	158
I	1500–1540	1400–1540	1000–1540	40	140	540

Period I is the terminal prehistoric time unit in this chronology (Table 11). Based on seriations, I assigned forty-nine components to this period. Although there are twenty-four dates for the period, only two components with absolute dates (Upper Nodena and Lake George) are ordered by one of the seriations. In all three temporal models, the terminal date of Period I is 1540, immediately before De Soto's entry into the region, but origin dates vary. For the minimum estimate, I employed Morse's origin date (1500) for the Parkin phase (1981). Phillips's 1970 origin date for the Late Mississippi period is employed in the mean estimate (1400) and for the maximum estimate, Phillips' 1970 date for the Mississippi period is used (1000). While certain pottery types (for example, Neeley's Ferry Plain, Bell Plain, Barton Incised, and Parkin Punctated) occur throughout the period, other pottery types (for example, Owens Punctated, Avenue Polychrome, Rhodes Incised, Ranch Incised, Kent Incised, and Vernon Paul Applique) are more spatially restricted and have shorter durations. No European material is reported for the period.

Period II, coincides with Spanish and French exploration of the Lower Mississippi Valley, and begins with the De Soto *entrada* of 1541. The minimum

Table 11 Characteristics of Chronological Periods in the Lower Mississippi Valley

PERIOD I	
Radiocarbon Dates:	27 (See Appendix A, Table 57)
Minimum Time Range:	A.D. 1500–1540
Mean Time Range:	A.D. 1400–1540
Maximum Time Range:	A.D. 1000–1540
Ceramics:	Shell tempered types including Neeley's Ferry Plain, Bell Plain, Barton Incised, Parkin Punctated, Kent Incised, Rhodes Incised, Ranch Incised, Vernon Paul Applique, Avenue Polychrome, Owens Punctated.
European Trade:	Absent
Components:	49 identified by seriations (Appendix A, Tables 56, 61–66)
PERIOD II	
Radiocarbon Dates:	0
Minimum Time Range:	A.D. 1541–1673
Mean Time Range:	A.D. 1541–1682
Maximum Time Range:	A.D. 1541–1699
European Trade:	Present; Clarksdale Bells, Glass Trade Beads.
Components: (n = 10)	Satartia, Clay Hill, Parkin, Wallace, Menard, Oliver, Clarksdale, Haynes Bluff, Rice, Dead Oak.
PERIOD III	
Radiocarbon Dates:	0
Minimum Time Range:	A.D. 1700–1730
Mean Time Range:	A.D. 1700–1750
Maximum Time Range:	A.D. 1700–1764
Ceramics:	Not well known.
European Trade:	All classes of European function present.
Components: (n = 7)	Lockgard, Portland, Fatherland, Bayou Goula, Trudeau, Greenfield, Thoroughbred

estimate of period duration covers the time between the exploration of De Soto and that of Marquette and Jolliet (1541–1673). While the mean estimate extends from the De Soto baseline to the first La Salle exploration (1541–1682), the maximum estimate lasts until the beginning of French colonization (1541–1699). During this period, limited quantities of European materials, "Clarksdale" bells and glass trade beads, are found. Pottery is not well reported. Ten components, four of which are ordered by seriations, are assigned to Period II.

Period III coincides with French colonization and settlement and is represented by seven components. European products from this period are fundamentally different from those of Period II. All types of metal products as well as European crockery, glass bottles, and quantities of trade beads are present in aboriginal assemblages. Although period duration varies from thirty to sixty-four years, all three temporal models employ the same origin date, A.D. 1700. The minimum estimate (1700–1730) terminates with the Natchez War; the mean estimate (1700–1750) terminates in the middle of the century, and the maximum estimate (1700–1764) terminates with the abandonment of the Tunica settlement of Trudeau.

This chronology is superficially similar to some other chronologies in that my Period II occupies the same temporal position as I. Brown's (1985) Emerald phase and Williams and Brain's (1983) Wasp Lake phase. Although it would be convenient to treat the new unit as the protohistoric expression of the Late Mississippi period, I choose not to do so because of the use of either term implies a kind of continuity with earlier expressions that may not be justified. If examination of the record reveals catastrophic change in population beginning with Period III, then these attributions are justified. If, however, catastrophic population loss is an event of Period II, then terms that imply continuity in population or culture must be seriously questioned.

To recapitulate, Period I marks the terminus of the aboriginal prehistoric record, ending just before De Soto enters the valley. Period II, the first historical period, begins with the De Soto *entrada* and continues through French exploration of the region. While European material is not reported for any Period I site, European bells and glass trade beads are present at Period II sites. Period III dates to the eighteenth century and coincides with French settlement in the valley. The aboriginal assemblages of European material from Period III are functionally more diversified than those from Period II. Finally, the empirical evidence suggests that European contact begins during Period II. Whether this catastrophic decline begins with Period II will be determined by analysis of aboriginal population.

Analysis of Population Change

Settlement counts (S_c), the most biased of archaeological estimators, are the only archaeological measure of population available in the Lower Mississippi Valley. I cannot, therefore, employ archaeological formulas of population developed in Chapter 3 to estimate population change in the region. I limit analysis to consideration of S_c and to changing distributions of settlements. Although I attempt to make use of counts to assess hypotheses regarding the initiation of collapse, biases implicit in the measurement of S_c are expected to produce ambiguous results (see Appendix A, Table 70 for settlement list).

SETTLEMENT COUNTS (S_c) Table 12 summarizes changes in S_c across temporal units. Actual counts in column 2 (n = 66) are higher than those summarized on Table 6. This difference is because some settlements have multiple occupations. Presented in subsequent columns are counts normalized to a standard period duration.

Table 12 Lower Mississippi Valley Settlement Counts and $[S_c/(T/100)]$

Period	Raw Counts	Adjusted Counts $[S_c/(T/100)]$ Minimum	S_c	Mean	S_c	Maximum	S_c
III	7	0.3	23.3	0.5	14.0	0.6	11.6
II	10	1.3	7.5	1.4	7.1	1.6	6.3
I	49	0.4	123.0	1.4	35.0	5.4	9.1

The actual mathematics of adjusting counts are straight forward. A minimum estimate of a period duration of 200 is normalized to 2 when 200 is divided by the temporal term 100. This figure is then divided into the actual settlement count for that period. For instance, a settlement count of 10 becomes a normalized count of 5 in the above example.

Despite differences in the temporal dimension, $[S_c/(T/100)]$ shows similar changes in direction. (See Figure 7 for graphical display of settlement trends.) Between Periods I and II, counts precipitously decrease, followed by a slight increase between Periods II and III. Before evaluating these trends, biases due to archaeological sampling and residental instability must be considered.

As described previously, prehistoric and historic records have not been sampled equally. The importance of ethnohistory, archaeological reliance on the direct historical approach, and judgmental sampling of the prehistoric

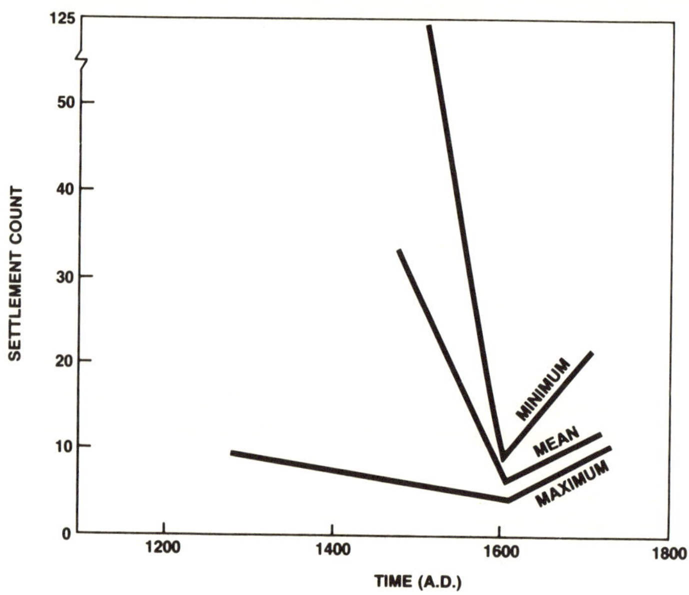

Figure 7. $[S_c/(T/100)]$ Measured against Estimates of Period Duration

record have skewed archaeological knowledge in favor of historic periods. Consequently, archaeologists are more likely to have identified a larger fraction of aboriginal settlements occupied during Periods II and III than those of Period I. This known bias should inflate historic counts relative to prehistoric counts.

The question of residential instability needs to be considered. Although there is considerable evidence that groups were abandoning and relocating villages by the late seventeenth century, the onset of this pattern is not reliably placed in time. I. Brown's recent work in the Natchez Bluff area (1982, 1985), however, suggests a pre-French origin.

Relying heavily on historical documents, I. Brown (1985) explicitly attempted to locate specific settlements that the Grigra and other groups occupied during the late seventeenth and early eighteenth centuries. These attempts were unsuccessful, not because the documents were in error regarding the locations of settlements, but because Brown assumed continuity of occupation throughout the temporal period. I. Brown (1985) stated that his assumption was wrong and suggested that other populations had settled and abandoned the Natchez area before the eighteenth-century settlements of the Grigra.

The pattern of abandonment and relocation is well established by the late seventeenth century, the end of Period II. In 1682, La Salle recorded four Quapaw villages at the mouth of the Arkansas River. Between 1690 and 1700, two of these villages were abandoned, one had moved downriver, and a new hybrid community was founded (Kellogg 1917). Between 1698 and 1700, the Tunica resided in the Yazoo Basin. Between 1706 and 1731, they migrated downriver, and either settled with or replaced the Houma at one of the latter's villages. After 1731, the Tunica established residence at Trudeau, located at the mouth of the Red River (Brain 1975b). Between 1699 and 1706, three different groups were living with the Bayagoula (Quimby 1957), and between 1720 and 1730, remnants of the populations of Yazoo, and Tioux were absorbed by the Natchez.

These data suggest that from the latter part of Period II through Period III aboriginal populations of the Lower Mississippi Valley were continually shifting residences. Even though the origin of the movement cannot be identified, it seems probable that French exploration does not mark the origin of the pattern, but rather, the documentation of a preexisting pattern.

The effects of archaeological emphasis on historic period settlements and instability of population should lead to a situation in which S_c steadily increases during Periods II and III. Since between Period I and II counts decrease rather than increase and since the pattern of change is comparable in all temporal models, it is reasonable to assume that the change represents catastrophic population loss that begins with Spanish contact. The question is whether the suggested increase between Periods II and III represents a demographic recovery or is a reflection of sampling and cultural bias. As described below, available information suggests that the increase in counts is a function of bias, not of population increase.

Of the seven Period III settlements, five were new communities (Portland, Lockgard, Trudeau, Greenfield, Thoroughbred) with founding dates ranging from 1708 to 1731. The two other communities (Fatherland and Bayou Goula) were continuations of settlements from earlier periods; amalgamation of smaller remnant groups in part explained the survival of both. None of the seven communities persisted for the maximum duration of Period III (1700–1764). By 1764, Trudeau was the only surviving community, but Trudeau was not founded until 1731.

In summary, the decrease in $[S_c/(T/100)]$ between Periods I and II suggests a precipitous population decline that predates French settlement of the valley. While Period III counts suggest a population increase, counts cannot be taken at face value. In fact, while settlement counts are increasing, population may be declining.

SETTLEMENT DISTRIBUTION Changes in the distribution of settlements across the three temporal periods demonstrate progressive downriver movement. In Period I, all counties on both sides of the Mississippi River from Memphis through the Yazoo Basin are occupied (Figure 8A). During Period II, populations abandon the area north of the southern end of the Yazoo Basin; and northern settlements that persist are spatially discontinuous (Figure 8B). By Period III, except for two new settlements at the mouth of the Yazoo River, the northern part of the valley is unoccupied (Figure 8C). Population has migrated south, clustering into settlements in the vicinity of Fatherland and Bayou Goula.

CONCLUSIONS I expected archaeological analysis of population change in the Lower Mississippi Valley to produce ambiguous results regarding the initiation of aboriginal collapse. Settlement counts were the only archaeological measure of population, and counts were extremely biased in favor of the historic periods. Despite these problems, data were not ambiguous, and conclusions were, in fact, strengthened because the initial direction of change so completely contradicted expectations.

As demonstrated by the changes in settlement counts, aboriginal collapse did not begin with sustained French presence in the valley, but rather with the De Soto *entrada* more than 150 years earlier. Consequently, I conclude that the beginning of European contact also marks the onset of aboriginal population loss. Several important consequences follow from this conclusion.

Although the De Soto chronicles may describe pristine populations, French documents do not. The latter are important descriptions of populations in the process of adapting to new environmental conditions, especially catastrophic reduction of people. As suggested by Phillips (Phillips, Ford and Griffin 1951), a comparison of Spanish and French sources may prove very fruitful in determining the nature and direction of these changes.

Furthermore, since the loss predates sustained European presence, infectious disease is causal. This conclusion, in turn, supports Dobyns's hypothesis of the sixteenth century as the disease century in the Southeast.

There are, however, several problems with the archaeological data. While I have argued that the normalized increase in settlement counts of the eighteenth century, Period III, is a function of sampling bias rather than of recovery of population, the archaeological record is insufficient for indicating how population is behaving relative to the increase in counts. Fortunately, there are eighteenth-century census records for aboriginal populations; and these records can be analyzed to determine whether or not the loss, beginning with the De Soto *entrada*, continues into the period of French settlement.

Lower Mississippi Valley History, 1541–1764

In this section, I shall review European exploration and colonization, aboriginal settlement counts and relocation, and aboriginal population estimates. Following these discussions, I shall consider epidemic history of the Southeast.

EUROPEAN EXPLORATION AND COLONIZATION Spain was the first European nation to explore and to attempt colonization of the Southeast in general. The primary motive in these ventures was the acquisition of wealth. Since native populations had largely disappeared from the Spanish West Indies by 1510, trafficking in aboriginal human populations was the earliest southeastern resource to be exploited (Sauer 1971) (Table 13). Attempts at colonization began shortly thereafter; in 1526, Lucas Vasquez de Ayllon with about 500 settlers established a colony near Winyah Bay, South Carolina. Within six months, the colony had failed; and the 150 survivors returned to the West Indies (Hudson 1976).

The Panifilo de Navaez and Cabeza de Vaca expedition (1527–1536) was the first major Spanish attempt at inland exploration from the west coast of Florida. The party, including 400 men and some 150 horses, explored north from Tampa Bay. Indian resistance was so great that the party never traveled farther inland than northwest Florida. Survivors were forced back to the coast where barges were built in hopes of following the Gulf coast to Mexico. While traveling west, the expedition made a brief foray up the Mississippi delta; and by 1528, ninety survivors, including Cabeza de Vaca, had reached Galveston Bay. For the next six years, survivors lived among native populations in east Texas; by 1536, only four of the original 400 were still alive (Fernandez 1975; Sauer 1971).

The De Soto *entrada*, initially comprised of approximately 600 men, 4 or 5 women, 200 horses and 2500 swine (Swanton 1939), was not only the first

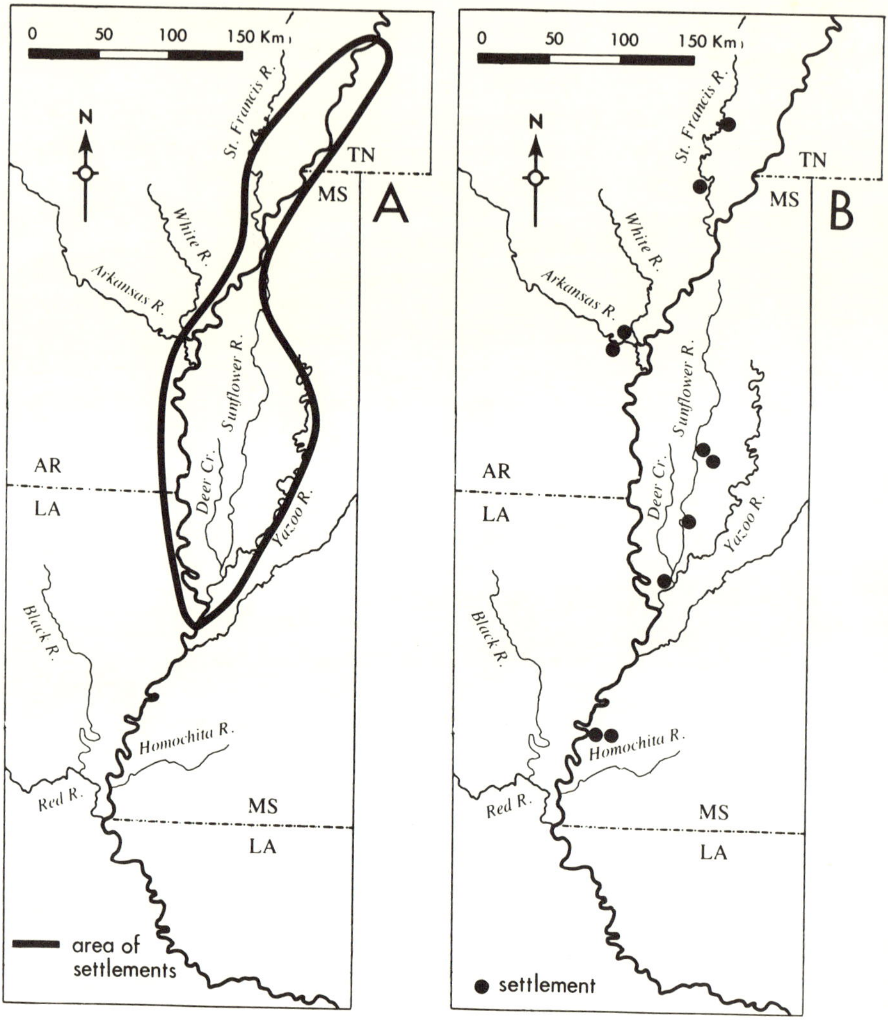

successful inland exploration of much of the Southeast, but also recorded the first contact in the Lower Mississippi Valley. During the four-year journey (1539–1543), the party traveled a circuitous route through parts of west Florida, the Carolinas, Tennessee, Alabama, Louisiana, Mississippi, Arkansas, and Texas (Hudson et al. 1985; Swanton 1939). In May 1541, they reached the Lower Mississippi Valley, somewhere between the Yazoo and Sunflower drainages. After approximately six weeks, they pushed into Arkansas and then turned south crossing into Louisiana before reaching Texas. Four narratives by the Gentleman of Elvas, Hernandez de Biedma, Rodrigo Ranjel (Bourne 1904),

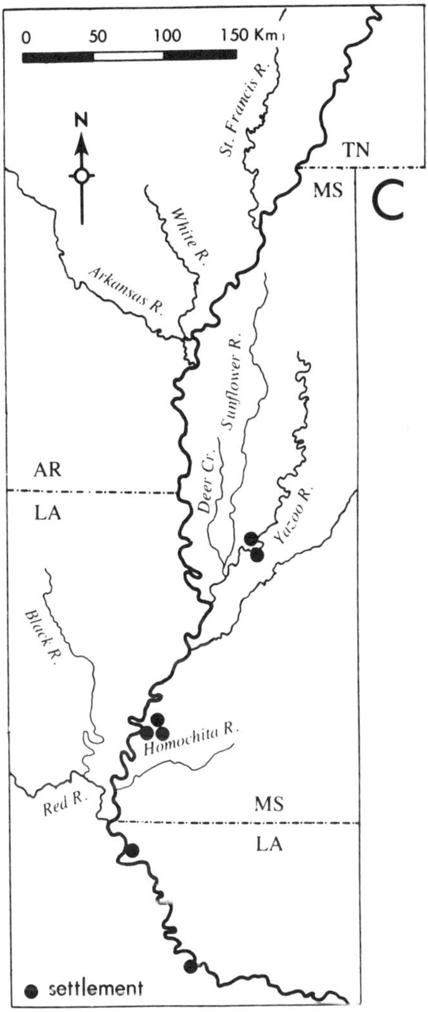

Figure 8. Distribution through Time of Settlements in the Lower Mississippi Valley

and Garcilaso de la Vega, El Inca (Varner and Varner 1951) described the expedition. According to Bourne (1904) and Swanton (1939), the first three chroniclers were the most reliable sources since they were part of the expedition. El Inca was not part of the exploration, and his account was based on the account of a participant made forty years after the event.

Between the De Soto *entrada* and 1673, there were no recorded contacts of Lower Mississippi Valley populations. In that year, Marquette and Jolliet traveled down the Mississippi as far south as the Arkansas River. Although extensive notes were made, many were later lost (Nasatir 1952; Shea 1903). The

Table 13 Some Historical Events in the Southeast and Lower Mississippi Valley

1510	Spanish begin slave raids along east coast of Florida.
1527–1536	Panifilo de Navaez and Cabeza de Vaca explore the Gulf Coast from Florida to east Texas.
1539–1543	De Soto *entrada* explores the Southeast from Florida to east Texas.
1541	De Soto reaches the Lower Mississippi Valley.
1673	Father Marquette and Jolliet explore the Mississippi from its headwaters to the Arkansas River.
1679–1682	La Salle explores the Mississippi as far as its delta.
1686, 1687–1691, 1698–1699	Tonti makes three expeditions in the Lower Mississippi Valley. In 1686 he establishes a small trading post near Osotouy on the Arkansas River. In 1698, he guides French Jesuits into the valley.
1699	Iberville establishes the first French colony at Biloxi Bay.
1698–1710	French religious efforts (Recollets and Jesuits) begin among populations of the Lower Mississippi Valley.
1718	Bienville establishes New Orleans.
1718	French establish Fort Rosalie at Natchez.
1719	Fort St. Pierre established on the Yazoo River.

La Salle and Tonti expedition followed the initial French exploration by roughly ten years (Shea 1903). Their exploration had lasting effects in terms of French control of Louisiana: In the wake of their journey, independent French traders (*Coureurs de Bois*) began exploiting the region. Small forts and colonies such as La Salle's colony in east Texas founded in 1695 (Joutel 1906; Kellogg 1917) and Tonti's fort on the Arkansas River founded 1686 (Kellogg 1917) sprang up. Jesuit missionaries took up residence with native populations.

The push toward permanent French colonies in the Lower Mississippi Valley was triggered by France's desire to expand her empire in America, to increase her revenues, and to curtail British expansion from the rapidly developing colonies along the Atlantic seaboard. To these ends, Iberville established the first colony at Biloxi Bay in 1699. Although the colony persisted, existence was precarious. Given France's financial difficulties in the early eighteenth century, funds and raw materials were always in short supply. Although the colony aimed at self-sufficiency, the low population density and lack of farmers prevented attainment of that goal. Near starvation conditions prevailed more often than not (Giraud 1974).

Gradually, the situation began to change. Between 1715 and 1720, New Orleans was established and military forts began to spring up. French military requested assignment in Louisiana, and the colonial population also began to increase (Giraud 1974; Nasatir 1952). The development came too late. By 1740, French colonies had been pushed south of the Illinois River, and by 1763, France had lost her American empire.

The sequence of events of the early contact period in the Lower Mississippi Valley suggests that archaeological conclusions regarding the loss of aboriginal populations may be correct. Direct interaction with Europeans began in 1541. Although French settlement was established in the early eighteenth century, colonies did not gain a secure foothold until after 1720. As seen in the archaeological record, initial population loss may have predated French settlement by several hundred years.

ABORIGINAL CENSUS COUNTS As described previously, Phillips (Phillips, Ford, and Griffin 1951) argued that population loss was the most dramatic aboriginal change he could identify in the archaeological and historical records of the Lower Mississippi Valley. This archaeological analysis supported Phillips's position and pointed to an initial catastrophic loss that began in the second half of the sixteenth century and continued through French colonization. By the time France had lost her political position in North America, native populations and cultural systems of the Lower Mississippi Valley were essentially extinct.

Although there were no aboriginal census counts contained in the De Soto chronicles from the Lower Mississippi Valley, the impression one receives from these narratives was that of a sizable population. The impression is entirely consistent with the known archaeological record from 1540. Between the Yazoo Basin and the St. Francis Lowlands, the region was densely populated and divided into four provinces: Quizqui, Aquixo, Casque, and Pacaha (Bourne 1904; Swanton 1939). Aquixo was the smallest province, consisting of only a single town. All other provinces were composed of two or three major towns. While building *piraguas* for the crossing of the Mississippi, Spaniards observed the warrior potential of Pacaha: ". . . about seven thousand warriors . . . with more than two hundred canoes" (Ranjel in Bourne 1904:2:137) traveled onto the river and showered the Spaniards with arrows. When the attack failed to drive the intruders away, the natives themselves withdrew.

The earliest French records described an aboriginal population of the valley that was quite different. In 1682, La Salle and Tonti encountered no resident groups between the St. Francis Lowlands and the Yazoo Basin. The Quapaw were their first aboriginal contacts, and this group lived in four villages at the mouth of the Arkansas River (Kellogg 1917; Shea 1903). Although below the Quapaw, La Salle encountered aboriginal groups such as the Taensa, Natchez, and Bayagoula, the distribution of population was not continuous.

Changes in population density or distribution match the pattern of warrior estimates summarized in Table 14. Except for the Natchez who were actively absorbing smaller remnant populations, initial estimates were low and continued to decrease throughout the eighteenth century.

Variability in Natchez estimates between 1686 and 1722 cannot possibly reflect intrinsic population growth. Although a temporal interval of 36 years is

Table 14 Warrior Counts of Some Aboriginal Groups in the Lower Mississippi Valley[a]

Year	*Natchez*	*Taensa*	*Tunica*	*Bayagoula*	*Houma*	*Yazoo*
1682		700				
1686	1500					
1699				200–250	350	
1700		300				
1715	4000					
1716	800					
1721	2000					
1722	600					
1729	700					
1730	500					40[e]
1731	200–300					
1735	180					
1739				90–100[c]	90–100[d]	
1758			60		60[d]	15[f]
1764	150[b]					
1784					25[d]	12[f]
1799	50[b]					
1805			25			

[a]After Swanton 1911.
[b]With Creek.
[c]Includes Houma and Acolapissa.
[d]Includes Bayagoula and Houma.
[e]Includes Koroa.
[f]Includes Ofo.

longer than a generation, the period is still too brief to allow for a population increase of 166% followed by a decrease of 50%. Consequently, the pattern in the Natchez estimates must be reflecting cultural practices or observer biases. For instance, the 1715 estimate was made shortly before Ft. Rosalie was established at Natchez and may have served to justify the establishment of the post.

Besides showing continuing loss of population, estimates are of interest for demonstrating amalgamation processes. All Yazoo counts and most of those for the Houma and Bayagoula include several other groups. Although not indicated in the table, counts for the Yazoo and Tioux are part of Natchez counts for the period 1720–1730.

In addition to recorded depopulation trends, there are more general descriptions of population loss during the eighteenth century. In 1704, De La Vente wrote:

> The Natchez . . . assure us that they came here to the number of more than 5,000. The other ones say that many centuries ago they were, some 3,000,

> others 2,000, others a thousand, and all that is reduced now to a very moderate number. What is certain is that our people in the six years in which they have been descending the river, know certainly that the number has diminished a third, so true is it that it seems God wishes to make them give place to others (from Swanton 1911:39).

Charlevoix also described aboriginal population loss, attributing the cessation of mound-building activity to the disappearance of people:

> The greatest part of the Nations of Louisiana, had formerly their temples as well as the Natchez . . . But the temple of the Natchez is the only one subsisting at present, and is held in great veneration by all the savages inhabiting this vast continent, the decrease in whose numbers is as considerable, and has been, still more sudden, then that of the people of Canada, without it being possible to assign the true reason of this event. Whole nations have entirely disappeared within the space of forty years at most; and those who still remain, are not more than the shadow of what they were, when M. De Salle discovered this country (Charlevoix 1977 [1761]:256).

Finally, census counts are invaluable for pointing out that Period III settlement counts [$S_c/(T/100)$] are, indeed, biased. While I argued that the increase in Period III counts did not represent a genuine population increase, I was unable to determine whether population was stable or declining. This question can now be addressed. Although settlement counts show an increase, population is declining. Consequently, any attempt to measure prehistoric aboriginal changes in population from historic counts of settlements must be viewed with considerable suspicion.

In summary, then, comparison of Spanish and French sources indicate that at the time De Soto entered the Lower Mississippi Valley, large and dense populations were divided into a number of polities. Following De Soto, populations declined, and the decline continued through the French period. Amalgamation processes were a response to decline.

ABORIGINAL SETTLEMENT HISTORY From the beginning of consistent documentation, aboriginal populations were in such a state of flux that it is difficult to trace relocations of particular groups or to identify a uniform pattern of movement among all groups. The process of abandonment of the north part of the region continued into the eighteenth century. By 1720, remnant groups were clustered into few villages at the Homochito River or farther south.

Table 15 summarizes what can be gleaned from historical sources. Because these data are in dramatic contrast to the settlement counts and density of Period I, they, like warrior estimates and archaeological trends in population,

Table 15 Village Counts, Lower Mississippi Valley[a]

			Ethnic Group		
Year	*Natchez*	*Taensa*	*Quapaw*[b]	*Tunica*	*Bayagoula*
1686	9	8–9	4		1*
1699		1–7	3	1*	
1706		Abandonment following war with Houma		1*	Abandonment following war with Taensa
1710					
1720	5				
1731	Abandonment			1*	
1764				Abandonment	

[a]Except for Quapaw, all village counts taken from Swanton 1911.
[b]Shea 1903; Kellogg 1917.
*Settlement relocated.

support the argument that catastrophic population loss preceded French settlement. As a consequence, French documents describe the terminus of aboriginal sequences. Moreover, historic records contain descriptions of population instability and offer a number of insights into adaptive strategies that were emerging in response to drastically changed demographic structures.

Of the five groups it is likely that the Bayagoula, Natchez, and Taensa were present in the valley before 1680. Natchez and Bayagoula employed a strategy of amalgamation to survive. They remained in the same area and persisted by absorbing remnants into their ranks. Tunica migrated into the valley after 1680; their survival depended on relocation rather than amalgamation (Brain 1975b, 1980).

The Quapaw strategy is difficult to define largely because there is no agreement about the identity or origin of this ethnic unit (Hoffman 1983). Linguistic affiliation of the Quapaw with Siouan speakers suggests that the group entered the valley after 1680. At the same time, archaeological material from the Lower Arkansas Valley suggests the presence of some group(s) in this area prior to 1650 (Morse and Morse 1983). The question is whether the historically defined Quapaw were a postdisease amalgamation who took up residence in a recently abandoned area or whether they were autochthons of the area who developed other survival strategies.

It seems that residential instability and/or village reduction coupled with amalgamation processes were adaptive responses to new selective pressures. (See Dobyns 1983 for a similar discussion.) When village population fell below a threshold necessary for defense and maintenance, mobility or amalgamation developed as attempts to correct the situation. Although the cause(s) of these responses were obviously complex, population loss was clearly a significant factor. In the end, all such attempts were short-lived since population levels never stabilized.

EPIDEMIC HISTORY My brief historical summary has been quite consistent with archaeologically defined trends in population. The collapse began in the late sixteenth century and continued until aboriginal group sizes were too small to sustain previous cultural adaptations. Had the historical record demonstrated trends of stability or increase in population, the hypothesis of collapse would have been less convincing. Since this was not the case, it is appropriate to consider the epidemic disease record from the Southeast.

Although there are very few direct references to disease outbreaks in the sixteenth and seventeenth-century documents from the lower valley, a considerable body of historical data suggests that the disease contact began in the sixteenth century.

The earliest and only direct documentary evidence of the consequences of disease contact are contained in the De Soto chronicles. Upon reaching Cofitachequi, located on the South Carolina side of the Savannah River or at the headwaters of the Santee River, both Elvas and Biedma described the consequences of some disease on this seemingly impressive town:

> About this place, from half a league to a league off, were large vacant towns grown up in grass that appeared as if no people had lived in them for a long time. The Indians said that two years before, there had been a pest in the land, and that the inhabitants had moved away to other towns (Elvas in Bourne 1904:1:66).

There is some disagreement regarding the timing of this event. At the Cofitachequi temple, Spaniards found "two wood axes of Castilian make, a rosary of jet beads, and some false pearls . . . all of which we supposed they got in exchange, made with those who followed Licentiate Ayllon" (Biedma in Bourne 1904:II:13–14). Although the Spaniards did not see a link between the disease outbreak and trade goods, I think it likely that the two products were simultaneous introductions, diffusing from the Ayllon colony in 1526.

Although Dobyns (1983:262–264) cited the above description, he placed the origin of the epidemic between 1535 and 1538. (See Table 16.) Because maize was still present in the abandoned towns and because the southeastern climate did not facilitate long-term preservation of organics, Dobyns suggested that the epidemic diffused from Mexico shortly before De Soto began his exploration.

Without a finer temporal resolution of the archaeological record, there is no way to resolve the timing of the epidemic episode. It is clear, however, that

Table 16 Known or Probable Epidemics in Florida and the Lower Mississippi Valley

Lower Mississippi Valley	*Florida (Dobyns 1983)*
	1513
	1519–1524
	1528
	1535–1538
	1545–1548
	1549
	1550
	1559
	1564–1570
	1585–1586
	1586
	1596
	1613–1617
	1649
	1653
	1659
	1672
	1675
	1686
1698	
	1716
1718–1734	1726–1728

disease affected southeastern aboriginal populations prior to De Soto's exploration.

One sixteenth-century reference to disease is slim evidence to argue for a century of decimation. The lack of direct historical evidence does not mean, however, that native populations did not experience the ravages of such infections as smallpox or malaria simultaneously or sequentially. Sixteenth-century Europeans were unaware of their microbial imports. Further, since parasites that erupt in disease have incubation periods prior to the expression of illness, it is possible that explorers simply did not observe the consequences of microbial introductions. Another possibility is that disease introductions, independent of European presence, diffused like spatial waves.

Spatial diffusion is Dobyns's point of departure. Table 16 summarizes Dobyns's known or suspected epidemics of peninsular Florida. With the exception of the 1535 date, Dobyns thinks all disease episodes prior to 1596 were the result of diffusion from Cuba (Wright 1970) or Mexico (Gerhard 1972) or both. Seventeenth-century epidemics were a different matter. Since documents were a common feature in seventeenth-century Florida, direct historical observations were the sources for epidemic episodes identified by Dobyns.

The question raised by examining Table 16 is whether some or all of Dobyns's reconstructed epidemics for sixteenth-century Florida are applicable to other parts of the Southeast. Without independent evidence, Dobyns's synthesis stands as plausible speculation. When judged by the archaeological record from the Southeast, the synthesis becomes highly probable.

My population analysis from the lower valley was dramatic support of catastrophic population loss that dated to the late sixteenth and early seventeenth century. The magnitude of the loss suggested disease. Caddoan populations in east Texas seem to have experienced a similar and equally dramatic attrition at approximately the same time (Perttula 1984; Perttula and Ramenofsky 1981). Smith (1984), working in the interior Southeast, has also suggested a population collapse of Coosa Chiefdoms during the sixteenth century.

The timing and similarity of demographic events from different areas suggests not only that a single cause is responsible but that the decline postdates De Soto. Given that Dobyns suggests that twelve epidemics spread to Florida before 1600, disease is most likely, if diffusion pathways from outside the continent and across the Southeast can be demonstrated.

Fortunately, mechanisms of spread between the Caribbean or Mexico and the Southeast as well as throughout the Southeast are not difficult to infer. Dobyns (1983:247–289) has provided ample evidence of sixteenth-century contact between European centers outside the continent and the peninsula of Florida. Travel by boat was frequent, and parasites spread as people moved.

Within the Southeast, stylistic similarities across large areas such as the Pensacola complex of the Gulf Coast (Davis 1984; Knight 1984) suggest that southeastern groups were not isolated. Interaction, expressed as a veneer of style overlying regionally distinct systems, was a common feature during later periods. Although stylistic sharing does not necessarily imply disease sharing, it does suggest that pathways existed by which infectious parasites could have diffused from Europeans to uncontacted groups.

In summary, the archaeological record provided the necessary support for Dobyns's hypothesis of a sixteenth-century collapse throughout the Southeast. If the record had been limited to one region or if archaeological styles had suggested isolation, the case in support of sixteenth century disease would have been much weaker. Consequently, although I cannot stipulate specific diseases or precise times of epidemics, I can state that, in light of current evidence, the sixteenth-century is the disease century in the Southeast.

A consequence of consistent documentation is a much improved record of epidemic events. The seventeenth and eighteenth-century documents from the lower valley show that disease and population loss continued after French contact.

St. Cosme was one of the French missionaries whom Tonti guided down the Mississippi. In 1698, he described the consequences of smallpox among the Quapaw:

> We were deeply afflicted by finding this nation of the Arkansas, formerly so numerous, entirely destroyed by disease. Not a month has elapsed since they had rid themselves of smallpox, which had carried off most of them. In the villages are now nothing but graves, in which they were buried two together, and we estimated that not a hundred men were left. All of the children had died, and a great many women (Kellogg 1917:359).

One of the most complete descriptions of native experience of Old World diseases was that of Le Page du Pratz, who lived with the Natchez from 1718 until 1734. Among the Natchez, du Pratz found that both smallpox and colds were particularly devastating:

> Two distempers, that are not very fatal in other parts of the world, make dreadful ravages among them; I mean smallpox and a cold, which baffle all the arts of their physicians, who in other respects are very skillful. When a nation is attacked by the smallpox, it quickly makes great havoc; for as a whole family is crowded into a small hut, which has no communications with the external air, but a door about two feet wide and four feet high, the distemper, if it seizes one, is quickly communicated to all. The aged die in consequence of their advanced years, and the bad quality of their food; and the young, if they are not strictly watched, destroy themselves, from an abhorrence of the blotches on their skin. . . .
>
> Colds, which are very common in winter, likewise destroy great numbers of the natives. In that season they keep fires in their huts day and night; and as there is no other opening but the door, the air within the hut is kept excessively warm without any free circulation; so that when they have occasion to go out, the cold seizes them, and the consequences of it are almost always fatal (Le Page du Pratz 1975 [1758]:305–306).

The discussion of epidemic history has emphasized several points. Disease contact in the lower valley began in the sixteenth century. Some of these contacts may have been the result of direct interactions with Europeans; others were the result of diffusion. In either case, as the archaeological record demonstrated, the attrition in population was catastrophic. Finally, the process of population loss from infectious diseases that preceded colonization continued after the onset of French settlement.

Summary and Conclusions

I presented two hypotheses to account for the European contact record in the Lower Mississippi Valley. The first proposed that while the De Soto *entrada* marked the origin of European contact in the valley, the onset of aboriginal collapse was a later phenemenon, not tied to the initial contact. Either warfare or disease could have caused the collapse. The second hypothesis suggested that the onset of aboriginal decline occurred in the sixteenth century. The timing and magnitude of the loss implicated infectious disease as the primary factor in the change. I stated that resolution of these issues would clarify previous interpretations of the contact record and effectively test the Cook-Dobyns model.

The independent evaluation of both archaeological and historical records supported the second hypothesis: Catastrophic population loss began in the sixteenth century. Based on this evidence, several conclusions are warranted: The De Soto *entrada* was not a "false dawn" in the Lower Mississippi Valley, but marked the beginning of both European contact and the onset of aboriginal population loss; the beginning of history and aboriginal population change were simultaneous events. French records described reduced populations in the process of adjusting to a drastically changed population structure.

Besides offering a new interpretation of the contact period, this analysis has been exceptionally useful in other regards. Despite biases present in the archaeological record, conclusions were not ambiguous. The southeastern test case, thus, supported the position argued first by Cook and most recently by Dobyns. Disease was the earliest European introduction, drastically changing aboriginal demographic profiles and cultural systems long before consistent documentation. Consequently, archaeology, not history, must be the primary basis for developing descriptions of "pristine" aboriginal systems.

Of equal importance has been the demonstration of biases in the historic archaeological record. Although archaeological settlement counts from the eighteenth century suggested that aboriginal populations were increasing, counts were biased by sampling practices and residential instability of native groups. While counts showed an increase, population was, in fact, decreasing. If archaeologists ever want to employ settlement counts for population research more specific than those considered herein, the record must be sampled systematically.

CENTRAL NEW YORK

As used in this analysis, central New York is a roughly oval area that includes a number of major drainage systems as well as the Finger Lakes (Figure 9). The area is bounded on the west by an arbitrary line that crosses the Genessee River; on the eastern edge, the confluence of Schoharie Creek with the Mohawk River

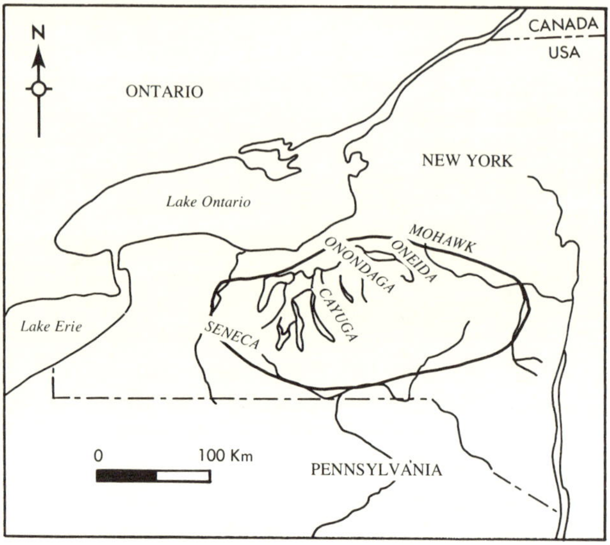

Figure 9. Central New York Study Area

is the boundary. A line parallel to the Seneca River and running just north of Oneida Lake marks the northern boundary. In the south, the boundary is more irregular and crosses several major rivers including, from west to east, the Cohocton River, the Chemung River, and the Susquehanna River.

At the beginning of the historic period (*circa* 1613), the five Iroquois tribes—Seneca, Cayuga, Onondaga, Oneida, and Mohawk—who formed the nucleus of the Iroquois confederacy occupied central New York. The origin of the confederacy is not known precisely (Morgan 1851), but Tooker (1978) suggests that founding dates follow initial contact along the St. Lawrence River, falling somewhere between 1570 and 1663. Although a collective movement, the confederacy was not a single political or economic organization. Each tribe sought its own policy, and no tribe dictated the activities of others.

Significance of the Test Case

Like the Southeast, European contact in the Northeast was a sixteenth-century event. Consequently, the New York Iroquois, like Southeastern groups, could have experienced the effects of disease during that century. Unlike the southeastern groups, New York Iroquois have demonstrated a kind of cultural continuity through nearly 500 years of European contact. With the possible exception of some southwestern Pueblo societies, this continuity is unique in North America. They have persisted as a biological unit; they played a crucial political role during the colonial period; they were obviously successful in manipulating and controlling numerous other tribes of the Northeast. Although these facts justify an assumption of stability rather than catastrophic decline of population during the early centuries of European contact, ethnologists, historians, and archaeologists are not in agreement on this point.

Researchers who hold the conservative view (for example, Fenton 1985; Lenig 1977; Ritchie and Funk 1973; Tooker 1978; Trelease 1971) argue for stability of population and culture into the eighteenth century. If considered at all, the introduction of disease postdates European settlement near Albany, in 1614. Certain consequences follow.

Census counts of the Iroquois describe pristine populations that remained stable from initial contact until the American Revolution. As Trelease states:

> The tremendous military power of the Iroquois and the widespread influence which resulted from it were out of all proportion to the league's population. Although Mooney's estimates of 5,500 for 1600 is probably too small, it can be said that from the coming of the white man until very recent times their combined population never exceeded 15,000 persons. They never had a fighting force of more than 2,500 men, and at no time did they put this number in the field at one time. An estimate of 1660 gave the Mohawk no more than 500 warriors, the Oneida less than 100, the Onondaga 300, the Cayuga 300, and the Seneca no more than 1,000—a total of 2,200 men. These figures are perhaps as accurate as any available for a fairly early period, and they reflect the relative size of member tribes (1971:6).

Excluding the possibility that diseases had reduced populations before the earliest census counts means that the qualitative and quantitative assessments of trade goods mark the beginning of European contact *circa* 1525. Because trade goods increased steadily through time, earlier postcontact components have fewer trade items than later components. Archaeologists use counts or frequencies of trade goods to place historical aboriginal settlements into temporal intervals of twenty-five to thirty years (Table 17).

Since researchers assume that the consequences of European contact on native populations are additive or acculturative, it follows that historic settlement duration pertains to prehistoric periods. (See Starna 1980 for a similar discussion.) During the historic period, duration of Iroquois settlement was relatively short, ranging from fifteen to thirty years (Beauchamp 1900; Bradley 1979; Lenig 1977; Wray 1983; Wray and Schoff 1953). Using single radiocarbon dates for prehistoric villages that have superimposed structures, Pratt (1976) and Tuck (1971), for instance, bracket occupations into intervals of twenty-five years.

Dobyns (1983) has also considered the case of the Iroquois in central New York. While not presenting a specific estimate of Iroquois, Dobyns thinks

Table 17 Temporal Referents of Some Postcontact Iroquois Components

Component	*Number or Percentage of Trade Items*	*Temporal Designation (AD)*
Clock[a]	1	1525–1550
Garoga[a]	3	1550–1575
Pagerie[a]	5	1575–1600
Dutch Hollow[b]	25%	1590–1616
Factory Hollow[b]	25%	1590–1616
Fuegle[b]	25%	1590–1616
Vita-Taft[b]	25%	1590–1616

[a]Lenig 1977.
[b]Wray and Schoff 1953; counts not available.

previous estimates are postepidemic. He argues that, beginning with the smallpox epidemic of 1520, some of the epidemics of Florida diffused into New York. Other epidemics originated from northeastern centers. As a result, population size and settlement organization fundamentally changed. One of these changes was village location. Using Wray and Schoff's summary of historic Seneca village movements (1953), Dobyns correlates relocations with infectious disease episodes in the Northeast and elsewhere. The outcome is an epidemic chronology that Dobyns thinks may be applicable to central New York and other regions of North America.

There is a logical inconsistency in the use of Wray and Schoff's estimate of Seneca settlement duration that contradicts the original definition. Whereas some archaeologists think that historic settlement intervals apply to the prehistoric period, Dobyns links these intervals to episodes unique to the historic period. Wray and Schoff developed the interval by dividing their estimate for number of years by village counts within those years. "The Senecas . . . moved seven times in approximately 150 years. . . . They must have remained from 15 to 25 years at each location" (1953:53). Had the interval been shorter or the settlement count higher, their settlement interval would have been different.

A third perspective on Iroquois population has recently begun to appear in the literature (F. Jennings 1984; Snow 1980; Snow and Starna 1984; Starna 1980; Trigger 1976, 1978, 1981a, 1981b, 1985) (See Chapter 2). Iroquois and Huron populations seemed to have been in a state of flux throughout the colonial period, and the diffusion of infectious disease into the Northeast is a major factor in that instability. The lack of hard evidence on sixteenth-century epidemics coupled with the documentary evidence of epidemics during the seventeenth century leads to several conclusions.

Epidemic mortality is a seventeenth-century phenomenon in both central New York and Huronia, postdating the appearance of trade goods and European settlement, but predating the first census counts. Since initial population estimates postdate the decline, they represent only a fraction of the precontact population. Conversion factors are necessary to estimate precontact population.

In summary, the persistence and success of the Iroquois through the colonial period make this test case particularly important. Of significance is whether the success was a consequence of stability or whether it occurred despite fundamental changes in populations and systems. There is no consensus on this issue. While such scholars as Fenton (1985) assert that historical documents are accurate guides to the past, Dobyns argues that they are not. The sixteenth century is the terminus of the aboriginal condition. Still other scholars who, like Dobyns, support a position of fundamental change, suggest that population begins its downward spiral in the seventeenth century. Although the timing of disease contact is a century later than Dobyns would have it, the effect is the same.

To determine which, if any, of these perspectives is correct, alternative views are framed into specific hypotheses:

Hypothesis 1 (H1) states: Iroquois populations and cultural systems are stable up until the American Revolution. Although earlier disease outbreaks may have occasionally affected segments of the New York Iroquois, these were strictly local events. A larger population and a stable cultural system explains the persistence and success of the New York Iroquois.

Hypothesis 2 (H2) states: Epidemic mortality is a seventeenth-century event in central New York, postdating trade goods and colonization. Exogenous factors explain the persistence of the Iroquois.

Hypothesis 3 (H3) states: Iroquois suffered bouts of epidemic illness, losing significant parts of their population base during the sixteenth century. Their biological survival and cultural florescence is due to exogenous historical factors.

Chronologies

The assumption of demographic and systemic continuity is the oldest of the three approaches to European contact in central New York, and it has guided the formation of traditional culture-historical units. Before presenting my chronology, I consider limitations of existing temporal frameworks.

OWASCO-IROQUOIS TRADITIONS In central and eastern New York, the Late Woodland stage is divided into the Owasco and Iroquois traditions. Although Owasco-Iroquois are currently accepted as indigenous developments in New York, this was not always the case.

In the nineteenth century, a common belief was that native populations had not substantially changed. The purpose of archaeology was to provide temporal depth for historically identified tribes and institutions (Trigger 1981a, 1985). This assumption also allowed prehistoric antiquities to be assigned to historic tribes. Accordingly, the mounds of western New York became the product of the Iroquois (Squire 1851).

The gradual development of chronology began to change this perspective. Since Iroquois assemblages differed from and postdated Owasco assemblages (Ritchie 1944), different groups were responsible for each. The Algonkins were an earlier group (Beauchamp 1900; Parker 1907) that were expelled by the infiltration of the Iroquois (Parker 1916; Ritchie 1944).

MacNeish (1952) debunked the migration hypothesis. By means of ceramic seriations, he demonstrated that Iroquois ceramics grew from Owasco ceramics and that both were *in situ* developments. Since MacNeish's work, archaeologists have expended considerable effort in delimiting the ceramic traditions of individual tribes.

Table 18 contains a summary of current Owasco-Iroquois chronologies. Areal designations are from culture historical divisions. In this analysis, both central and eastern New York are treated as one region, central New York. Field work in both central and eastern areas of New York were the basis of Ritchie and Funk's synthesis. Lenig worked in the Mohawk River Valley, and his focus was on the Oak Hill horizon. Lenig (1965) and others perceive the horizon as transitional between Owasco and Iroquois traditions. The purpose of Tuck's work (1971) was to define changing settlement patterns in the area of the historic Onondaga occupation.

All authorities agree that differences between these traditions are largely a matter of degree rather than of kind. On the basis of radiocarbon dates and stylistic analyses, Ritchie (1980) placed the Owasco tradition between A.D.

Table 18 Comparison of Owasco-Iroquois Chronologies from Central New York

TIME (AD)	RITCHIE & FUNK (1973) PHASES	LENIG (1965) HORIZONS	TUCK (1971) PHASES	RAMENOFSKY PERIODS
1775				V
1700				
1650		LATE COLONIAL MOHAWK	HISTORIC	VI
1600		MID-COLONIAL MOHAWK		
1550	GAROGA	EARLY COLONIAL MOHAWK	PROTOHISTORIC	III
1500	CHANCE	PRE-COLONIAL MOHAWK	GAROGA	
1450				II
1400			CHANCE	
1350	OAK HILL	CHANCE		
1300			OAK HILL	
1250	CASTLE CREEK			
1200		OAK HILL	CASTLE CREEK	I
1150	CANANDAIGA			
1100	CARPENTER BROOK			
1050				
1000				

1100–1300. Domesticates including corn (*Zea mays mylacea*) and (*Zea mays indurata*), beans (*Phaseolus vulgaris*), squash (*Cucurbita pepo*), and gourd (*C. pepo* var. *ovifera*), constituted the criteria for separating Owasco from the earlier Point Peninsula tradition; at the more recent end, aspects of settlement and ceramics separated the Owasco and Iroquois traditions. The subsistence strategy of the Owasco tradition was diversified including agriculture, fishing and hunting (Ritchie 1980). Closer to contact, hunting seems to have become less important (Ritchie and Funk 1973).

Owasco settlements contained few houses (Ritchie and Funk 1973), and were located on relatively accessible topographic features in the uplands. Houses were small, and either oval, round, or rectangular structures; early in the tradition, settlements showed no evidence of palisades. Palisades appeared with the Castle Creek phase and increased in frequency through the historical period (Ritchie 1980; Ritchie and Funk 1973).

Owasco ceramics were grit tempered with large concoidal jars predominating. Exteriors were corded, fabric impressed, and later check stamped. Lips were everted and flattened or thickened; rims tended to be cord impressed. Although vessel shapes remained basically the same through the tradition, collared and castellated rims began to be manufactured in the Castle Creek phase. Later, these rim shapes came to dominate the ceramic field. Finally, Owasco clay pipes tended to be stylistically simple, and projectile points were small and triangular (MacNeish 1952; Ritchie 1980; Ritchie and MacNeish 1949).

Traditional chronologies carry an assumption of continuity between prehistory and history. This assumption is expressed in naming the latest unit Iroquois; the temporal duration of the unit, A.D. 1300–1776; and the use of the direct hisorical approach. As stated by Ritchie and Funk:

> At the upper (late prehistoric to early contact) segment of the Late Woodland continuum, the direct historical approach has proved highly valuable . . . especially with regard to the better documented Iroquoian tribes. This is a consequence of the unbroken continuity of tribal units into the seventeenth and eighteenth centuries prior to the reservation period. . . . The direct historical approach is most useful at the recent terminus of the Late Woodland column, since the late prehistoric components display very close affinities to historic material (1973:358)."

Typical Iroquoian material traits included palisaded villages made up of oval or rectangular longhouses, separated into smaller sleeping compartments and storage areas (Hayden 1976; Ritchie 1952; Ritchie and Funk 1973; Tuck 1971). The settlement pattern was one of a few large villages and satellite hamlets (Ritchie and Funk 1973). Villages were located on tongues or ridges in relatively inaccessible upland locations; and settlement duration may be relatively brief. New settlements located within a kilometer of abandoned settlements suggested abandonment and relocation (Wray and Schoff 1953).

Although still grit tempered, Iroquoian pottery was different from Owasco ceramics in decoration, surface treatment, and shape. Vessels were large and caldron-like, and rims were collared and included castellations. Incised or punctated geometric designs were located on collars and below castellations. In addition, human and nonhuman effigy forms appeared (Lenig 1965; MacNeish 1952; Pratt 1976). During Oak Hill and Chance phases, pipe styles diversified in both form and shape; in the Garoga Phase, diversity of shapes decreased (Lenig 1965; Tuck 1971).

Most northeastern archaeologists think that European contact in central New York began when trade goods filtered south from the St. Lawrence area. The majority of dates for the beginning of this diffusion are 1550 (Engelbrecht 1972; Ritchie 1954; White 1961; Wray and Schoff 1953), but there is some disagreement. Kidd and Kidd (1970) placed the beginning of contact when Europeans began to trade along the Grand Banks 1492 ± 50. Grassman (1969), on the other hand, uses 1614, the date that corresponds to the first documents in New York and the founding of Fort Orange near Albany.

In summary, archaeologists have separated late prehistoric and historic time in central New York (A.D. 1100–1776) into two traditions. Owasco is the earlier and shorter of the two and is followed by the Iroquois tradition. The best estimates for the beginning of contact are *circa* 1550; and, as suggested by this culture history review, Iroquois population and culture are seen as extending in an uninterrupted manner from roughly A.D. 1350 to the American Revolution.

ALTERNATIVE CHRONOLOGY AND PERIODIZATION New chronological work is necessary because the existing framework is a product of different archaeological goals and assumptions. Since MacNeish's demonstration of the *in situ* hypothesis, archaeologists have accepted continuity of archaeological traditions from *circa* 1000 to 1700. Although such an assumption may be warranted, it cannot be assumed *a priori*. To do so ignores the question of catastrophic decline.

Much chronological work has been directed toward delimiting the culture history of specific tribes, i.e., Mohawk, Oneida, Onondaga. While these pursuits are admittedly important, the chronology of one tribe cannot be applied to the entire region. The only way to correlate settlement change of the Mohawk Valley with that from Oneida Lake is to develop one temporal scale applicable to the whole region.

Using component assemblages, I employed eight temporal orders (Table 19) to develop periods. Four of these orders (identified by an asterisk in the table) were based on new classifications. Only two pottery seriations and the fre-

Table 19 List of Temporal Orders for Central New York

Radiocarbon Dates
Pottery Occurrence Seriation 1
Pottery Frequency Seriation 1
*Pottery Occurrence Seriation 2
*Occurrence Seriation of Pipe Bowls
*Occurrence Seriation of Metal Objects
*Cumulative Frequency Curves of European Functional Classes
Frequencies of Glass Trade Beads

*New classifications developed to order components.

quency analysis of glass trade beads were based on culture historical classifications or descriptions. (See Appendix B for details.)

Based on stylistic changes and historical records, I divided my chronology into five periods (Table 18). Since temporal assignments of periods are not known in any absolute sense, I placed greater weight on relative methods. Consequently, multiple orders were necessary for creating a reasonably accurate sequence; and components were ordered by as many of these methods as possible. For the two prehistoric periods, change in pottery styles constituted the primary criterion for period separation; I established historical periods, by measuring the nature and frequency of European trade goods in the archaeological record against the written record of contact in New York (Appendix B). Fortunately, since some of the seriations crossed the boundary of European trade goods, I could compare the temporal position of settlements ordered two different two ways.

I estimated period duration for each period as minimum, mean, and maximum lengths of time (Table 20) which produced temporal overlap within and between periods, thus demonstrating the lack of precision in the temporal dimension. The approach was useful, nonetheless, because it provided three separate estimates of period duration against which changes in S_c could be judged. Bias in the measurement of S_c was thus more clearly identified.

Table 20 Length of Archaeological Periods in Central New York

	Time Range (A.D.)			*Period Duration (Years)*		
Period	*Minimum*	*Mean*	*Maximum*	*Minimum*	*Mean*	*Maximum*
V	1700–1775	1700–1775	1700–1775	75	75	75
IV	1613–1700	1613–1700	1609–1700	87	87	91
III	1550–1609	1525–1613	1498–1613	59	88	115
II	1460–1537	1382–1549	1227–1638	77	167	411
I	1186–1275	1098–1382	1010–1489	89	284	479

For periods with radiocarbon determinations, I based the maximum estimate on the largest differences in standard deviations of the earliest and latest components within the period. The mean time estimate was taken from mean radiocarbon dates of these components, and I used the smallest differences in deviations of these same components to establish minimum dates. In historic periods, I employed a variety of dates including estimates for the beginning of contact, European exploration of New York, or initial historical descriptions.

Of the five periods, only I through IV are known archaeologically. Period V is known only from ethnographic and historical sources, and is, thus, fundamentally different from previous periods. This temporal unit marks the terminus of prereservation settlement types. Table 21 summarizes characteristics of each period.

I have placed seven components in Period I, with estimates of duration ranging from 89 to 479 years. Pottery styles during this period include classes 1122, 2122, 3122, 4111 (Appendix B, Tables 71, 72, 76, 77). Everted rims are cord impressed, and incisions are completely absent. Collars and castellations are present only in the latest components. European trade is absent; a variety of pipe bowl shapes are present.

Four radiocarbon dates suggest that Period II may begin as early as 1227 and terminate as late as 1638. Estimates of period duration range from 77 to 411 years. Six components are in the period. Pottery classes include 2422, 2522, 3122, 4111, 4211, 4212, 4411, 4412 (Appendix B, Tables 76, 77). Although everted rims are still present, incised, or incised/gouged, collared rims are more common. Cord impression is minimally represented. Effigy collared pipe bowls appear for the first time; trade goods are absent.

Period III marks the beginning of European trade goods in central New York. Since European products precede documentation, there are no absolute dates for any components in this time unit. Estimated time ranges are drawn from historical events in New York or along the St. Lawrence. Based on these considerations, Period III may begin with initial European contact along the St. Lawrence (1498) and terminate immediately prior to the founding of Fort Nassau (1498–1613). The mean time range uses the same terminal date, but begins with a slightly later entry of European material into New York (1525–1613). The minimum range is drawn from Ritchie's temporal determination for the origin of European material in central New York (1550), and a terminal date coincident with Hudson's exploration of the Hudson River (1609). Thus, period duration may be as brief as 59 years or as long as 115 years. Although pottery classes are the same as in the previous period, metal trade, including copper/brass and iron scrap, and copper/brass shaped objects are present; glass beads are absent. Seven components are placed in this period.

During Period IV, historic documentation of central New York aboriginal populations begins. If Period III terminated in 1609, then maximum time range

Table 21 Characteristics of Chronological Periods in Central New York

PERIOD I	
Radiocarbon Dates:	6 (See Appendix B, Table 72.)
Maximum Time Range:	A.D. 1010–1489
Mean Time Range:	A.D. 1098–1382
Minimum Time Range:	A.D. 1186–1275
Pottery Styles:	Cord impressed everted rims; absence of incisions. Collars and castellations are present but rare.
Pipe Bowl Shape:	Straight sided, conical, barrel, vasiform, square and trumpet.
Components: (n = 7)	Maxon Derby, Round Top, Sackett, Chamberlain, Furnace Brook, Howlett Hill, Kelso
PERIOD II	
Radiocarbon Dates:	4 (See Appendix B, Table 72.)
Maximum Time Range:	A.D. 1227–1638
Mean Time Range:	A.D. 1382–1549
Minimum Time Range:	A.D. 1460–1537
Pottery Styles:	Cord impressed and incised and/or gouged designs on collared rims. Everted rims continue; castellations present.
Pipe Bowl Shape:	Conical, trumpet, collared, effigy
European Trade Goods:	Absent
Components: (n = 6)	Getman, Nahrwold #1, Temperance House Fort, Buyea, Goff, Burke
PERIOD III	
Radiocarbon Dates:	0
Maximum Time Range:	A.D. 1498–1613
Mean Time Range:	A.D. 1525–1613
Minimum Time Range:	A.D. 1550–1613
Pottery Styles:	Cord impression continues; incising and/or gouged designs on collars; castellations present.
European Trade Goods:	Trade items including scrap copper/brass and iron and shaped copper and brass present. No glass trade beads.
Components: (n = 7)	Garoga, Barnes, Atwell Fort, Chase, Quirk, Diable, Bach
PERIOD IV	
Radiocarbon Dates:	0
Maximum Time Range:	A.D. 1609–1700
Mean Time Range:	A.D. 1613–1700
Minimum Time Range:	—
Pottery Classes:	Not well known
Pipe Bowl Shape:	None recorded
European Trade Goods:	Scrap and shaped copper/brass and iron objects; glass beads present in significant numbers.
Components: (n = 5)	Cameron, Beecher, Thurston, Marshall, Caughnawaga
PERIOD V	
Mean Time Range:	A.D. 1700–1775
Components:	2

for Period IV is from 1609–1700. If Period III terminates with Dutch settlement, then mean time range for Period IV is 1613 to 1700. The range in period duration is from 87 to 91. No minimum dates are suggested. Knowledge of the pottery samples from this period is insufficient for suggesting the nature or direction of stylistic change. European trade goods, including glass trade beads, occur in abundance. Five components are placed in Period IV.

Since there is very little data of any kind for Period V, I suggest only a mean time range, 1700 to 1775. Two ethnographic components are known, one of which is next to Fort Hunter (Fenton and Tooker 1978; Grassman 1969).

As summarized in Table 21 this chronology is different from other late prehistoric and historic central New York chronologies. I have based divisions between temporal units on archaeological criteria that includes all available archaeological materials from A.D. 1000 to the terminus of aboriginal systems. Period I synthesizes several cultural historical phases or horizons, including Oak Hill, which is considered the traditional origin of the Iroquois tradition. Period II also includes several phases or horizons. Rather than perceiving European introductions as a gradual addition of nonnative items to native assemblages within the same tradition, the use of periods separates prehistory from history. Period III is the earliest of the postcontact periods and may be comparable to Ritchie and Funk's Garoga phase (1973). During Period IV, trade goods show a dramatic increase in frequency, and documentation begins. Several phases or horizons are synthesized into Period IV. Period V is a wholly ethnographic period.

Analysis of Population Change

The archaeological analysis of population change has several sections. First, settlement parameters, S_c , $\overline{S_a}$, and $\overline{S_{ra}}$, necessary for estimating regional population are calculated by period. Then, I employ equations (4) and (5) (see Chapter 3) to develop the pattern of regional population change (P_{ar}) through time with which I evaluate the three hypotheses. (See Appendix B, Tables 88, 89 for data on individual settlements.)

SETTLEMENT COUNTS (S_c) I have limited analysis of settlement counts to the twenty-seven components ordered chronologically (Table 22). It was not possible to assign additional components to periods that were not involved in one or more of the seriations. Counts from central New York appear in column 2 of Table 22. The remaining columns present adjusted counts in terms of period duration.

Settlement counts from central New York are not a representative sample of the archaeological record. First, the post-European record of aboriginal settlements is better known than the pre-European record due to archaeological

Table 22 Central New York Settlement Counts by Period

Period	*Raw Settlement Count*	*Adjusted Counts [S_c/(T/100)]*					
		Minimum	S_c	*Mean*	S_c	*Maximum*	S_c
V	2	0.75	2.7	0.75	2.7	0.75	2.7
IV	5	0.87	5.8	0.87	5.8	0.91	5.5
III	7	0.59	11.9	0.88	8.0	1.20	5.8
II	6	0.77	7.8	1.70	3.5	4.10	1.5
I	7	0.89	7.9	2.80	2.5	4.80	1.5

reliance on historical documents (Beauchamp 1900; Bradley 1979; Grassman 1969; Pratt 1976; Tuck 1971). In Pratt's volume on the Oneida (1976), of fourteen settlements only one is prehistoric; in Tuck's Onondaga sequence (1971), of twenty-four settlements that date between 1400 and 1750, eighteen existed between A.D. 1575 and 1750.

Eighteenth-century settlements are known only from documentary evidence. Although the absence of eighteenth century archaeological data runs counter to expectations regarding the archaeological knowledge of the historic period, the absence is itself a consequence of history. There are numerous descriptions of Iroquois in eighteenth-century documents. Written knowledge of the Iroquois makes archaeology less important.

An additional source of bias in the calculation of S_c is the result of the difference between historic and prehistoric settlement duration. During historical periods, evidence suggests that the Iroquois relocated every fifteen to thirty years because of epidemics or depleted resources (Lenig 1977; Tuck 1971; Wray 1983; Wray and Schoff 1953). Grassman (1969), for instance, identified twenty-seven Mohawk villages between 1634 and 1693. Most of these were occupied no longer than fifteen years and some for less than ten years. If settlement duration during prehistoric periods was longer than thirty years, settlement counts for those periods will appear to be lower.

The problems of settlement duration combined with the biases in discovery or reporting settlements should artificially increase S_c values for later periods. Thus, if population trends do not show a precipitous decline historically, the collapse hypothesis is not falsified, nor the stability hypothesis confirmed. Such results must be interpreted as ambiguous so long as S_c is employed to calculate regional population. On the other hand, given biases in S_c, a result showing population loss does falsify the stability hypothesis. It is only this latter possibility that makes population estimation worthwhile under current conditions.

As shown in Table 22, the data produce an unexpected pattern. The estimates do not steadily increase in all later periods. Regardless of variations in period duration, maximum values of S_c occur in Period III, late fifteenth and early sixteenth centuries. During the seventeenth century estimates of settlements sharply decrease.

Since the direction of S_c in Periods IV and V is counter to expectations regarding the behavior of S_c, Iroquois must be in the process of collapse by the seventeenth century. The association of European trade goods and an increase in S_c during Period III suggest that these counts are also biased. If this is the case, then the origin of the collapse may date to the late sixteenth century.

The interpretation of the data, therefore, hinges on whether the apparent increase in S_c during Period III is real or merely a reflection of bias. Several lines of evidence support the evaluation that Period III counts are a product of sampling bias. Five of the seven settlements from Period III derive from Tuck's work in Onondaga County (1971); the emphasis of his work is clearly post-European. Consequently, for that county at least, the number of post-European settlements is greater than the pre-European settlements. Furthermore, Tuck (1974) treats these settlements as sequential occupations of the Onondaga during his Garoga phase. If his analysis is correct (and data limitations prevent evaluating this question), then during the phase, Onondaga make at least five moves. Individual settlement duration is no more than 15 years.

While it is probable that Period III counts are inflated and are contributing to the suggested increase in S_c, the magnitude of the bias cannot be evaluated. Consequently, I view these counts as ambiguous; they are of little utility in determining the question of the initiation of the decline. At the same time, the question of a population collapse during Period III is not a closed issue; I will consider it as other classes of settlement data are presented.

SETTLEMENT AREA (S_a) Although areal measurements are available for all settlements except those of Period V, measurements are drawn from different types of data. I have calculated eight areal measurements directly from published excavation maps. While six of these settlements represented areas within palisade lines or ditches, the remaining two represented house areas only. I have taken seventeen measurements of settlement areas from published descriptions. Although palisades were present at most of these settlements, I have not been able to determine whether estimates correspond to palisade lines or to some smaller area. Although this source of imprecision in calculating S_a makes it an intrinsically unreliable estimator of population, the bias occurs in all periods and is not systematic.

I have calculated estimates of S_a in two different ways (Table 23). Since some type of estimate is available for all settlements from Periods I through IV, S_a is first estimated as the sum of all settlements by period. I employ the mean and sample variance, however, in regional population estimates. Although values for the sum and mean are quite different, they show the same trend and agree

Table 23 Central New York Estimates of Settlement Area by Period (in hectares)

Period	*Settlements with Area Measured*	*Sum of S_a*	$\overline{S_a}$	*Sample Variance (S^2)*
IV	5	6.01	1.20	8.67
III	7	9.22	1.32	13.87
II	6	6.03	1.00	7.07
I	7	4.82	0.75	4.43

with that observed for $[S_c/(T/100)]$ values. $\overline{S_a}$ and S^2 increase to the early seventeenth century and then decrease. Maximum estimates of mean and variance are, thus, coincident with the earliest appearance of European trade goods and suggest a population increase through Period III.

Although there is an imprecision in the measurement of S_a, it is not subject to the biases associated with S_c; and there is no reason to assume that the tendency toward large areas observed in Period III is due to sampling biases or length of settlement duration. If the increase in S_a is not a function of bias, then regardless of how the measure is obtained, trends reflect first a genuine increase in size of settlements through Period III (or the sixteenth century) followed by a genuine decrease.

The results of this analysis are at variance with those suggested for Iroquoian communities in Ontario. Warrick (1983), using Dodd's data (1982), posits a steady increase in settlement area through the seventeenth century. He relates this trend to the development of planned communities and a cohesive sociopolitical organization. Whether the difference in conclusions is a function of cultural variability or sampling bias cannot be resolved from available data.

ROOFED AREA OF SETTLEMENTS (S_{ra}) I have based roofed area of settlements (S_{ra}) on measurements of roofed area of excavated houses ($\overline{H_{ra}}$). Although a total of fifty-seven houses from four periods can be reliably measured (Appendix B, Table 89), the total is not distributed evenly through time or across settlements (Table 24). Period I has the largest sample of excavated houses, and all settlements include at least one house that can be measured. Between Periods II and IV, the sample of settlements with excavated houses decreases. In Period III 80% (8/10) of the houses are taken from one settlement; and in Period IV, 92% (11/12) of excavated houses derive from one settlement.

A consideration of the sample variance suggests that the trend in mean values is not wholly a function of sample size. The largest sample of houses and settlements is in Period I, but Period III has the largest mean and variance. Because dispersion of values in greatest in Period III, intrasettlement variability

Table 24 Estimates of Roofed Area of Houses ($\overline{H_{ra}}$) for Central New York

Period	*Settlements with Roofed Area Measured*	*House Counts*	$\overline{H_{ra}}$ *(meters²)*	S_2
V	0	0	0.00	0.0
IV	2	12	182.80	434346.1
III	3	10	295.60	864961.1
II	4	9	148.60	221287.9
I	7	26	157.76	715925.7

is roughly equivalent to intersettlement variability. Estimates based on even small samples are here accepted as reliable.

Patterns indicated by $\overline{H_{ra}}$ and sample variance are comparable, and indicate two peaks. The peak during Period I is explained by the presence of one house from Howlett Hill, which Tuck (1971) estimated to be greater than 775 m^2. This house is some 300 meters larger than any other house in any other period. If the measurement is excluded from Period I, $\overline{H_{ra}}$ drops to 132.98 m^2. Although the inclusion of this house does affect the change between periods I and II, it does not affect the change from Periods I to III. The maximum in both $\overline{H_{ra}}$ and variance occur in Period III. Like S_a and $[S_c/(T/100)]$, $\overline{H_{ra}}$ indicates a population increase through Period III, followed by some magnitude of population loss.

Other New York archaeologists have interpreted the pattern of larger houses through time as the development of Iroquois longhouses, but peaks in house size differ from those suggested here. Tuck (1971) suggested that dimensions in longhouses were declining prior to European contact. When I calculated his house sizes, however, they showed an increase up to European contact and then a decline. Dodd (1982) and Warrick (1983) also thought that maximum dimensions of Ontario Iroquoian longhouses peaked prior to the beginning of European contact. Although Dodd's analysis was thorough and based on quite a large sample, it has not been possible to compare her conclusions with my own.

Table 25 $\overline{S_{ra}}$ by Period in Central New York

Period	*Excavated Houses*	$\overline{H_{ra}}$ *(meters²)*	*House Count Estimate*	$\overline{S_{ra}}$ *(meters²)*
V	0	0.00	0	0.0
IV	12	182.80	12	2193.6
III	10	295.60	17	5025.2
II	9	148.60	12	1783.2
I	26	157.76	30	4732.8

Her latest prehistoric period crosses the historic boundary, 1450–1609, and, as a result, could not be related directly to my archaeologicial periods.

To convert $\overline{H_{ra}}$ to $\overline{S_{ra}}$ requires that $\overline{H_{ra}}$ be multiplied by estimates of house counts from all settlements. Since house counts are not available for all settlements, I have calculated $\overline{S_{ra}}$ by period (Table 25). Like $\overline{H_{ra}}$, $\overline{S_{ra}}$ shows two peaks, with the maximum occurring in Period III. The magnitude of the change between Periods II and III reflects both the increase in $\overline{H_{ra}}$, and the relatively large number of houses.

REGIONAL ESTIMATES OF POPULATION (P_{ar}) I first calculate P_{ar} by Equation (4):

$$P_{ar} = [S_c/(T/100)] \times \overline{S_a}$$

Since estimates of S_c vary according to period duration (see Table 20), regional estimates of $\overline{S_a}$ are calculated according to the three temporal models (Table 26). Although differences in period duration affect the magnitude of changes, patterns based on regional estimates of $\overline{S_a}$ are quite consistent (Figure 10).

Settlement area gradually increases between Periods I and II, and then increases more abruptly between Periods II and III. By the onset of Period IV in

Table 26 P_{ar} Based on Estimates of $\overline{S_a}$ in Hectares

	Mean Settlement	*$[S_c/(T/100)] \times \overline{S_a}$*					
Period	*Area*	*Minimum*	*S_a*	*Mean*	*S_a*	*Maximum*	*S_a*
V	0.00	0.0	0.0	0.0	0.0	0.0	0.0
IV	1.20	5.8	7.0	5.8	7.0	5.5	6.6
III	1.32	11.9	15.7	8.0	10.6	5.8	7.7
II	1.00	7.8	7.8	3.5	3.5	1.5	1.5
I	0.75	7.9	5.9	2.5	1.9	1.5	1.1

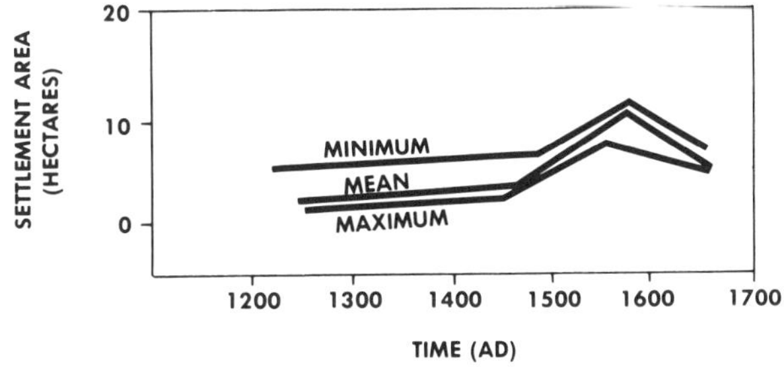

Figure 10. P_{ar} Based on $\overline{S_a}$

1613, regional estimates of $\overline{S_a}$ decrease; thus, I conclude that regional population shows some magnitude of loss by Period IV.

The major question raised by these data is whether the increase during the sixteenth century (Period III) is an artifact of bias or a genuine reflection of a population expansion. Although, as argued earlier, the trend toward larger settlement areas in Period III is not a product of bias, the same statement cannot be applied to values of S_c.

Sampling biases and potentially shorter settlement durations are contributing to estimates of settlement counts during Period III. If S_c values are inflated, then estimates of regional population that employ these values are also inflated. While the increase in settlement area does indicate a change, problems associated with S_c preclude interpreting the change as population increase.

The second estimate of P_{ar} employs Equation (5):

$$P_{ar} = [S_c/(T/100)] \times \overline{S_{ra}}$$

As in the previous equation, regional $\overline{S_{ra}}$ is estimated with all three temporal models (Table 27).

Table 27 P_{ar} Based on Estimates of $\overline{S_{ra}}$ in Square Meters

		$\overline{S_{ra}} \times [S_c/(T/100)]$					
Period	$\overline{S_{ra}}$	*Minimum*	S_{ra}	*Mean*	S_{ra}	*Maximum*	S_{ra}
IV	2193.8	5.8	12724.0	5.8	12724.0	5.5	12065.9
III	5025.2	11.9	59799.8	8.0	40201.6	5.8	29146.2
II	1783.2	7.8	13909.0	3.5	6241.2	1.5	2674.8
I	4732.8	7.9	37389.1	2.5	11832.0	1.5	7099.2

The pattern of these estimates through time (Figure 11) is comparable to that described for $\overline{S_{ra}}$. The first and smaller peak is in Period I, and the second peak occurs during Period III in the sixteenth century. Between Periods III and IV, regional estimates of population decrease. Like estimates of $\overline{S_{ra}}$ the decrease must be interpreted as indicating a population collapse.

Several different types of evidence suggest that population estimates in Period III do not reflect a population increase but are due to sampling bias. First, like regional estimates of $\overline{S_{ra}}$, settlement counts are probably biased by archaeological sampling practices and residential instability. The argument in favor of residential instability during Period III is, in fact, strengthened by considering the duration of this period. Even if the duration is 115 years (Table 20), the suggested magnitude of population increase is too great to be explained solely by intrinsic growth factors. Other processes, possibly a shorter settlement

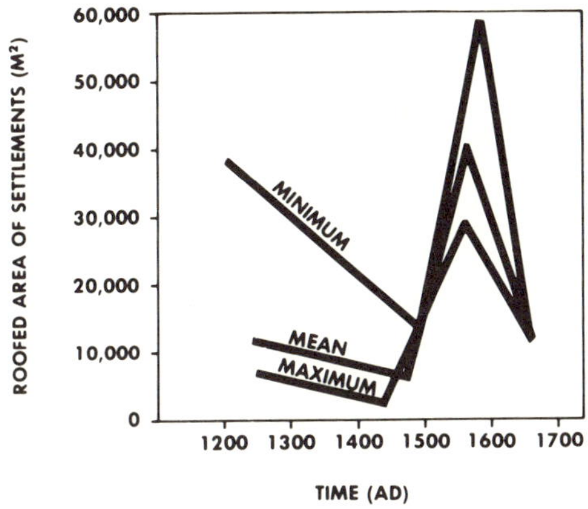

Figure 11. P_{ar} Based on $\overline{S_{ra}}$

duration or population amalgamation, are clearly creating a trend that, on the surface, appears to indicate intrinsic growth.

To recapitulate, regional estimates of archaeological population derived from $\overline{S_a}$ and $\overline{S_{ra}}$, suggested that the Iroquois were considerably reduced by the seventeenth century. Evidence for an earlier decline was ambiguous. Regional estimates pointed to an increase through Period III, but estimates were biased by inflated S_c values. Since population estimates based on $\overline{S_{ra}}$ argued that the purported increase could not be explained as a consequence of intrinsic growth factors, other processes must have caused the trend. Not only did biases present in the measurement of archaeological population support the thesis that population was not increasing during the seventeenth century, they prevented demonstrating the opposite argument of population collapse.

CONCLUSIONS Despite temporal imprecisions and biases present in the data, archaeological analyses of population are sufficient to reject H1. By the eighteenth century, Iroquois tribes of central New York were significantly smaller than they had been 100 years earlier. The decline was sufficiently great to suggest that Iroquois persistence and political power during the colonial period are due to other factors. Because the loss coincided with documented changes in the size and nature of settlements, it is clear that demographic processes of the postcontact period were major factors in changing the structure and organization of Iroquois towns and villages. Consequently, the assumption of continuity in settlement structure from prehistory through history is erroneous. The reverse assumption, that is, "upstreaming" (Fenton 1985:4) from historic to prehistoric periods must also be accepted as inappropriate.

Historical organization and structure of settlements were different than those of the prehistoric periods because of fundamental changes in population.

Unfortunately, settlement analyses were inadequate for differentiating between H2 and H3. While both equations for regional population showed that New York Iroquois were declining after 1613, biases present in the estimation of S_c precluded determining whether that century marked the origin of the loss. If, as stated in H2, the population collapse was a seventeenth-century event, then the disease would postdate the appearance of trade goods and be roughly contemporaneous with European settlement. In this case, the conclusions would support the work of Snow, Starna, and Trigger. If, as in H3, the collapse was a sixteenth-century phenomenon, then infectious disease becomes the most reasonable explanation of the loss. The simultaneous diffusion of infectious parasites and European trade goods would mark the European boundary in central New York. A consideration of the early history of central New York may help differentiate between alternative hypotheses.

Iroquois History, 1497–1775

Because the archaeological analysis of population has been sufficient for rejecting the hypothesis of demographic and cultural stability into the eighteenth century, I will focus this discussion on the sixteenth and seventeenth centuries. I will review subjects relevant for questions of disease and population collapse. These include a general description of the contact period in the Northeast, Iroquois-European interactions, Iroquois demographic and settlement trends. Following these summaries, I will consider causes of the decline.

EUROPEAN DISCOVERY The history of the region began along the St. Lawrence River more than 100 years before Hudson explored the Hudson River (Table 28). Between 1497 and 1534, five French or Portuguese exploring parties contacted populations along the Gulf of the St. Lawrence. After 1497, French, Breton, Portuguese, and English fishermen traveled yearly to the Grand Banks to recover cod and sturgeon (Biggar 1911; Sauer 1971; Trigger 1985). Barter was a common feature of these expeditions especially when the catch was dried on land rather than at sea (Ritchie 1954). Between 1540 and 1610, Portuguese whalers established seasonal fishing colonies along the Labrador coast. Colonies supported male populations of up to 1000 individuals (Tuck 1985). In 1534, Cartier discovered the St. Lawrence, and by 1541, he had made three voyages to the area. In the last two voyages in 1535 and 1541, small, impermanent forts were built (Biggar 1924; Burrage 1959a, 1959b, 1959c); and the third voyage included a few colonists.

French colonization began in 1603 with Champlain. The first settlement was on Isle de Saint Croix. After the founding of Quebec in 1608, until well into the

Table 28 Some Historical Events in New France and New York

Date (AD)	*Description*
1497	Contact and trade begin along the St. Lawrence.
1524	Giovanni Verrazzano discovers New York Bay.
1534–1541	Jacques Cartier explores the St. Lawrence, and establishes short-lived colonies.
1540–1610	Portuguese whaling colonies established along the coast of Newfoundland.
1608	Quebec is founded.
1609	Henry Hudson discovers the Hudson River.
1614	Fort Nassau established near Albany.
1664	New York becomes a British colony.

eighteenth century, the French played an active role in Iroquois history (Biggar 1925; Goldstein 1969; Morison 1972; Trigger 1976).

Although the coastline of New York had been known since 1524, the interior was not discovered until 1609 when Hudson sailed up the river named for him (Crouse 1933). Between 1609 and 1614, when Fort Nassau (later Fort Orange) was established, at least four Dutch trading ships sailed up the Hudson River for the purpose of obtaining beaver pelts from native populations (Lenig 1977). Between 1614 and the midseventeenth century, the Dutch controlled trade interactions with the Iroquois. In 1664, following the English take-over of New Amsterdam, the British became the primary recipient of Iroquois pelts.

The date 1609 marked the beginning of direct interaction between New York Iroquois and Europeans. Lenig (1977) suggested that New York Iroquois met and traded with Hudson in 1609. Others (for example, Trigger 1976, 1985) stated that Champlain was the earliest European to contact the New York Iroquois. In the summer of 1609, he, in association with Hurons and Algonkins, attacked the Mohawk at the south end of Lake Champlain.

Because European contact along the St. Lawrence preceded contact in New York, trade goods diffused to the Iroquois before there was any direct interaction. If European trade goods followed aboriginal trade networks, infectious diseases may have also diffused. If this was the case, then European trade goods and infectious disease reached native populations in New York at approximately the same time.

EUROPEAN-IROQUOIS INTERACTIONS Throughout the colonial period in the Northeast, the Iroquois dominated native interactions with the Dutch, the French, and later the English. Not only were the Iroquois strategically located between European colonies (first those of the Netherlands and France and then those of France and England), but they were also highly skilled diplomats. (See Leder 1956 for Iroquois diplomatic records.) Through a combination of aggression and shrewd political maneuvers the League remained politically independent through the seventeenth and most of the eighteenth century (Tooker 1978; Trelease 1971).

Motivations of the Iroquois during the colonial period have been discussed repeatedly. Hunt (1967) argued that the aggression of the Iroquois against Algonkins, Huron, Susquehanna, and others was directed toward establishing and maintaining their middleman position in the fur trade. Trelease (1971), rejecting this opinion, suggested that the Iroquois involvement in the fur trade was independent of their aggression. Their aggression stemmed from imperialistic tendencies, or the desire to extend their hunting territories. F. Jennings (1984, 1985) thought that the Iroquois wanted (and won) their leadership role of all Northeastern Indians.

Dutch, French, and British differed in their treatment of the Iroquois. The Dutch were primarily a trading nation (Crouse 1933; F. Jennings 1984) who lacked a grand political scheme in North America. The Dutch settled conflicts with Indians on a case-by-case basis with the result that they never developed strong Indian allies. Ultimately the overriding mercantilism of the Dutch worked against their survival on American soil. They were frankly commercial with the Iroquois, wanting to maximize monetary returns, to control trade interactions, and to remain aloof from French-Iroquois conflicts even though these conflicts reduced the flow of peltry into Fort Orange (Trelease 1971).

The French, on the other hand, had both economic and political ambitions. Because the French exchange rate on furs was always two to four times lower than English exchange rates (Trelease 1971), France had to support her colonial investments by continually extending trade networks. The Iroquois posed the greatest single political threat to French expansion; but they were the most important physical buffer to English economic control of the St. Lawrence River and the upper Mississippi River (F. Jennings 1984; Trelease 1971). The French could not resolve the conflict which led to simultaneous policies of subjugation, warfare, and expansion. As F. Jennings (1985) noted, it was the French who imposed neutrality on the Iroquois. The French needed to keep their Indian allies out of Albany and British traders away from imperial holdings.

Although the British, like the French, needed the Iroquois as a structural buffer, they approached the problem differently. The British and the Five Nations of the Iroquois became partners; for at least seventy-five years, the symbiotic relationship was very successful (F. Jennings 1984).

According to F. Jennings (1971, 1984, 1985), the covenant chain was the vehicle of interaction. It was basically an Indian institution that may have grown from the Iroquois confederacy. There were two primary parties within the chain: Indian tribes under the leadership of the Iroquois and the British colonies under the direction of the Department of Indian Affairs, which was established soon after British ascendency at Albany (Leder 1956; Trelease 1971). Throughout Iroquois history, the function of the chain changed (F. Jennings 1971).

Initially, neither the Iroquois nor the British lost their sovereignty; and all decisions were achieved through consultation and treaty. The Five Nations of the Iroquois provided protection for tribes who joined the chain and were spokesmen during negotiations. To the British, they were aggressive political and economic allies.

Because the British recognized that "if we lose the Iroquois, we are gone" (Leder 1956:26), they helped the Iroquois to maintain their position. They estabished a hands-off policy toward Iroquois lands. Until the eighteenth century, a concerted effort was made to keep traders and soldiers out of Iroquoia (Tooker 1978; Trelease 1971). Moreover, because westward expansion was seen as a threat to the fur trade, colonial incursions into Iroquoia stopped at Schenectady (Trelease 1971). To protect Virginia colonists and accommodate Iroquois imperial policies, the Carolina Road was moved east of the Blue Ridge Mountains in the Shenandoah Valley (Leder 1956). In addition, the Five Nations became the largest recipient of British ammunitions and were given access to Albany gunsmiths (Trelease 1971). The Iroquois also used these guns for invasions of Illinois or the Carolinas.

In the eighteenth century, the function of the chain began to change (F. Jennings 1971, 1984). The Iroquois took on a policing function for the British, and tribal negotiations were done on an individual basis. The Mohawk Valley was settled in 1723; and by 1760 Fort Hunter (1712) and Fort Stanwix (1758) had been built in Iroquoia (Fenton and Tooker 1978; Tooker 1978).

The mutual support that was crucial to Iroquois survival collapsed after the French and Indian War (1756–1763). After the war, Spanish colonies on the other side of the continent were the only obstacles to British expansion, and the Iroquois no longer played such a crucial role in British diplomacy. By 1768, all Iroquois holdings south of the Susquehanna River had been ceded to the British. The American Revolution followed shortly thereafter, resulting in major political and social changes. Iroquois loyalties were divided: the Oneida supported the Americans; all others, especially the Mohawk, supported the British. Each tribe pursued its own course with the result that Iroquois were pitted against each other (Tooker 1978). The Treaty of Paris (1784) included no provision for Iroquois lands; and, by 1794, the American government had established four reservations in New York (Tooker 1978).

Although the position of the Five Nations of the Iroquois during the colonial period will be debated for many years to come, enough is currently known to suggest that historical factors are, indeed, important in any explanation of

Iroquois persistence and success. Iroquois aggression and diplomacy worked to their advantage in the struggle between European nations. Simultaneously, without adequate support their story may have been very different, more comparable perhaps to that of the Huron.

IROQUOIS POPULATION TRENDS St. Lawrence Iroquois, known to history as the Stadaconans and Hochlegans, disappeared earlier than any other recorded northeastern group. The Stadaconans lived in a number of settlements near Quebec City, and the Hochlegans were farther up river near modern Montreal (Pendergast and Trigger 1972; Trigger 1976, 1985). Cartier met both groups on all three voyages; and although no population estimates were made (Biggar 1924; Burrage 1959a, 1959b, 1959c), descriptions suggest that the St. Lawrence Valley supported a sizable population. By 1600, the aboriginal population of the valley was gone (Trigger 1976). Hypotheses including war with neighboring Algonkins (Innis 1956) or Mohawk (Lenig 1977; Trigger 1962, 1976) for control of the St. Lawrence, increased reliance on hunting in response to European demand for furs (Hunt 1967), or introduced disease (Fenton 1940) have been suggested to account for the disappearance.

The first estimate of a New York Iroquois group was made in 1643, roughly 143 years after Europeans began trading along the St. Lawrence, and 34 years after Hudson sailed as far north as Albany. Recently, all Iroquois population estimates for the period between 1643 and 1763 were summarized by Michelson (1977) (Table 29). Unfortunately, estimates do not suggest a clearly definable pattern. While Mohawk, Cayuga, and Onondaga warrior counts suggest population decline, Seneca estimates indicate a decrease through 1698 followed by gradual increase.

Table 29 Warrior Estimates of the Five Nations of the Iroquois

Period	*Date (AD)*	*Seneca*	*Cayuga*	*Onondaga*	*Oneida*	*Mohawk*	*Total*
	1643						700
	1660	1,000	300	300	100	500	2,200
IV	1677	1,000	300	300	150	200	2,150
	1685	1,200	200	300	150	200	2,050
	1689	1,300	320	500	180	270	2,570
	1698	600	200	250	70	110	1,230
V	1712	1,000	150	350	120	180	1,900
	1721	700	130	250	200	160	1,440
	1763	1,050	200	150	250	160	1,950

[a]After Michelson 1977.

Observer bias or Iroquois cultural policies explain lack of agreement among tribal estimates. Most seventeenth-century estimates were by French Jesuits who not only were irregularly present among the Five Nations (no outsiders were welcomed in Iroquoia), but may have increased the number to win favor from the French crown. In this regard, Mohawk estimates may be the most accurate: they were in close proximity to the British, and they had the most frequent visitation (Grassman 1969).

Furthermore, Iroquois demographic policies affected the direction of population trends. During the colonial period, Iroquois actively sought to expand their population and used the confederacy and the covenant chain as formal structures for integrating population. Some groups, like the Tuscarora, migrated to New York to join the Iroquois "tree of peace." Trigger (1976) noted that between 1648 and 1650 several thousand Huron joined Iroquois society. In 1657, no less than seven nations were present at Onondaga; in 1668, two-thirds of the Oneida residents were Algonkin or Huron (F. Jennings 1984). Besides voluntary assimilation, Iroquois adopted captive children and young men into their system (Hunt 1967; F. Jennings 1984).

Although biased, population estimates are nonetheless important. Like the archaeological record, some census counts are inflated and give the impression of population increase. The increase may have come about because of Iroquois' policies of population expansion, which may have been promulgated because population was falling. The steady decrease in Mohawk, Onondaga, and Cayuga counts seem to suggest this interpretation. Furthermore, the link between population loss and amalgamation was not unique to the Northeast.

My discussion of population trends from the Lower Mississippi Valley suggested that this was the case. Dobyns (1983 especially) argued that the amalgamation of remnant groups was continental in scope and due to catastrophic decline from disease. Although cause of Iroquois amalgamation has yet to be considered, there is no reason to suppose that it was not a response to declining population.

Unfortunately, limits imposed by historical documents preclude determining whether decline and amalgamation were sixteenth- or seventeenth-century processes. If they date to the sixteenth century, then the Period III peak in the archaeological curve of population may be reflecting this process. The disappearance of the St. Lawrence Iroquois coupled with an increase in their pottery on late sixteenth-century Huron sites (Trigger 1984) increases the plausability of this interpretation. Clearly, however, the suggestion requires further documentation.

In summary, although trends in census counts were not comparable among the Five Nations, they were sufficient to suggest that the Iroquois were declining during the seventeenth century. Slight increases in population were attributable to either observer bias or Iroquois policies of population assimilation. Limits of historical documentation precluded determining whether the origin of the decline was a sixteenth- or seventeenth-century phenomenon.

SETTLEMENT HISTORY Historical descriptions of Iroquois settlements are surprisingly meager. Such data as do exist support the interpretation of population loss and amalgamation. Since there are no sixteenth-century descriptions of Iroquois settlements in New York, discussion is limited to the seventeenth (Period IV) and eighteenth (Period V) centuries.

The seventeenth-century record is more complete than the eighteenth century largely because seventeenth-century settlements of the Iroquois were still relatively intact. During Period IV, Iroquois populations were sedentary, and settlements, termed castles, were spatially discrete and bounded by palisades. As Lenig (1977) stated and Grassman (1969) documented, settlements tended to have a riverine orientation.

Settlement history of the Mohawk in the seventeenth century has been particularly well documented by Grassman (1969). Grassman has identified seven individuals who estimated Mohawk village counts between 1634 and 1666. The range in village counts was from one to eight, the largest of which was made by the Dutch early in the period (between 1634 and 1635). The average number of houses across the eight settlements was twenty-three. Between 1667 and 1693 three individuals visited Mohawk castles, and estimates ranged from two to four. The largest estimate was made in 1677, and included a description of houses for each village. Average house count in the four villages was twenty-two. Between 1694 and 1780, the average Mohawk village count was two (Fenton and Tooker 1978; Grassman 1969).

Changing location of villages and travelers knowledge of Mohawk territory explains variability between estimates from the same period. Despite variability, these figures implied a pattern. If maximum village counts are employed, then between 1634 and 1677 village counts showed a 50% decrease; and house counts a 4% decrease. Between 1677–1780, Mohawk village counts dropped another 50%. The downward trend in Mohawk villages matches that of Mohawk warriors (See Table 29) over roughly the same period.

Although Period IV settlement structure persisted up until the American Revolution (terminus of Period V), documentary evidence suggested that another settlement type was also evolving. The community of Otsiningo (1737–1780) was composed of house clusters that were unbounded by palisades, which stretched out along the banks of the Chenango River (Elliott 1977). Bartram (1751) described a similar rambling pattern for the Onondaga, whose unbounded town covered more than three kilometers along Onondaga Creek. Cabins, rather than multifamily longhouses, were scattered along both sides of the creek and were separated by swaths of grass and agricultural plots.

As the structure of settlements changed, the composition of population within settlements also changed. Elliott, for instance, described Otsiningo as a "refugee center" (1977:94); during its 53-year history, the community included Shawnee, Onondaga, Tuscarora, Conoy, Mohikan, Cayuga, Nanticoke, and Ontager.

Although reasons for the progressive loss of settlements and shift in settlement structure were obviously complex, population loss from disease and warfare was unquestionably the major variable. By the seventeenth century, Iroquois were declining; the decline coincided with the decrease in the number of inhabited villages. In the eighteenth century, when there were too few people to maintain older settlement structures, new structures evolved. These were associated with hybridization of population.

CAUSES OF DECLINE Since definite evidence of population loss dated to the seventeenth century and coincided with sustained presence of Europeans in New York, warfare or disease could be causing the loss. The goal of this discussion is to determine whether disease, warfare, or some combination of the two was most likely responsible.

At least two types of warfare were possible: aggression between native groups or between Europeans and Iroquois. Since native attacks against each other were mentioned more frequently in historical documents than were epidemics (Jennings 1984; Trigger 1981b), it is reasonable to assume that this type of aggression drained the population. It is highly unlikely, however, that native warfare alone was responsible for the attrition seen in both archaeological and historical records.

Warfare had been a chronic problem in the Northeast for centuries. (See Finlayson 1985 for a discussion.) Evidence of the problem, including palisaded villages in defensive locations, human bone artifacts, and nucleation of population, preceded the arrival of European by centuries. Despite the persistent aggression, the aboriginal population continued to increase through the later prehistoric period. It was only after European contact that the Iroquois population levels fell, and that Iroquois reduced the Huron, Petun, Neutral, Erie, and Susquehanna (Hunt 1967). Because warfare predated and collapse postdated European presence, it is logical to argue that factors other than native aggression were responsible.

European aggression against the Iroquois is another alternative. In the seventeenth century, and especially after 1640, the French invaded Iroquoia quite consistently (F. Jennings 1984). Although single skirmishes had minimumum consequences on population levels, persistence of these raids impacted the size of Iroquois populations (F. Jennings 1984). In the eighteenth century, Iroquois suffered attacks from both the French and the British.

It appears likely, therefore, that some magnitude of Iroquois population loss that postdated 1640 was due to European aggression. How much of the attrition could be attributed to death by war cannot be determined from available evidence. With a clearer chronological record of archaeological settlement, it might be possible to approach this problem.

Implication of warfare as causal in decline of the Iroquois does not exclude disease. As suggested by the archaeological record, the onset of Iroquois decline in 1613 preceded sustained European aggression by a number of decades. Since native warfare has already been excluded as a factor, disease is the only other possible explanation. Furthermore, historical documents suggest that population loss from disease may be linked to success in war. The Iroquois, for instance, destroyed the Huron in 1649; but the destruction postdated several major epidemics recorded between 1634 and 1641. Estimates of Huron population loss from that epidemic interval ranged from one-half (Trigger 1976) to two-thirds (Starna 1980). The disease record from the Northeast, therefore, must be considered (Table 30).

If taken at face value, Table 30 gives the impression of early and repeated epidemics. Unfortunately, only the 1535 episode is recorded in the sixteenth-century documents of the Northeast. In December 1535, some fifty Stadaconans and twenty-five Europeans died of an unknown illness (Biggar 1924). Although it is likely that European deaths were due to scurvy, Indian deaths were probably due to an introduced infection.

All other sixteenth-century epidemics are from Dobyns's epidemic chronology of the Seneca. In the Northeast, Dobyns based his sixteenth-century epidemic history on a 1630 document by Roger Williams (1863 [1638]). Williams stated that Narragansett connected earthquakes with episodes of illness. Dobyns, in turn, uses Williams's earthquake chronology as an epidemic chronology, linking the latter to Wray and Schoff's historical Seneca relocations (1953). The case in favor of sixteenth-century epidemics was strengthened by timing of disease events in Florida.

In the southeastern test case, the archaeological record demonstrated significant population loss during the sixteenth century; it was possible, therefore, to suggest that Dobyns's epidemic history for that region was correct. This is not, possible however, in the Northeast.

The archaeological record from central New York suggested that population was increasing through the sixteenth century. Although the increase may have been due to amalgamation processes that, in turn, were caused by population loss, this interpretation demands systematic archaeological investigation. Consequently, this analysis has not confirmed Dobyns's sixteenth-century epidemic hypotheses.

Tabulation of seventeenth-century epidemics are probable since they are recorded in local histories and are confirmed by this archaeological analyses of population. The earliest seventeenth-century epidemic is taken from Gookin

Table 30 Recorded or Suspected Native Epidemics in the Northeast[a]

New France	*New England*	*New York*
1535[b]		
	1568[c]*	
	1574[c]	
	1586[c]*	
	1592[c]	
	1612–1613[d]	
	1616[e]	
	1617[c]*	
	1633–34	1634
1634–1641		
		1637–1638
1647		
	1649[c]	1649
	1654[c]	1662
	1666	
1668	1669–1670	1669
	1678	
		1679[f]
	1689	1690

[a]after Stearn and Stearn 1945 except where noted.
[b]Biggar 1924.
[c]Dobyns 1983; * also present in Florida.
[d]Gookin 1806 [1792, 1674].
[e]Cook 1973a.
[f]Leder 1956.

who described the illness and resulting loss some sixty years after the event. He stated that the Pawtuckett or

> A very great number of them, were swept away by an epidemical and unwanted sickness, A. 1612–1613, about seven or eight years before the English arrived in those parts to settle the colony of New Plymouth (1806 [1792, 1674]:143).

Cook (1973a) suggested that the 1616–1617 New England epidemic was plague. If the identification is correct, then it may not have spread from Massachusetts to New York. Plague, an acute bacterial infection, is communicated to human populations through a flea that typically affects rats (Benenson 1976b). The diffusion of the disease would depend on migration of rats. All other recorded seventeenth-century epidemics were smallpox (Stearn and Stearn 1945).

The seventeenth-century compilation (Table 30) demonstrates several important points:

(1) Between 1613 and 1690, northeastern groups, including the Iroquois, experienced no less than 24 epidemics. The effect of this loss was seen in both the archaeological and historical records of the seventeenth century.

(2) As argued by Starna (1980), the earliest estimates of Iroquois population were postepidemic estimates and cannot be presumed to represent pristine populations or systems.

The only logical conclusion is that the earliest census counts represented populations already drastically reduced by disease.

(3) If temporal priority of disease indicates the point of origin, then the Northeast constituted a single disease "interaction sphere." The 1633–1641 epidemic may have originated in New England, spreading north and west. The 1668–1670 epidemic originated in New France and diffused east, south, and west. The 1678 epidemic originated in New England and spread west. Although no origin is indicated, it is probable that the recorded Massachusetts outbreak of 1612–1613 derived from Dutch trading vessels on the Hudson.

In summary, it seems that initial attrition of the Five Nations was due to disease rather than warfare. After 1640, however, both factors contributed to the downward spiral of population that continued to the American Revolution. Further, timing and geography suggest that seventeenth-century disease events were diffusing between groups. Two implications follow from this proposition.

Table 30 must be seen as minimal list of diseases, representing only those that occurred when Europeans happened to be present. Secondly, if disease was diffusing in the seventeenth century, it certainly could have been happening a hundred years earlier. Again, Dobyns's sixteenth-century epidemics must be taken as hypotheses that require additional archaeological testing.

Summary and Conclusions

In the significance section, three hypotheses were presented to account for the sequence of events of the contact period in central New York. The archaeological analysis of population rejected H1, the proposal that the Iroquois were demographically stable into the eighteenth century. The settlement record from central New York showed that Iroquois population was drastically reduced during the seventeenth century. The question then became whether the onset of Iroqouis demographic collapse was a sixteenth- or seventeenth-century event. Unfortunately, the archaeological record was ambiguous on this point. A biased archaeological record demonstrated population increase through Period III (the sixteenth century); the archaeological record of decline was a seventeenth-century event.

Because of the ambiguity, the goal of the historical analysis was to differentiate between H2 and H3. This was only a partial solution since historical records in central New York did not exist until the seventeenth century. Consequently, if documentary evidence from the seventeenth century showed that Iroquois groups were declining, they could support H2 but could not disprove H3. The latter could be rejected or confimed only through archaeology.

The historical record supported H2, the seventeenth-century hypothesis. The earliest, clearly accepted, disease outbreak anywhere in the Northeast occurred along the St. Lawrence in 1535. Seventeenth-century epidemics preceded signficant attrition from warfare, and were of primary importance in explaining Iroquois population collapse. Furthermore, by documenting hybridization of communities and the final breakdown of multifamily dwellings and bounded settlements, available seventeenth- and eighteenth-century descriptions supported and extended the archaeological pattern of collapse and amalgamation.

Absence of well-documented disease episodes from the sixteenth century does not disconfirm Dobyns's position. Disease diffusion was occurring in the seventeeth century, and there is the enigmatic disappearance of the St. Lawrence Iroquois during the sixteenth century. Consequently, two interpretations of archaeology and history of central New York are possible.

If the data are taken at face value, then the population increase during the sixteenth century was independent of contact events along the St. Lawrence. In this case, as argued by Snow, Starna, and Trigger, epidemics resulting in Iroquois collapse were seventeenth-century phenomena, that coincided with sustained colonization at Albany. Presence of European trade materials which first occurred anywhere from 1500 to 1550 marked the origin of European contact in New York.

A second interpretation assumes a wave-like pattern between contact events along the St. Lawrence River and central New York. Due to accidents of proximity, St. Lawrence Iroquois experienced consequences of disease earlier than New York Iroquois; and by 1600, they had disappeared. Remnant populations from the St. Lawrence were absorbed by New York communities, creating the record of apparent population increase in the New York area. Since individuals carried disease, amalgamation processes meant to maintain stability resulted in the catastrophic decline visible by the seventeenth century. The simultaneous appearance of disease and trade goods between 1500 and 1550 define, in this case then, European contact in central New York. Seventeenth century trends in population mark the terminus, not the onset of collapse.

Current evidence supports the conclusion that the New York Iroquois experienced a catastrophic decline that certainly was underway by the early seventeenth century. Since the onset of significant demographic change preceded documentation and census counts, historical records, like those from the Mississippi Valley, are descriptions of populations developing new, adaptive strategies. The confederacy and covenant chain were expressions of that strategy. These institutions were not rooted in prehistory but developed under new selective pressure.

At the same time, the sixteenth-century hypothesis cannot be discounted. Since the proposed change preceded written records, archaeology is the only means by which the hypothesis can be tested. Consequently, obtaining settlement data that are reasonably free of bias must become a priority in northeastern research. Only then can the question of a sixteenth-century decline in the Northeast be evaluated.

THE MIDDLE MISSOURI

Because the archaeological sample from the upper Missouri Trench is a product of the River Basin Surveys (J. Jennings 1985; Petsche 1968), it is concentrated in those areas of North and South Dakota impounded by dam construction and reclamation projects. The region, including the Missouri River floodplain and terraces, is defined as the Middle Missouri, a geographic division of the northern Plains (Lehmer and Caldwell 1966) that is approximately 805 kilometers long. In North Dakota, the confluence of the Knife and Missouri rivers defines the northern boundary, while the White River of South Dakota marks the southern boundary (Figure 12).

Within this section of the Missouri trench, a number of secondary drainages enter into the Missouri channel from the West. Structural alterations that occurred during the Pleistocene produced the current pattern (Flint 1955, 1957; Todd 1914). Older terraces above the floodplain are dissected and eroded by fluvial action and have a general north to south slope. Elevations along the floodplain range from 425 to 550 m; terraces may be 100 meters higher. Most of the human habitation is confined to lower terraces and floodplain of the Missouri.

Historic Aboriginal Occupation

Although European contact with Plains groups began in 1540 with the Coronado expedition, the historic period in the Middle Missouri was considerably later. Documentation of aboriginal groups preceded sustained European presence which began in the early eighteenth century (1738) with the explorations of La Verendrye and his sons (Burpee 1927; Smith 1980). Sustained European presence occurred in the early decades of the nineteenth century when the French, Spaniards, and later Americans, established fur trading posts in the region.

In the eighteenth century, three groups of sedentary horticulturalists inhabited the area between the Knife-Heart rivers in North Dakota and the Grand

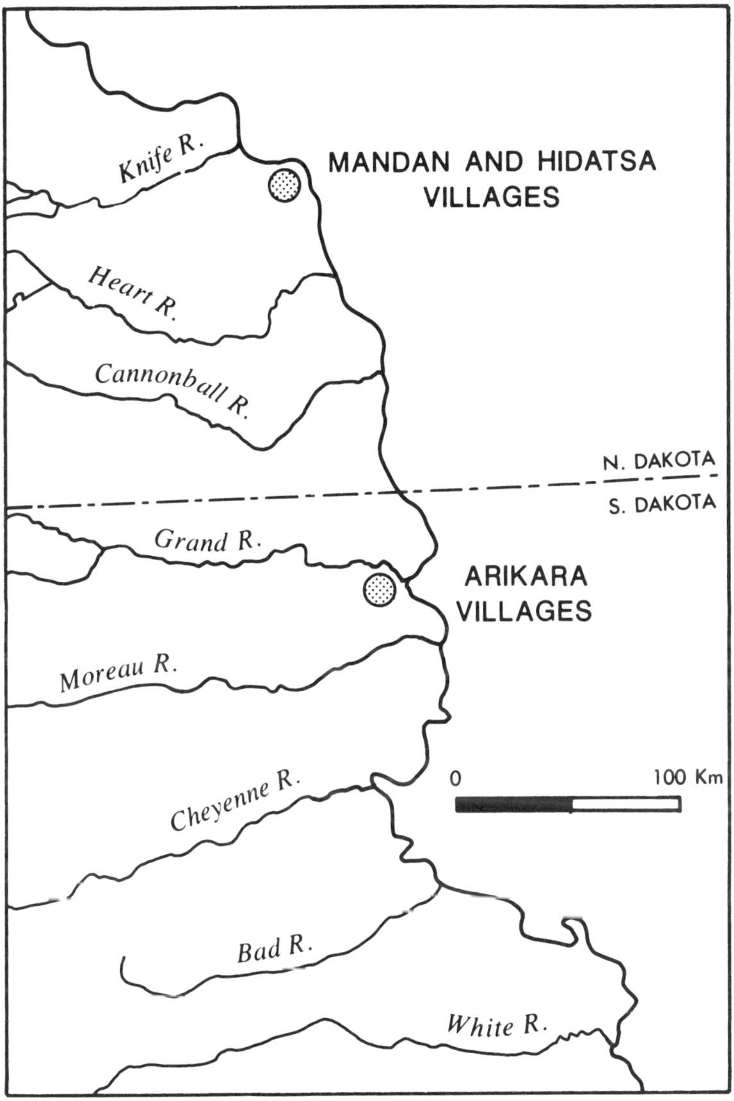

Figure 12. Middle Missouri Study Area

River in South Dakota (Figure 12). The Mandan and Hidatsa were clustered into several villages in the Knife-Heart area, and the Arikara were located at the mouth of the Grand River (Smith 1980). Between these two clusters of villages, and south of the Grand River, the area was uninhabited.

Four smaller units, the Nuitadi, Nuptadi, Awigaxa, and Isotopa comprised the Mandan, who, according to tradition, had been long-term residents in the area (Stewart 1974). Bowers (1965) suggested that the three Hidatsa bands, the Awaxawi, Awatixa, and Hidatsa proper, immigrated to the Knife-Heart area sometime after 1780; prior to their immigration, they may have been migratory hunters. Ahler (Ahler and Swenson 1985) suggested that this date was incorrect, and that the Hidatsa proper may have been present in the Knife River area by 1600. The Arikara, related to the Pawnee, reached the Middle Missouri around A.D. 1300 (Deetz 1965).

All three groups shared the same basic settlement-subsistence strategy. Villages were palisaded; houses were substantial earth-covered lodges; and subsistence was based on horticulture, hunting, and trade. The trade network, described by early explorers, has been particularly well treated by anthropologists (for example, Ewers 1955, 1968; Jablow 1951; Orser 1984; Wood 1980).

The geographic position of the three tribes made them ideal middlemen for the movement of aboriginal and European goods between the high plains or the Southwest and the eastern woodlands. According to Ewers (1955), the aboriginal network involved the exchange of garden produce for products of the hunt. Following European contact, the pattern continued and expanded to include the movement of horses from the Spaniards in the Southwest and metal products from the French and British in the Northeast.

The persistence of the Mandan, Hidatsa, and Arikara as independent cultural entities lasted only 100 years after the beginning of historic documentation. Between 1738 and 1845, there was considerable instability of population marked by village abandonment and relocation. The instability was attributed to population loss from disease, warfare with mobile Plains groups, and the continuing demand for wood. Beginning in 1845, remnants of the three groups consolidated into a single community at Like-A-Fishhook near Fort Berthold, North Dakota. In 1868, the first agent of the U.S. Bureau of Indian Affairs was established at Fort Berthold (Smith 1972).

The disappearance of settled, independent, horticultural tribes prior to the development of anthropology has had significant repercussions on the perception and analysis of the aboriginal record. In constructing ethnographies, ethnologists (for example, Bowers 1965; Ewers 1955, 1968; Lowie 1954) have relied on historical documents (Wedel and DeMallie 1980), and especially on explorers' journals. Archaeologists have also relied on the historical record, but they have not assumed stability of populations through the contact period.

Significance of the Test Case

Since Middle Missouri groups remained isolated from direct contact with Europeans until the eighteenth century, disease contact in earlier centuries could have reached native people only by diffusion. This case, therefore, is a robust test of the disease hypothesis. If the analysis from the Middle Missouri demonstrates that disease and population collapse preceded European exploration and settlement, then that part of the Cook-Dobyns hypothesis that suggests diffusion of diseases as preceding direct contact is strengthened. At the same time an eighteenth-century introduction of infectious pathogens coincident with the presence of Europeans in the region would tend to confirm the Kroeberian position regarding disease and demographic stability. Archaeologists have not previously considered this particular dichotomy; they have, because of the nature of the record from the Middle Missouri, blended assumptions of both positions.

Although Plains archaeologists were largely responsible for developing the twentieth-century version of the direct historical approach (Strong 1935, 1940; Wedel 1938), the use of the method has followed a course slightly different from in other test cases. Certainly, archaeologists have employed historical records to identify historical locations, which in turn, have biased archaeological knowledge of settlements toward those of the historical periods. For example, a historic village of the Hidatsa, 32 ME 11, was known by 1883 (Wood 1978); Will and Spinden (1906) used Lewis and Clark's journals to locate historic Mandan sites of the historical periods. By 1924, Will had identified a large percentage of currently known post-European aboriginal components.

At the same time, Plains archaeologists have not assumed demographic or cultural continuity through the historical period or from history to prehistory. This departure in perspective (see Strong 1933 for this discussion) was partially a reaction to the ethnological focus on culture areas (Wissler 1917). Since this approach assumed long term stasis and since the historical record of the Plains populations demonstrated anything but stability, the ethnological perspective was simply inappropriate. Consequently, the direct historical approach was regarded with considerable skepticism. (See Wylie 1985 for a similar view.)

Strong, for instance, argued that the similarities between historical and archaeological traits suggested ethnic continuity of the Pawnee in the historic period. He, however, was circumspect regarding continuity from the prehistoric to the protohistoric period:

> With the protohistoric period the need for a general methodology to supplement and extend the direct historical approach becomes acute. Once beyond the historic period specific tribal organization merges into the complex stream of culture history. The known tribal terminations of these streams are essential to link history and prehistory. They convert archaeological sequence into historic reality and anchor archaeology to social science. Yet, from the protohistoric to earlier periods, all tribal and linguistic appellations become increasingly fallacious (Strong 1940:377).

The recognition of historical aboriginal change and caution regarding the applicabililty of the direct historical approach has continued into the present. In a cultural reconstruction study, Deetz (1965) analyzed historical ceramics of the Arikara in order to suggest changes in their social organization of the eighteenth century. While assuming that archaeologically defined styles correlated through time with the Arikara, Deetz did not assume that their social organization was stable. Using change in pottery styles, he attempted to describe a change in the social organization of the Arikara from a matricentered pattern to one based on generational principles.

Although Ahler's work in the Knife River Indian Villages National Historic Sites (Ahler 1978, 1979; Ahler and Benz 1980; Ahler and Swenson 1980, 1985; Ahler et al. 1980) has a strong historical component, it is not strictly ethnohistorical. His interests are primarily archaeological, and he employs disparities among documentary sources to identify archaeological problems.

Not only have archaeologists assumed instability in population size but, beginning with Strong (1940), they have considered the role of diseases in aboriginal population decline. Lehmer was influential in developing this perspective. During the last years of his life, Lehmer devoted considerable time to the archaeological study of the consequences of smallpox epidemics on the Mandan, Hidatsa, and Arikara. Although much of his work remains unpublished (Lehmer n.d.), Lehmer incorporated several of his ideas into his last few publications.

(1) He argued (1971, 1977) that disease began in 1780, despite the possibility of earlier smallpox epidemics. Disease introduction, thus, postdated both the appearance of European trade goods in 1675 and European exploration of the region in 1738 and was roughly contemporaneous with sustained European presence among the Mandan.

(2) In response to the diffusion of smallpox, epidemics resulted and population sharply declined. Village counts dropped; remnant populations abandoned South Dakota, migrated upriver, and ceramic traditions deteriorated (Lehmer 1977). In North Dakota, for instance, the Knife River Phase (1780–1837) was the postepidemic cultural complex. Pottery types of the phase contrasted sharply to those of ceramics from earlier phases and were "obviously the product of less sophisticated and adept potters. Recognizing that the term is distinctly value-laden, Knife River Phase pottery can nevertheless be aptly described as decadent" (Lehmer et al. 1978:83).

Because of Lehmer's position regarding the role of disease among aboriginal populations, Ahler has tried to incorporate the question of decimation into his Knife-River research. At least one archaeologist has also used ethnohistorical sources to describe the smallpox epidemic of 1837 (Trimble 1979). This epidemic so reduced the Mandan and Hidatsa that remnants of these groups were forced to amalgamate at Like-A-Fishhook village.

In summary, since archaeologists have already shown disease to be a major factor in the destruction of aboriginal populations, only the timing of population collapse needs to be considered. The timing of the collapse has implications for the larger, more fundamental issues of cultural disruption or continuity. Three hypotheses are suggested:

Hypothesis 1 (H1) states: The sequence of events suggested by Lehmer is essentially correct. Catastrophic population loss attributable to infectious disease is an eighteenth-century phenomenon, postdating the diffusion of trade goods and European exploration.

Hypothesis 2 (H2) states: Disease contact is a seventeenth-century event, predating European exploration but roughly equivalent in time to the diffusion of European trade goods into the region.

Hypothesis 3 (H3) states: Disease contact dates to the sixteenth century and is the earliest European introduction into the Middle Missouri.

Middle Missouri Late Prehistoric and Historic Chronologies

The culture historical framework of the Middle Missouri is largely the work of Lehmer. For more than 20 years, Lehmer not only was actively involved in excavating settlements in the Middle Missouri, but continually attempted to integrate the empirical record into a chronology. The results of this work and the development of his system appeared in a number of publications (Lehmer 1952, 1954a, 1954b, 1971; Lehmer and Caldwell 1966).

Lehmer's system is basically a modification of the Willey and Phillips system (Table 31). The largest cultural-temporal unit is the tradition, and within the Plains Village period (A.D. 900–1720), there are three traditions: Plains,

Table 31 Late Prehistoric and Historic Chronologies of the Middle Missouri

TIME(AD)	TRADITION & VARIANTS (LEHMER, 1971)							(RAMENOFSKY)
	MIDDLE MISSOURI TRADITION			COALESCENT TRADITION				PERIODS
							DISORGANIZED VARIANT	V
1850								
1800						—1780—	—1780—	IV
						POST-CONTACT VARIANT		
1700			—1675—		—1675—	—1675—		III
			TERMINAL VARIANT		EXTENDED VARIANT			
1600								II
		—1550—	—1550—	—1550—	—1550—			
1500				INITIAL VARIANT				
1400	—1400—			—1400—				
		EXTENDED VARIANT						
1300								
1200								I
	INITIAL VARIANT							
1100		—1100—						
1000								
900	—900—							

Middle Missouri, and Coalescent (Lehmer 1954a, 1954b; Spaulding 1956). Only the Middle Missouri and Coalescent traditions are found in the Middle Missouri region. Variant, rather than horizon, is the largest spatial unit and is larger than a phase and distinguished by "its geographic distribution, age, and/or cultural content" (Lehmer 1971). Each tradition, thus, includes a number of variants.

Major criteria employed to assign components to phases, variants, and traditions include: geographic distribution, village plan, house type, and stylistic attributes of pottery (Lehmer and Caldwell 1966). Since many excavations of Middle Missouri settlements postdated the application of the principles of radioactive decay to archaeological dating methods, radiocarbon-dates are added to the list of other criteria.

Certain general characteristics separated the Plains Village period from the previous Plains Woodland period and the subsequent Equestrian period. Subsistence was based on horticulture and hunting, and settlements were sedentary and located on first terraces and the heavily wooded floodplain. Houses were semisubterranean earthlodges with enclosed entryways. Pottery was grit tempered with paddle marked bodies and cord impressed or incised rims and lips. Projectile points were small and either notched or unnotched.

The Middle Missouri tradition (A.D. 900–1675) was an indigenous development of the Middle Missouri region, beginning earlier than the Coalescent tradition, and terminating before the appearance of European trade goods. The tradition is thought to represent the ancestors of historical period Mandan. Early, the tradition overlapped with the Plains tradition, located south and east of Middle Missouri complexes. Lehmer (1971) established three variants within the Middle Missouri tradition. Markers of the tradition included rectangular semisubterranean houses and coarse, friable, grit-tempered pottery. The initial Variant tended to have cord roughened exteriors, but this trait was absent from both later variants. Pottery rims were S-shaped or flared. Lithic remains included grooved mauls, celts, small notched or unnotched projectiles, and snubnose scrapers. During the tradition, houses not only increased in size, but more houses were present in each village. In the Initial Variant, house counts ranged from 20 to 30; while at Huff, a Terminal Variant, there were more than 100 houses (Lehmer 1971; Wood 1967). Although palisades were present, no consistent temporal pattern in the presence or size of palisades was recorded (Lehmer 1971).

The Coalescent tradition, supposedly a blend of *in situ* traits of Middle Missouri tradition with those of the Plains tradition, was interpreted as a physical migration of Plains populations into the region. As indicated in the Table 31, the tradition overlapped the Middle Missouri tradition by several centuries. It appeared first in South Dakota, but by the Post Contact variant, it was found throughout the Dakotas. Typical characteristics included circular, semisubterranean earthlodges with centrally located fire basins. In early variants, roof supports were irregularly placed about the perimeter of structures; in later variants, the pattern changed to four main posts centered around the fire pit. Because of the ubiquitous occurrence of circular structures in the Central Plains tradition, its appearance in the Middle Missouri was seen as a cultural mixing of two previously separate peoples (Lehmer 1971; Spaulding 1956). Palisades or ditches, considered a Central Plains trait, were present, but they did not form a consistent pattern. Between the Initial and Extended variants, houses increased in size. At Arzberger, an Initial Coalescent Variant, the largest circular structure had an area of 157 m^2 (Spaulding 1956); while at Molstad, an Extended Variant, the largest habitational structure was 336 m^2 (Hoffman 1967).

Like houses, pottery was described as a blend of Middle Missouri and Plains styles. Many vessel exteriors were plain, cord roughened, simple stamped, smoothed over simple stamped, and ocassionally check stamped surfaces were also found. S-rims, popular during the Middle Missouri tradition, disappeared during later Coalescent variants and were replaced by flared, collared, braced, or vertical rims. In later variants, incised rim decorations were more common than cord impressed ones although both persisted to the end of the tradition.

There were two post-European units in Lehmer's chronology. European contact began with the Post Contact Variant (1675–1780). Besides the presence of European trade goods that marked the onset of the variant, no other material changes were recorded. Historic documentation of Middle Missouri populations began during the middle of this unit. Disease, and specifically the diffusion of smallpox from the Southwest to the Dakotas, was the last European introduction and constituted the basis of separating the Disorganized Variant (1780–1862) from the earlier Post Contact Variant. As stated by Lehmer:

> The village tribes of the Middle Missouri . . . rode the wave of prosperity and cultural elabortion through the third quarter of the eighteenth century. Then another European introduction, epidemic diseases, came close to wiping out the population, and left the survivors with a badly disorganized remnant of their former culture. This phase of village development . . . deserves recognition as a separate configuration (1971:172).

Markers of population loss included the nearly complete abandonment of South Dakota and smaller, or fewer, villages in North Dakota. By the time Lewis and Clark explored the Middle Missouri, the Arikara were confined to two or three villages in the Grand River area; and the Hidatsa and Mandan were located in five villages in the Knife-Heart area (Coues 1893; Thwaites 1904). Concommitantly, pottery styles deteriorated.

ALTERNATIVE CHRONOLOGY Since, according to Lehmer, disease was the latest European introduction, his scheme could not be employed in this analysis. By developing a new chronology all three hypotheses could be tested and confirmed or rejected by archaeological and historical data.

I have employed five temporal methods to develop the Middle Missouri chronology. Methods included radiometric assays, frequency seriations of aboriginal ceramics, occurrence seriations of metal objects, and cumulative frequency analysis of European functional classes. Although dendrochonological dates of some components were available, the method did not provide useful information in constructing this chronology. Seriations and cumulative frequency analysis were based on new classifications (see Appendix C for discussion of individual orders).

Orders were synthesized into a chronology consisting of five periods (Table 31). Given biases in radiometric determinations, I placed greater weight on relative methods, necessitating verification of sequences through multiple orders. To seriate pottery samples, the region was separated into three smaller areas (Appendix C, Figure 21). Area 1 extended from the Knife River to the South Dakota border; Area 2 extended from this border to the north bank of the Cheyenne River; and Area 3 was from the south bank of the Cheyenne to the White River. In all cases, seriations crossed the European trade goods boundary. Comparable stylistic changes in rim attributes were observed in all three seriations, leading to the identification of three stylistic pottery periods. Two of the periods occurred before European trade reached the Middle Missouri; the third period was coincident with European trade. The occurrence seriation for metal products and cumulative frequency analysis of European materials refined the later part of the sequence. Finally, historical documents were employed to confirm the relative assignment of late eighteenth- early nineteenth-century components.

Duration of periods was not sharply defined in this chronology. As in the other test cases, minimum, mean and maximum definitions of periods were employed to estimate the magnitude of error arising from imprecision in dating (Table 32). This approach provided independent assessments against which the value of S_c could be judged. Since there were no reliable radiometric determinations for Periods III through V (see Ahler and Swenson 1985 for a possible exception), estimates of period duration for these periods were based on historical documents.

Components assigned to Periods I through IV were ordered through archaeological methods and historical sources. The single Period V component could not be assigned a relative position but founding (1845) and abandonment dates (1885) were known from documents. Period characteristics including areas occupied are summarized in Table 33.

Table 32 Length of Archaeological Periods in the Middle Missouri

	Time Range (A.D.)			*Period Duration (Years)*		
Period	*Minimum*	*Mean*	*Maximum*	*Minimum*	*Mean*	*Maximum*
V	1845–1885	1845–1885	1845–1885	40	40	40
IV	1804–1837	1780–1837	1738–1837	33	57	99
III	1680–1738	1649–1780	1612–1780	58	131	168
II	1497–1612	1416–1649	1335–1686	115	233	351
I	1078–1295	1030–1359	982–1423	217	329	441

I have assigned eleven components from Areas 1 and 3 to Period I; and some components from both areas have ^{14}C dates. Estimates of period duration vary from 217 to 441 years. In Area 1, S-rims decorated by incision or cord impression are most popular; in Area 3, only one S-rim class is popular, but straight/flared rims that are either cord impressed or tool impressed/punctated are present. No European material is present.

All three areas are occupied during Period II, represented by 10 components. There are nine radiometric dates for this period. According to dates, period duration ranges from 115 to 351 years. Straight/flared rims that may or may not have a brace are popular in all three areas. All decorative modes are present on rims, but specific types of decoration vary by area. No European material is present during this temporal interval.

Period III was the most difficult period to date largely because there are no reliable radiometric dates for components of this temporal unit. Problems in the radiocarbon reservoir as well as biased sampling contributed to this problem.

Period III incorporates the sixteenth century and part of the seventeenth. Estimates of period duration range from 58 to 168 years and are based on a combination of sources. In the minimum estimate, Lehmer's date for the introduction of European trade in the region (1680) is the origin and La Verendrye's exploration (1738) marks the terminus. In the mean estimate, the origin date (1649) is the same as the mean terminal date of Period II; the terminal date (1780) coincides with the first recorded smallpox epidemic in the Middle Missouri. The maximum estimate has the same terminal date as the mean estimate (1780), but the origin date (1612) is the upper limit of the Period II minimum estimate.

Traditional evidence of European contact begins during Period III. European trade goods appear followed by historical documentation of aboriginal populations. Only components from areas 2 and 3 (seven total) are ordered chronologically and assigned to Period III. Although Area 1 is certainly occupied during at least part of this general temporal range (Ahler and Swenson

Table 33 Characteristics of Chronological Periods of the Middle Missouri

PERIOD I	
Radiocarbon Dates:	12 (Appendix C, Table 91)
Maximum Time Range:	A.D. 982–1423
Mean Time Range:	A.D. 1030–1359
Minimum Time Range:	A.D. 1078–1295
Areas Occupied:	1, 3
Components:	Area 1 (n = 3) 32 ME 1[a], 32 SI 4, 32 SI 19[a] Area 3 (n = 8) 39 ST 16[a], 39 ST 11[a], 39 LM 209, 39 ST 238[a], 39 ST 30 (Anderson Phase), 39 ST 223[a], 39 LM 208, 39 LM 232[a]
Pottery Classes: (Frequencies ≥15%)	Area 1: 135, 231, 232 Area 3: 133, 135
European Trade Goods:	Absent
PERIOD II	
Radiocarbon Dates:	9 (Appendix C, Table 91)
Maximum Time Range:	A. D. 1335–1686
Mean Time Range:	A.D. 1416–1649
Minimum Time Range:	A.D. 1497–1612
Areas Occupied:	1, 2, 3
Components:	Area 1 (n = 4) 32 MO 11, 32 EM 10, 32 OL 14[a], 32 OL 16[a] Area 2 (n = 2) 39 CO 1, 39 DW 234 Area 3 (n = 4) 39 ST 9(A)[a], 39 ST 9/232(B)[a], 39 HU 1[a], 39 HU 6
Pottery Classes: (Frequencies ≥15%)	Area 1: 113, 135, 232 Area 2: 131, 135 Area 3: 121, 133, 134, 135
European Trade Goods:	Absent
PERIOD III	
Radiocarbon Dates:	0
Maximum Time Range:	A.D. 1612–1780
Mean Time Range:	A.D. 1649–1780
Minimum Time Range:	A.D. 1680–1738
Areas Occupied:	2, 3
Components:	Area 2 (n = 3) 39 DW 2, 39 WW 7 (C/D), 39 WW 7 (B) Area 3 (n = 4) 39 ST 30 (Stanley Phase), 39 ST 15, 39 ST 6, 39 LM 215
Pottery Classes: (Frequencies ≥15%)	Area 2: 111, 112, 133, 134 Area 3: 113, 114, 115
European Trade Goods:	Present: brass, copper, and iron scrap and shaped objects.

(*continued*)

Table 33 (*Continued*)

PERIOD IV	
Radiocarbon Dates:	0
Maximum Time Range:	A.D. 1738–1837
Mean Time Range:	A.D. 1780–1837
Minimum Time Range:	A.D. 1804–1834
Areas Occupied:	1, 3
Components:	Area 1 (n = 6) 32 ML 39, 32 ME 5, 32 ME 8, 32 ME 11, 32 ME 12, 32 ME 15 Area 3 (n = 2) 39 ST 14, 39 HU 26
Pottery Classes: (Frequencies ≥15%)	Area 1: 112, 115 Area 3: 112, 113, 114, 115, 135
European Trade Goods:	Present: copper, scrap, brass scrap and shaped objects, iron shaped objects, European crockery.
PERIOD V	
Radiocarbon Dates:	0
Time Range:	A.D. 1845–1885
Areas Occupied:	Area 1 (n = 1)
Components:	32 ML 2 (Like-A-Fishhook)

[a]Ordered only by radiometric dates.

1985), there is insufficient information to incorporate the available data into a chronological scheme. Consequently, for Period III, I assign Area 1 a zero value. In areas 2 and 3 straight/flared rims classes with or without bracing are most popular.

Duration of Period IV ranges from thirty-three to ninety-nine years. As documented historically, some Area 1 components survive through the entire interval, but components from Area 3 do not. Since the smallpox epidemic of 1837 very nearly annihilated the Mandan and Hidatsa, all three estimates of period duration have the same terminal date. Origin dates are, however, based on different considerations. The Lewis and Clark expedition (1804) marks the lower boundary for the minimum estimate (1804–1837). The 1780 smallpox epidemic marks the lower limit of the mean estimate (1780–1837); and La Verendrye's expedition in 1738 is the lower boundary for the maximum estimate (1738–1837). Styles of pottery are dominated by classes of straight/flared rims that are braced. The character of European trade changes dramatically during Period IV, largely because of the development of the fur trade and establishment of trading posts in the region.

Like-A-Fishhook is the only component assigned to Period V. Since dates of founding (1845) and abandonment (1885) are known (Smith 1972), all estimates of period duration are the same, forty years. Although other settlements, for example Crow-Flies-High (Malouf 1963), were presumably occupied during Period V, they were excluded because published information was insufficient for my analyses. Like-A-Fishhook was a large permanent village established by traders near Fort Berthold. Ethnic composition of the village included Mandan, Hidatsa, and Arikara survivors from the 1837 smallpox epidemic.

In summary, I developed this chronology which synthesized much of the published record for the Middle Missouri primarily through relative dating methods, including seriations and cumulative frequencies. Since different problems and assumptions guided this investigation, the resulting structure was quite different from that developed by Lehmer. Stylistic and functional change was the basis of integration rather than culture historical notions, such as migration of people or diffusion of ideas. Consequently, terms and concepts such as variants or traditions were unnecessary.

Period I of this chronology included some components Lehmer assigned to Initial and Extended variants of the Middle Missouri tradition. Period II, which terminated prior to the diffusion of European trade into the Middle Missouri, included components from four variants of both the Middle Missouri and Coalescent traditions. Except for period duration, Period III was quite similar to Lehmer's Post Contact Coalescent variant. Period IV may also be comparable temporally to Lehmer's Disorganized Coalescent variant, but in contrast to that variant, Period IV included components from both North and South Dakota. Finally, Period V covered the terminus of the historical aboriginal record and persisted throughout the beginning of reservations in the Middle Missouri.

Analysis of Population Change

Settlement parameters necessary for estimating regional change in population are presented first, after which Equations (4) and (5) are employed to establish patterns of population change through time. These patterns are then used to evaluate alternative hypotheses regarding the origin of disease introduction and population collapse in the Middle Missouri. (See Appendix C Tables 105 through 107 for measurements of individual settlements).

SETTLEMENT COUNTS (S_c) I have limited settlement counts to the thirty-seven components ordered chronologically (Table 33). Table 34 lists, by period, raw settlement counts and $[S_c/(T/100)]$ counts, estimated in terms of minimum, mean, and maximum period duration. Despite differences in period duration, adjusted counts have the same trend: an increase between Periods I and IV followed by a decrease in Period V. Consideration of the early recorded epidemic history of the Middle Missouri is sufficient evidence for rejecting part of this pattern. Population is not increasing during Period IV, the late eighteenth and early nineteenth century.

Table 34 Middle Missouri Settlement Counts by Period

Period	Raw Counts	Adjusted Counts $[S_c/(T/100)]$ Minimum	S_c	Mean	S_c	Maximum	S_c
V	1	0.40	2.5	0.40	2.5	0.40	2.5
IV	8	0.33	24.2	0.57	14.0	0.99	8.1
III	7	0.58	12.1	1.30	5.4	1.70	4.1
II	10	1.20	8.3	2.30	4.4	3.50	2.9
I	11	2.20	5.0	3.30	3.3	4.40	2.5

Terminal dates for Periods III (1780) and IV (1837) mark the diffusion of two major smallpox epidemics that decimated Middle Missouri populations. Since native populations typically did not experience a growth spurt following an epidemic and since the time lapse was not long enough to facilitate population recovery, the increase in Period IV counts must have been due to factors other than an expanding population. Evaluation of biases suggests that the increase in Period III counts is also in error.

First, archaeological sampling practices have inflated counts. As previously described, historical documents have guided the location of historic period settlements, and counts of these settlements have not changed substantially since 1924 (Will 1924). While it can be assumed that the sample of settlements with trade goods is quite accurate, the same assumption cannot be made for counts of prehistoric settlements.

Population mobility and residential instability relative to period duration are the second major bias inflating S_c during Periods III and IV. Because there are historical sources that describe populations of the Middle Missouri after 1780, the record of instability is better documented for Period IV than for Period III. Nonetheless, there is some evidence that aboriginal populations are relocating during both periods. As documented by this chronology, South Dakota was largely abandoned sometime during Period III. Furthermore, horses were present in the Middle Missouri by 1738. Besides providing a new trade item for the Mandan and Arikara, they also facilitated the harassment of sedentary groups by mobile Plains groups. Evidence of this harassment is suggested by Arikara relocations that began sometime during the eighteenth century (Chomko 1977; Stewart 1974).

By the late eighteenth century, the pace of this process had quickened. Writing in 1804, Tabeau commented that the Arikara changed residence every five or six years because of the continuing demand for wood (Abel 1939). Whether this process operated prehistorically as well is not known.

The settlement history of Mandan and Hidatsa between 1780–1837 is well known (Ahler and Swenson 1985; Coues 1897; Stewart 1974). Of eight historically described villages that date to this interval, three were abandoned before the Lewis and Clark expedition. These villages had a mean settlement duration of thirteen years. Three other villages that date to this interval were established in 1798 and had a mean settlement duration of forty years. Only one settlement, 32 ME 12, persisted throughout the entire interval.

In short, the only reasonable evaluation of these data is that Period III and Period IV counts are inflated relative to prehistoric counts and that they will seriously influence regional estimates of population. Furthermore, these data demonstrate more clearly than any other test case the disparities between the known archaeological record and processes of population change. While populations were precipitously falling, settlement counts were increasing. Only when populations were near extinction do settlement counts decrease (Period V).

Although sampling practices and historical records are sufficient for documenting biases in Periods III and IV, they are insufficient for indicating biases in earlier periods. Since Period II crosses not only the disease boundary in the Lower Mississippi Valley, but the historic boundary for the western Plains, Southwest, and Northeast, there is some question whether disruptions of the contact period in adjacent areas are influencing Middle Missouri populations during Period II. Obviously, S_c is inadequate for indicating whether or not there were such influences, but the question will remain open as other classes of settlement data are considered.

SETTLEMENT AREA (S_a) A series of factors, for example, incomplete excavation, multiple occupations, and inconsistent presence of structural boundaries, have limited S_a measurements to 54% (20/37) of the known settlements. Since measurements describe different types of space and are taken from different sources that are restricted particular periods, S_a is both a biased and unreliable estimator of population. Regional population estimates that employ these data, therefore, may be of little utility.

I calculated eleven measurements of S_a from maps; and while seven of these were areas within palisades or ditches, four were limited to house areas only. The preponderance of palisades occurred in later periods, while measurements of house areas were more common earlier. Although some settlements where only house areas had been measured also had palisades, these features either did not surround the entire village or did not correlate temporally with the component used in this analysis. Eight settlement areas, largely confined to Periods I and II, were taken directly from published descriptions and were not calculated independently.

Between Periods I and II, $\overline{S_a}$ increases followed by a decrease in Periods III and IV, and a final increase in Period V (Table 35). (See Appendix C, Table 107 for individual measurements.) The huge size of the single Period V settlement is

Table 35 Middle Missouri Estimates of Settlement Area in Hectares

Period	*Settlements With Area Measured*	$\overline{S_a}$	S^2
V	1	16.0	
IV	4	1.3	8.04
III	3	2.9	32.78
II	6	6.1	258.57
I	6	2.3	37.58
TOTAL	20		

the result of a fundamentally new structure developed by Europeans. The community, composed of two villages and two fur trading posts, continued to grow during its forty-year history. In 1858, Fort Berthold II was built south of the original post and the native village; in 1862, the Arikara added their own extension to the north (Smith 1972). The size of the Period II estimate of S_a was a consequence of the estimated size of Arzberger, 17.2 hectares (Spaulding 1956). This figure was more than three times larger than any other estimate for a known settlement area during Period II.

Although the correlation between the type of description and the estimate of S_a may well be affecting the magnitude of change between mean estimates, there is no reason to assume that the direction of change is fundamentally in error. The increase between Periods I and II coincides with the largest number of S_a estimates that are not calculated independently, but since both mean and variance showed the same pattern, variability is comparable between periods. Furthermore, S_a is not subject to sampling biases that so skew S_c during periods III and IV. Consequently, the decrease in S_a during these periods can be accepted as correct in outline.

ROOFED AREA OF SETTLEMENT (S_{ra}) Roofed area measurements of settlements (S_{ra}) are based on roofed area measurements of houses (H_{ra}) and estimates of house counts per settlement. The total sample of excavated houses for the Middle Missouri is quite large (n = 159) facilitating a thorough discussion of both H_{ra} and S_{ra}.

Data pertinent for estimating $\overline{H_{ra}}$ appear in Table 36 and, except for Periods III and V, the distribution of the total sample across periods was quite even. Although the Period V sample was from one settlement, the size of the variance suggested that intrasettlement variability was comparable to intersettlement variability.

The mean and sample variance for roofed area of houses are bimodal and

Table 36 Middle Missouri Roofed Area of Houses ($\overline{H_{ra}}$)

Period	*Settlements With H_{ra}*	*House Count*	*$\overline{H_{ra}}$ (meters²)*	*S^2*
V	1	9	216.1	467186.1
IV	6	49	56.2	158163.5
III	6	18	72.1	98691.9
II	10	44	125.4	707152.4
I	10	39	94.8	358206.2
TOTAL	33	159		

comparable to trends in $\overline{S_a}$. The first peak occurs in Period II followed by a decrease in Periods III and IV. The second peak occurs in Period V, but this value is skewed. Although earthlodges and log cabins are present at Like-A-Fishhook (Smith 1972), measurements are limited to earthlodges which are typically much larger than log cabins. Consequently, the Period V estimate does not represent total variability in house area, even within a single settlement; is biased in favor of large structures.

Since measurements of roofed area are the most reliable estimator of population and since H_{ra} is not subject to biases affecting S_c, the pattern of increase and decrease from Periods I through IV is assumed to be accurate. Evaluation of variance supports this contention and offers additional information to changes in population size.

As seen in the values of S^2 and demonstrated differently in Table 37, the greatest spread in house sizes occurs in Periods II and IV. The size of the sample variance of Period V is due to the nature of the sample, large earth lodges. Had

Table 37 House Count by Size Class and Temporal Period

	House Size Class							
Period	*1*	*2*	*3*	*4*	*5*	*6*	*7*	*8*
V	0	0	2	1	5	0	1	0
IV	27	18	2	1	0	0	1	0
III	4	11	3	0	0	0	0	0
II	3	16	15	6	1	0	2	1
I	1	28	7	2	1	0	0	0

1 = 0–49 m²
2 = 50–99 m²
3 = 100–149 m²
4 = 150–199 m²
5 = 200–249 m²
6 = 250–299 m²
7 = 300–349 m²
8 = Greater than 350 m²

the sample included a few smaller structures, the mean would have been smaller and the variance larger.

Temporal factors are definitely contributing to the size of the variance during Period II; and these factors may, in turn, imply some type of disruption in population size. The three Period II houses with measurements greater than 300 m^2 are from two components (DW 234 and ST 9/232(B)) both of which have radiocarbon dates. The dendrocalibrated date for DW 234 is A.D. 1586 ± 53. ST 9/232(B) is too recent for calibration, but the uncorrected mean date is AD 1604 ± 37 (Appendix C, Table 91). Although biases in the radiocarbon reservoir cast serious doubt on the reliability of the dates, the best available evidence suggests that the three large houses were confined to the latter part of the sixteenth or the early part of the seventeenth century.

Furthermore, although the stratigraphy at ST 9/232 is particularly complex, there is some indication that larger and smaller houses were temporally sequential. ST 9/232(B) was followed by ST 9(A) with an uncorrected mean date of A.D. 1649 ± 37 (Appendix C, Table 91). From this latter component seven houses were excavated; and the range in measurements of roofed area is 57.8 m^2 to 148.6 m^2 (Hoffman 1968). (See Appendix C, Table 106.)

The times of the changes in roofed area of houses overlaps with European colonization and settlement in the Southwest and with disease contact in the Lower Mississippi Valley. Given the extent of prehistoric trade networks, it is possible that events in adjacent regions were having repercussions on populations of the Middle Missouri.

In summary, maxima in the sample variance of $\overline{H_{ra}}$ were a consequence of several factors. The size of the Period V variance was related to the nature of the sample; the Period II variance is larger than that of Period IV and may be explained by changes in house size that clustered in the late sixteenth or early seventeenth century. Changes in house size may have reflected population loss, whose origin may be attributed to the diffusion of infectious diseases from populations in adjacent regions.

Because the calculation of $\overline{S_{ra}}$ required that a settlement have both excavated houses and estimated total house counts, sample size of houses and settlements is smaller for $\overline{S_{ra}}$ than for $\overline{H_{ra}}$. This requirement has excluded any estimate of $\overline{S_{ra}}$ for Period V. Excluding Like-A-Fishhook has consequences on resulting trends.

In estimating $\overline{S_{ra}}$ by period, $\overline{S_{ra}}$ for each settlement was first calculated by multiplying settlement $\overline{H_{ra}}$ by estimated total house count (Appendix C, Table 108). Period means and variances are based on the sum of individual means.

Table 38 summarizes $\overline{S_{ra}}$ by period. $\overline{S_{ra}}$ and variance are bimodal with peaks occurring in Periods II and IV. The mean value is smaller in Period II than in IV, but the reverse holds true for values of S^2. Several factors account for this curious reversal. Sample size is influencing the estimates. Period II has twice the

Table 38 Middle Missouri Measurement of $\overline{S_{ra}}$ in Square Meters

Period	Settlements Counts	Excavated Houses	House Count Estimate	$\overline{S_{ra}}$	S^2
V	0	0			
IV	3	19	96	5625.5	2693297.9
III	3	6	121	3342.1	744658.9
II	6	32	280	4931.1	3050370.8
I	6	20	123	1768.9	897683.1
TOTAL	18	77	620		

[a]All estimates in square meters.

number of settlements with houses and 66% more house counts. The size of the mean value in Period II reflects the requirement for calculating $\overline{S_{ra}}$. For instance, the very large houses from 39 DW 9/232 were excluded because there were no estimates of unexcavated houses.

In addition, the mean value of Period IV is likely too large due to the incomplete excavation of 32 ME 11 (Appendix C Table 108). There were forty houses estimated but only one, measuring 314.2 m², was excavated. This bias in terms of an excavation of a single house coupled with the size of that house produced a $\overline{S_{ra}}$ of 12,568.0 m². This estimate was roughly four times larger than the next largest $\overline{S_{ra}}$ for the period. If this estimate is excluded, Period IV $\overline{S_{ra}}$ would drop to 2154.8 m², making trends in $\overline{S_{ra}}$ comparable to $\overline{H_{ra}}$.

REGIONAL ESTIMATES OF POPULATION (P_{ar}) In the first equation of regional population change, $\overline{S_a}$ is measured against minimum, mean, and maximum estimates of S_c:

$$P_{ar} = [S_c/(T/100)] \times \overline{S_a}$$

According to Table 39, trends in these data are different from estimates of $\overline{S_a}$ by period (Table 35) and vary by temporal model. Minimum and maximum estimates of period duration produced the same pattern: regional population increases between Periods I and II; decreases between Periods II, III and IV; and peaks again in Period V. While the mean estimate of period duration also produced peaks in Periods II and V, the pattern between Periods III and IV was different. Regional population shows some magnitude of loss between Periods II and III, and then some recovery between Periods III and IV (Figure 13).

Biases inherent to the estimates of S_c, as well as biases and imprecisions in the measurement of S_a seriously affected regional estimates of population based on

Table 39 P_{ar} Based on Estimates of $\overline{S}_a$ in Hectares

		$[S_c/(T/100)] \times \overline{S}_a$					
Period	$\overline{S}_a$	*Minimum*	S_a	*Mean*	S_a	*Maximum*	S_a
V	16.0	2.5	40.0	2.5	40.0	2.5	40.0
IV	1.3	24.2	31.5	14.0	18.2	8.1	10.5
III	2.9	12.1	35.1	5.4	15.7	4.1	11.9
II	6.1	8.3	50.6	4.4	26.8	2.9	17.7
I	2.3	5.0	11.5	3.3	7.5	2.5	5.8

$\overline{S}_a$. While certain patterns can be evaluated, general trends in population size cannot be determined.

The increase in population in Period V is a function of the community structure developed by Europeans to accommodate survivors of the 1837 smallpox epidemic. The increase in settlement size, thus, reflects European influence and amalgamation of aboriginal populations, not an actual increase in population size. Further, the magnitude of population increase during Period II is partially explained by the estimated settlement size of Arzberger (Appendix C, Table 107).

Despite problems in estimating S_a, the pattern of population change between Periods I and III is consistent across all temporal models and can be assumed to be reasonably accurate. Between Periods I and II, population appears to be increasing followed by a decrease in Period III. The decrease during the sixteenth and seventeenth centuries coincides with the appearance of European trade goods in the Middle Missouri. The population loss in Period III is particularly significant because the direction of the change is counter to expecta-

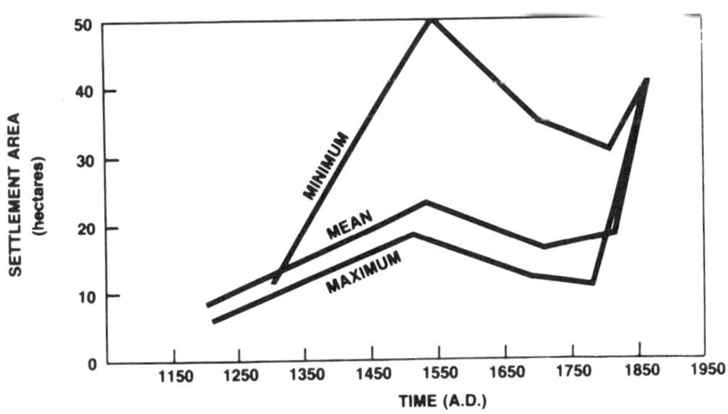

Figure 13. P_{ar} Based on $\overline{S}_a$

tions regarding the behavior of population after the appearance of European trade goods in the region.

The second equation for estimating regional change in population employs S_{ra} and adjusted counts:

$$P_{ar} = [(S_c/(T/100)] \times \overline{S_{ra}}$$

Bimodal trends in regional estimates of population are consistent among temporal models (Table 40) and with trends developed for $\overline{S_{ra}}$ (see Table 38.) The first and smaller population peak occurs in Period II, and the maximum estimate of regional population occurs in Period IV, the late eighteenth and early nineteenth centuries (Figure 14). Before evaluating regional trends, biases affecting estimates of periods II through IV are considered.

Inflation of S_c during historic periods should be reflected as a steady increase in population during Periods III and IV. This is not, however, the case. Since, between Periods II and III, population demonstrates a decline despite estimates of period duration, the change is assumed to be accurate. Only in Period IV do regional estimates of population increase. Because during this period, documented smallpox epidemics are known to have decimated Middle Missouri groups, archaeological estimates of population cannot be taken at face value. While estimates suggest an increase in population size, population is actually falling.

Whether regional estimates of population during Period II are also biased is more difficult to evaluate. Although there was undoubtedly some population growth between the tenth and fifteenth centuries A.D., the question is whether this growth continues into the sixteenth and seventeenth centuries.

Archaeological trends suggest this was the case, but isolated pieces of data suggested that the increase may not have been uniform. As previously shown, the $\overline{S_{ra}}$ for Period II was based on roofed area of houses and, during the last 100 years of the period, house size was variable (see Table 37). By the end of the period, no house was greater than 150 m^2.

Table 40 P_{ar} Based on Estimates of $\overline{S_{ra}}$ in Square Meters

		$[S_c/(T/100)] \times \overline{S_{ra}}$					
Period	$\overline{S_{ra}}$	*Minimum*	S_{ra}	*Mean*	S_{ra}	*Maximum*	S_{ra}
V	0						
IV	5625.5	24.2	136,137.1	14.0	78,757.0	8.1	45,566.6
III	3342.1	12.1	40,439.4	5.4	18,047.5	4.1	13,702.6
II	4931.1	8.3	40,929.8	4.4	21,696.8	2.9	14,300.8
I	1768.9	5.0	8,844.5	3.3	5,837.4	2.5	4,422.5

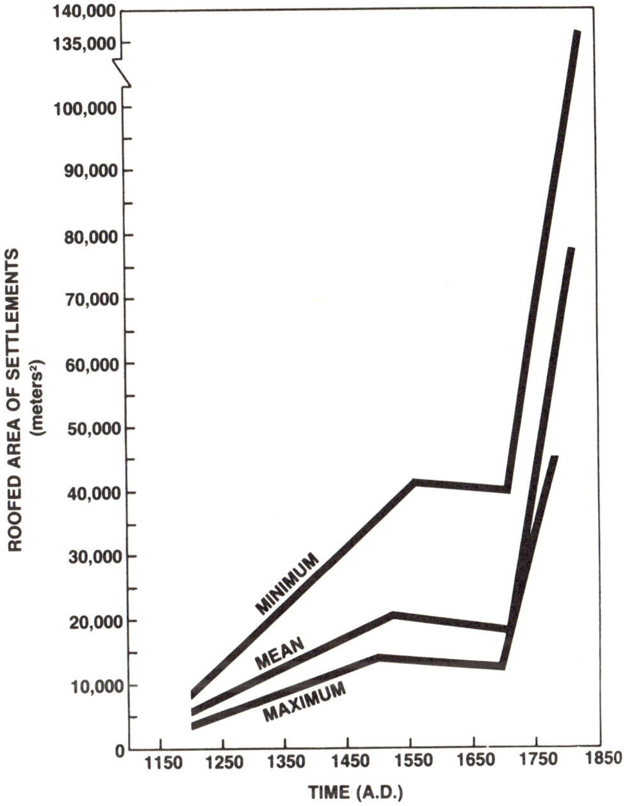

Figure 14. P_{ar} Based on $\overline{S_{ra}}$

Thus, while regional estimates of population based on $\overline{S_{ra}}$ were more reliable than estimates based on S_a, trends cannot be accepted at face value. Population appears to be increasing between Periods I and II, but the increase may not have continued throughout the entire period. Furthermore, although population estimates for Period IV suggested an increase, historical records contradict this interpretation. Regional estimates of population suggested a sizable population loss in Period III and historical sources demonstrated that the loss continued through Periods IV and V.

CONCLUSIONS Analyses of the Middle Missouri settlement record are sufficient for rejecting H1. Lehmer's hypothesis that marked the beginning of disease contact as a late eighteenth-century event can no longer be supported. According to this chronology, disease introduction and resulting catastrophic loss of population occurred in Period III. Since estimates for the beginning of that period ranged from 1612 until 1680, the decline began at least 100 years earlier than suggested by Lehmer and coincided with the appearance of European trade goods in the region. Diffusion of infectious parasites and European products were simultaneous introductions into the region.

The rejection of Lehmer's hypothesis is also a rejection of the Kroeberian position of continuity. The arrival of Europeans did not mark the onset of change. Consequently, the nature of even the earliest historical records have to be reevaluated. While documents are appropriate descriptions of populations adjusting to a sizable loss, they cannot be assumed to represent the aboriginal condition.

The question of whether Period II or III marked the origin of the population decline cannot be resolved unambiguously by these data. While the bulk of the settlement record argued for an increase in population until the mid to late seventeenth century, some house size data from late sixteenth and early seventeenth centuries (Period II) suggested that disruptions date to the late sixteenth or early seventeenth century. If these disruptions were related to population decline, then Hypothesis 3, which presented infectious disease as the earliest European introduction into the Middle Missouri, is correct. If disruptions in settlement are not a function of population loss, then Hypothesis 2 that viewed disease and European material as simultaneous diffusions becomes more likely.

Middle Missouri History, 1738–1845

This section focuses on European exploration and colonization, aboriginal population estimates, and settlement history. Following the discussion of these topics, the issue of the timing of disease contact is considered in light of known and suspected epidemics.

EUROPEAN DISCOVERY AND COLONIZATION This discussion of European exploration is multi-regional. Even though the earliest recorded contact of Middle Missouri groups by Europeans was an eighteenth-century event (Table 41), historical records suggest that the Mandan, Hidatsa, and Arikara were familiar with Europeans and their products long before that time. When La Verendrye entered the Middle Missouri, he found Indians mounted on horseback and others who spoke Spanish (Nasatir 1952). The role of the Mandan, Hidatsa, and Arikara in aboriginal trade networks and the fact that European contact in regions adjacent to the Middle Missouri occurred centuries earlier partially explain why native populations knew about Europeans before the onset of direct interaction.

In 1541, following exploration of the Rio Grande area, Coronado and a party of perhaps 1500 traveled onto the Plains as far as Kansas where they contacted the Quivira (Bolton 1906, 1949). At approximately the same time, De Soto and

Table 41 Some Historical Events in the Plains including the Middle Missouri

1541	Coronado's incursion into the western Plains.
1541	De Soto and Moscoso explore east Texas.
1723	Bourgement reaches Arikara villages from the south.
1738	La Verendrye reaches Mandan and Arikara villages from the north.
1762	St. Louis is founded.
1780–1795	Spanish and French traders along the Middle Missouri.
1797	David Thompson contacts the Mandan from the north.
1802	Loisel's Fort established in South Dakota.
1804–06	Lewis and Clark explore the Missouri for the United States.
1826	Fort Kipp established in North Dakota.
1845	Fort Berthold established in North Dakota.

Moscoso were making incursions into the eastern periphery of the Plains in their travels through Oklahoma and east Texas (Perttula and Ramenofsky 1981; Swanton 1939). After Onate's colonization of Santa Fe in 1598, Spanish products began to trickle onto the Plains. Since Spanish colonists in New Mexico received European supplies by pack trains from Mexico and three years could elapse between contacts (Scholes 1930), there was little European surplus in the New Mexico colony.

Horses, one of these items, were the earliest Spanish product to reach aboriginal populations. The Ute acquired the horse by 1640; Kiowa and Kiowa Apache were trading horses to Pawnee by 1682; and the Caddo were mounted by 1690 (Ewers 1955).

French influences spread into the Middle Missouri from Canada and the Mississippi. The center of diffusion in the Northeast was earlier because colonization of the St. Lawrence preceded that along the Mississippi. As suggested by Ewers (1955), metal was the primary commodity diffusing east from Canada. Horticulturalists of the Middle Missouri were the middlemen in the westward movement of metal and the eastward movement of horses.

Although French traders may have occasionally contacted Middle Missouri populations in the seventeenth century, definite contacts began in the eighteenth century. In 1723, moving north from Fort Orleans, Bourgement reached the Arikara villages where he may have spent several years (Nasatir 1952). Slightly later, in 1738, La Verendrye traveled south to the Mandan villages from forts established in Manitoba. La Verendrye left two of his party at the Mandan villages to learn the language; and in 1742, his sons returned to the area for a second exploration. They traveled south from the Knife River area, and after following a circuitous route, arrived at the Arikara villages (Burpee 1927; Smith

1980). By the time of the French and Indian War (1754), the only section of the Missouri that remained unexplored was between the Bad-Cheyenne rivers and the Platte River (Nasatir 1952).

Following the American Revolution, European contact along the Middle Missouri intensified. Although by that time, France had lost all her holdings in North America, French traders, working independently or for Spanish companies, continued to exploit fur resources of the Middle Missouri and to live among aboriginal groups (Nasatir 1952). Spain, concerned about the British in Canada and wanting to defend her colonies, established trading companies, based in St. Louis, and sent traders to the Mandan villages (Abel 1939; Chittendon 1954; Nasatir 1952). At the same time, British traders were pushing south and west from Hudson's Bay and were contacting Middle Missouri groups. David Thompson, who reached the Mandan in 1797, was the first recorded British trader (Coues 1897; Wood 1977).

American political influence and economic exploitation of the region did not begin officially until the early nineteenth century. Lewis and Clark, instructed by Thomas Jefferson to chart and describe newly acquired lands and peoples, were the first official explorers (1804–1806) . Shortly thereafter, fur trading posts were established; but their primary economic function was short-lived. By 1845, when Fort Berthold was built, animals had largely disappeared. As the war offensive against mobile Plains groups escalated, fur trading posts were converted into military forts.

Thus, Middle Missouri populations were familiar with European products before recorded history of the region. Products initially flowed into the region from both the Southwest and Northeast and were incorporated into aboriginal trade networks. Europeans entered the area from both of these directions as well as from the Southeast.

ABORIGINAL POPULATION ESTIMATES Table 42 summarizes warrior counts of population between 1780 and 1845. Unfortunately, all estimates of aboriginal population size and change are biased. Although Schoolcraft (1853–1857) and Mooney (1928) projected head counts back to their assumed "demographic present," for reasons discussed in Chapter 2, their projections cannot be accepted as reliable.

Going to the earliest historical record does not improve the reliability of estimates. The first census counts of Middle Missouri groups postdated even direct contact by a minimum of fifty years. In the nineteenth century, the Office of Indian Affairs provided estimates of the Mandan, Hidatsa, and Arikara; but all too frequently, agents responsible for the figures did not reside in the area. For instance, the 1837 census by William Fulkerson was developed more from heresay than from actual observations (Letter from W. Clark to C. A. Harris, OIA 1838).

Table 42 Middle Missouri Warrior Estimates

Time (A.D.)	*Mandan*	*Hidatsa*	*Arikara*
1773[a]	15,000		
1790[b]		700	
1797[c]	220	400	
1802[d]	400	600	500
1804[e]	350	650	650
1804–05[f]	350	650	600
1827–30[g]		600	550
1829[h]	150	300	400
1842[i]	120	300	450

[a]Schoolcraft, 1853–1857, Part III.
[b]Schoolcraft, 1853–1857, Part III.
[c]David Thompson Estimates, Coues 1897.
[d]Le Rays 1908.
[e]Lewis and Clark Estimates, Coues 1893, Vol. 1.
[f]Lewis and Clark Estimates, Thwaites 1904, Vol. 1.
[g]James Halsey's Estimate, Robinson 1918.
[h]OIA 1829.
[i]OIA 1842.

Nonetheless, census counts are important for pointing out problems and assumptions of both Middle Missouri archaeology and history. All census counts fall within Period IV of this chronology. Although archaeological estimates of population suggested an increase in Period IV, this increase is now confirmed to be in error. Comparison of the earliest and latest census figures suggests a strong downward trend that is logical given the known epidemics of 1780 and 1837. Thus, the archaeological record is biased by problems of sampling, settlement duration, period duration, and processes of amalgamation.

Finally, because the archaeological record suggested that the collapse began in the seventeenth century (Period III), census data do not describe predisease populations. Estimates are postcolonization and postepidemic.

SETTLEMENT HISTORY The historic settlement record agrees generally with the downward trend in census data and offers a number of insights into processes of postcontact settlement change. Table 43 shows a gradual reduction in village counts, which culminated in the single village, Like-A-Fishhook, a hybrid community. Counts, however, describe only those villages that persisted; they contain no information about the number of abandoned settlements, or processes of village fusion. Such information is found in the historical literature.

Table 43 Mandan, Hidatsa, and Arikara Village Counts, 1773–1845

Time (A.D.)	*Mandan*	*Hidatsa*	*Arikara*
1773[a]	9		
1797[b]	2	3	
1802[c]			3
1804[d]			3
1804[e]	2	3	3
1804–05[f]	2	3	3
1827–30[g]	2	3	2
1837[h]	2		
1845[i]	1	1	

[a]Schoolcraft, 1853–1857, Part III. Thwaites (1904, 1) also mentions that previously there had been 9 Mandan villages.
[b]David Thompson Estimates, Coues 1897, Vol. 1.
[c]Le Rays 1908.
[d]Tabeau's Estimate, Abel 1939.
[e]Lewis and Clark's Estimates, Coues 1893, Vol. 1.
[f]Op. cit. Thwaites 1904, Vol. 1.
[g]James Halsey's Estimate, Robinson 1918.
[h]OIA 1837.
[i]Smith 1972.

According to archaeological data, village abandonment began early in the eighteenth century. The earliest historical references of this process dated to the late eighteenth century. In 1794, when Truteau sailed up the Missouri, the first inhabited villages were those of the Arikara who were located in the vicinity of the Grand River. The region between the Grand and White rivers was abandoned. More explicit descriptions of abandoned villages were found in the Lewis and Clark journals (Coues 1893; Thwaites 1904).

Like Truteau, Lewis and Clark encountered no populations residing south of the Grand River. In the vicinity of the Grand River, they found three recently abandoned Arikara villages. Between the Grand River and the Knife-Heart area, again no inhabited communities were encountered; and in the Knife-Heart area, they described at least six recently abandoned Mandan villages.

> I walked out on the L. side (right bank of the Missouri River) . . . I saw an old remains of a village . . . on the Side of a hill where the Chief with Too-ne tells me that nation lived in 2 villages . . . (Thwaites 1904:1:200).
> . . . passed the 2.nd village of the Mandans which was in existence at the same time as the 1.st (Ibid, 1:201).

. . . proceeded on to a point on the NE side (of the Missouri River) opposite the remains of an old Mandan village a little below the entrance of the Chiss-che-t-or (Ibid:5:364).

In one of the descriptions of three abandoned villages, Clark described scatters of human bone:

. . . The mounds, nine in number along the River within 20 miles that fallen down earth of houses, some teeth and bones of men and animals mixed in these villages, human skulls are scattered in these villages (Ibid:1:202).

Population amalgamation and village fusion were associated with village abandonment. Truteau commented that in 1795–1796, one band of Arikara were residing "with Pani-Mah, and another with the Mandan" (Nasatir 1952:299). Alexander Henry is more explicit about the Arikara-Mandan association:

Not many years ago, the Pawnee (Arikara) and Mandanes were allied to each other and lived together in the same villages, on the Missourie. . . . A misunderstanding happening, they separated . . . (Coues 1897:1:334).

The Arikara migration between the Knife-Heart area and the Grand River continued until 1837 when they established a village near Fort Clark, North Dakota. They remained at Fort Clark until their move to Like-A-Fishhook in 1862 (Chomko 1977). After the Hidatsa immigrated to the Knife-Heart area, they established a series of villages, one of which was composed of both the Hidatsa and the Mandan.

In short, descriptions of the histories of settlements support the interpretation of the record continually alluded to throughout this chapter. Substantial and rapid population loss was followed by a period of instability, in which survivors attempted to balance population scales and to maintain existing systems. Villages were abandoned, and survivors pulled together or amalgamated into a smaller number of communities. Areas opened because of population loss were probably filled by new immigrants. Finally, depending on magnitude of loss and preexisting social structures, family organization may have either fractured into nuclear units or fused into extended units. As seen in these archaeological data, both changes may have been reflected in changing roofed area measurements of houses.

This summary of Middle Missouri history has clarified some ambiguities of the archaeological record and provided considerable detail to processes operative during postcontact periods. Although direct contact occurred quite late in the Middle Missouri, diffusion pathways into the region explain the difference in dates between direct contact and first contact. This difference, in part, accounted for the significance of the test case.

Middle Missouri census counts and settlement records could not specify the onset of population collapse, but they were helpful in resolving the archaeological pattern of population increase in the late eighteenth century (Period IV). Since both historical demography and settlement agreed with each other and were contrary to archaeological trends, I conclude that the archaeological record is biased. The collapse was clearly underway by 1780; processes of amalgamation, abandonment, and relocation were well established as responses to the catastrophic attrition of population.

EPIDEMIC HISTORY The primary goal of this section is to determine whether Period III, or the seventeenth century, marked the origin or the continuation of an epidemic pattern. Unfortunately, since history in the Middle Missouri began in the eighteenth century, it is of little help in resolving the temporal problem. Eyewitness accounts of epidemics are, nonetheless, important and these data are presented first (Table 44). Then, because diffusion of European products is a known occurrence in the Middle Missouri, the possibilty of an earlier disease diffusion is considered by examining epidemic histories from adjacent regions.

Between 1738 and 1845, populations of the Middle Missouri experienced only two recorded smallpox epidemics. Although the first epidemic (1780–1781) was not actually observed, its consequences were described by explorers and traders. I have traced the source of this scourge to the Valley of Mexico, where between September and December 1779, estimated deaths from smallpox ranged between 18,000 and 22,000 (Cooper 1965). The pathogen reached New Mexico pueblos in 1780 and resulted in the deaths of some 5,000 Indians (Croix 1781). From New Mexico, smallpox diffused, presumably by horse, to the Middle Missouri where an unknown number of people died (Lehmer 1977; Stearn and Stearn 1945) (Figure 15).

In 1795, Jean Baptiste Truteau, a French trader, described the consequences of this epidemic (and perhaps others) on the Arikara:

> In ancient times the Ricara nation was very large; it counted 32 populous villages, now depopulated and almost entirely destroyed by the smallpox which broke out among them at three different times. A few families only, from each of the villages, escaped; these united and formed two villages (Nasatir 1952:299).

The Mandan were quite specific in their description of the 1780 epidemic. Big White told Lewis and Clark in 1805 that at one time his nation inhabited seven villages, but the "Sieoux and smallpox killed a great part of them, and made

Table 44 Probable Epidemics in the Middle Missouri, Southwest, Southeast, and Northeast

Middle Missouri	*Southwest*	*Southeast*	*Northeast*
		1513	
	1520–1524	1519–1524	
		1528	
	1531–1533		
		1535–1538	1535
		1545–1548	
		1549	
		1550	
		1559	
		1564–1570	1568*
			1574*
		1585–1586	
		1586	1586*
			1592*
		1596	
		1613–1617	1613–1617
	1635–1638		1633–1641
			1647
		1649	1649
		1653	
			1654
		1659	
			1662
			1666
			1668–1670
	1671	1672	
		1675	
			1679
		1686	
			1690
		1698	
		1716	
		1718–1734	
1780	1780		
1837			

*Not supported archaeologically.

them so weak that all that were left only made two villages. . . ." (Thwaites 1904:5:347). In another volume, Clark commented that after seeing several abandoned villages near the Chisscheter River (Heart River), he found out that they belonged to Mandan but were abandoned because of population loss from smallpox and warfare with the Sioux (Thwaites 1904:1:261).

The 1837 epidemic was documented and known to have reached the Mandan, Hidatsa and Arikara by a steamboat traveling up the Missouri from St. Louis (Trimble 1979). Pre-1837 estimates of population for all three groups ranged up

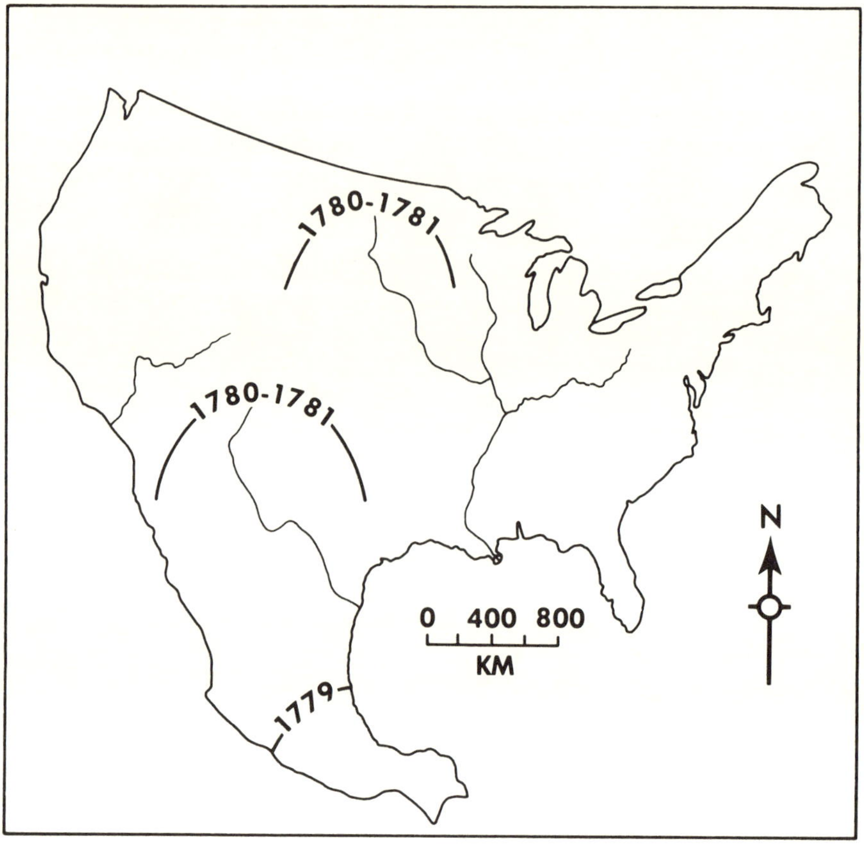

Figure 15. Diffusion of Smallpox from the Valley of Mexico into the Middle Missouri, 1779–1781

to 7,200. In 1842, the three tribes numbered no more than 1,100 (Lehmer n.d.). Despite biases common to all population estimates, the magnitude of aboriginal loss is obviously significant. Amalgamation of survivors at Like-A-Fishhook was the ultimate consequence of the epidemic.

Epidemic data from adjacent regions suggest that disease certainly could have been present prior to the eighteenth century (Table 44). Disease introduction and population collapse dated to the sixteenth century in the Southeast; despite Dobyns's claim to the contrary, archaeological evidence from the Northeast suggested that disease contact and population loss in that region was a seventeenth-century event. Only the southwestern data needs to be reviewed.

Dobyns (1981) suggested that the smallpox epidemic of Mexico between 1519 and 1524, reached southwestern populations in the sixteenth century. According-ing to Crosby (1972) and Dobyns (1981), the 1531 epidemic, which also diffused from Mexico, was measles. Both epidemics drastically reduced populations before the first Europeans entered the Southwest.

During the seventeenth century, two other epidemics were recorded in the New Mexico archives. In 1638, Fray Juan de Prado described the destruction of puebloan populations that he attributed to smallpox:

> The people that may be counted today in these settlements (Pueblos) will total 40,000 or a little less, for although, there must have been more than 60,000 baptized, today those conversions are diminished to that extent on account of the very active prevalence of smallpox (Hackett 1923–1937:3:107–108).

In 1671, following several years of reduced rainfall and crop yield, a second, and fundamentally different, disease struck New Mexico populations. In this instance, domestic livestock as well as European and aboriginal populations suffered (Hackett 1923–1937:3). Given preexisting environmental conditions, it is quite possible that the outbreak spread from domestic animals to humans.

Integrating these data with the known archaeological record from the Middle Missouri and epidemic histories of other regions leads to several important conclusions: The seventeenth century was certainly the disease century in the Middle Missouri. The archaeological record demonstrated a sizable loss during that period, and epidemic data support the trend. Between 1600 and 1700, a minimum of twenty epidemics were recorded in the Southwest, Southeast, and Northeast. Since horses were present among Plains groups by 1640, rapid mechanisms of communication were available to spread pathogens between regions.

The question of a sixteenth-century collapse is more ambiguous. Disease was certainly present in the Southeast during that century and could have diffused into the Middle Missouri through southern Plains groups, including the Pawnee. Archaeological evidence of population collapse in the Southwest has not been subjected to systematic testing, and the test case from the Northeast did not support the sixteenth-century disease hypothesis.

Although such negative evidence could lead easily to rejecting the sixteenth-century hypothesis, this is inappropriate. Despite all the problems in the known record from the Middle Missouri, there were intriguing fragments of data that suggested a fundamental change in population sometime during the late sixteenth or early seventeenth century. Further, if disease diffusion was occurring in the seventeenth and eighteenth centuries, why not in the sixteenth century as well? Until there is a more fine-grained chronology and a settlement record that is reasonably free of bias, the question of a sixteenth-century collapse must remain open.

Agreement between archaeological and historical records suggests that the seventeenth century marks the origin of the decline in the Middle Missouri. Although not as early as Dobyns would like, the conclusion still has major implications for the question of continuity held so tenaciously by the Kroeberians. Quite simply, as applied to the the Middle Missouri, Kroeber's position is untenable. Fundamental change in population and systems preceded even the earliest historical descriptions by 100 years. Such historical records must be approached from a perspective of fundamental and far-reaching change.

Conclusions

Since direct contact in the Middle Missouri occurred centuries later than in either the Northeast or the Southeast, this region was seen as particularly important for testing positions concerning the onset of disease contact and aboriginal population decline. In adjacent regions, where direct contact was early, disease contact was either a sixteenth- or seventeenth-century event. Consequently, if catastrophic loss preceded direct documentation, then a conclusion of spatial diffusion of epidemics was warranted. This conclusion, in turn, would be taken as support for Dobyns's, as opposed to Kroeber's, position. If the alternative was demonstrated, then Kroeber would be supported at the expense of Dobyns. To facilitate an accurate temporal resolution, three hypotheses were presented: the onset of catastrophic decline from disease could have occurred in the sixteenth, seventeenth, or eighteenth centuries.

The archaeological analysis of the complex and biased Middle Missouri settlement record demonstrated that H1, Lehmer's eighteenth century hypothesis, was in error. Although, Lehmer, unlike many of the North American archaeologists, integrated disease contact into his regional culture history, he tied the onset of epidemics to written records. Archaeological evidence of population demonstrated catastrophic decline at least a century earlier than written documents. Since Lehmer's temporal hypothesis was wrong, Kroeber's assumption of continuity is also wrong. The onset of demographic or cultural change did not begin with direct contact by Europeans.

The rejection of Kroeber's position tended to support Dobyns's position that epidemic diseases diffused into the Middle Missouri prior to European exploration, documentation, and settlement. The question of how early remained unresolved. The archaeological record suggested the seventeenth century, but imprecision in the temporal scale and sampling biases of archaeological record raised certain questions about the reliablity of that date. While it is clear that epidemics preceded the eighteenth century, its onset could have dated either to the sixteenth or seventeenth century. The temporal question can only be answered with better quality data.

Besides demonstrating that Dobyns's view of contact was essentially correct, the Middle Missouri records have been extremely fruitful in showing the nature and extent of archaeological biases. Since, in this region, archaeological work has been carried well into the historical period, it was possible to evaluate archaeology and history simultaneously. This evaluation clearly demonstrated the magnitude of the problem confronting archaeologists who attempt to use the archaeological record for demographic purposes. Because all archaeological estimators of population are biased, they cannot produce population estimates, especially during historic periods that reflect actual demographic trends. This problem can only be corrected by statistically based regional research designs that aim at equivalent sampling of all time periods.

COMPARISON OF TEST CASES

The purpose of the archaeological tests was to examine the Cook-Dobyns model of disease contact and aboriginal decline. Although a relatively straight-forward question, requiring only a yes or no answer, there were major problems that had to be dealt with before the question could be addressed.

Sampling biases of regional archaeological records were the most serious. Although the goal of a multi-regional approach was to compensate for this problem, grave doubts remained. It seemed more likely that the Kroeberian model would be supported and that aboriginal populations would appear to be either stable or increasing through the contact period.

This, however, was not the case. Despite the numerous biases present in regional records, there was considerable evidence of a major decline in populations present in all three regions. Unfortunately, it was not possible to translate demographic trends into rates of population loss. Biases present in the measurement of time would make such estimates meaningless. Nonetheless, the overwhelming impression from available data was that decline was rapid and catastrophic, not slow and gradual.

Besides documenting the presence or absence of catastrophic attrition in population, another important aspect of the general problem was timing of the loss. This, in turn, required reworking traditional chronological units.

Although Dobyns argued that the sixteenth century was the disease century in North America, I was not sure whether I could build such fine-grained chronologies. Further, even if I achieved precise temporal control and demonstrated catastrophic attrition of population, the question of why remained. Clearly, causes other than disease were possible. Since infectious parasites tend not to preserve in the archaeological record, I reasoned that the timing of the attrition carried implications as to cause. If the loss postdated initial European contact but predated sustained European presence at a regional scale, then infectious disease was the most likely explanation.

The results relative to time were variable. Only in the Southeast did the population collapse date to the sixteenth century. In the Northeast and the Middle Missouri, hard-won evidence from the archaeological record suggested that the collapse began in the seventeenth century. Reasons for differences will be considered in the last chapter; at this point, the major question must be whether disease was causal despite temporal variability.

In the Southeast and Middle Missouri, the role of disease was clear cut since depopulation preceded sustained European presence by more than a century. In the Southeast, my analysis provided the independent test of Dobyns's speculative epidemic history. Mutual confirmation of fundamentally different data bases synthesized by different researchers made the disease hypothesis most probable. In the Middle Missouri, where history began quite late, timing of the collapse coupled with epidemic histories from surrounding regions argued that disease was diffusing into the Middle Missouri prior to trade goods.

Only in the Northeast was the evidence ambiguous. Since decline postdated European settlement and French aggression against the Iroquois, warfare and disease must have contributed to the decline. If my chronology was correct, then disease contact preceded French aggression by several decades, significantly reducing aboriginal populations and making them more vulnerable to the European attacks.

In summary, then, these archaeological tests confirmed the essence of the Cook-Dobyns model at the expense of the Kroeberian model. Aboriginal North American populations experienced a demographic catastrophe that preceded the earliest census counts and sustained European presence by decades, and perhaps, centuries.

Since the case in favor of disease was supported, it is now appropriate to consider why native populations were at such risk from Old World pathogens and why these pathogens carried such a great diffusion potential. These problems are aired in the following chapter.

Five

The Disease Process and Patterns of Spread

When civilized nations come into contact with barbarians the struggle is short, except where a deadly climate gives its aid to the native race. New diseases and vices have in some cases proved destructive; and it appears that a new disease often causes much death until those who are most susceptible to its destructive influence are gradually weeded out (Darwin 1936 [1871]:543).

INTRODUCTION

Several approaches to the study of disease introduction to this or any other continent are possible. The most popular is ideographic, guided by the Principle of Uniformity (Gould 1977; Hooykas 1963). Here, the goal is to reconstruct a particular disease episode from historical records and to evaluate the effect of that episode on a particular culture (for example, Cook 1973a; Dobyns 1963b, 1981, 1983; Ewers 1973; Trimble 1979; Wood 1975). To accomplish this goal, scholars must be well grounded in the epidemiology of modern infectious diseases so that the modern syndrome can, in turn, be employed as an analogue for past historical descriptions.

Although these studies are important contributions to historical epidemiology, I shall use another approach in my discussion of disease. I do not want to duplicate the efforts of others who have dealt with this general topic in considerable detail (for example, Ackernecht 1965; Ashburn 1947; Cockburn 1963; Crosby 1972; Dubos and Dubos 1952; Duffy 1953; McNeill 1976; Stearn and Stearn 1945). In addition, the uniformitarian approach is subject to two logical difficulties.

First, employing modern diseases as analogues for past diseases violates evolutionary principles. As seen in the recent history of influenza (Jordan 1927;

Stuart-Harris 1981) or in the older history of syphilis (Crosby 1972; El-Najjar 1979; Youmans et al. 1980:495–499), microbes have changed through time. Consequently, there is no reason to presume that modern descriptions of smallpox or syphilis are applicable to sixteenth-century descriptions of "pox" or the "French Disease." Related to this first point is that historical descriptions of disease are questionable sources when trying to identify a particular disease. European medical knowledge was not well developed in the early centuries of European contact (Ashburn 1947; Creighton 1894), and colonists were naive regarding their microbial imports (Dubos 1971; Hariot 1973 [1589]). In fact, the earliest attempt to curtail the spread of European parasites to the Western Hemisphere occurred in the late eighteenth century with Captain Cook's voyage (1776–1780) to the Sandwich Islands. For that trip, all personnel were required to have been vaccinated against, or previously exposed to, smallpox (Beaglehole 1967).

In this discussion I shall employ an actualistic approach (Hooykas 1970). Because natural laws and processes are constant through time, current knowledge of both the infectious disease process and properties of spatial diffusion can inform on the nature of the epidemic environment in North America during the early centuries of European contact.

INTERACTIONS BETWEEN HOSTS AND PARASITES

Interactions between a microbe and host are a special case of interactions that characterize a predator and its prey (Burnet and White 1972; Fenner et al. 1974; Steele 1979). The microbe tries to invade the host and the host tries to repel the microbe. If the microbe invades and successfully reproduces in host tissues, the microbe becomes a *parasite*; and the host's condition is termed *infection*. The term parasite, rather than pathogen, is deliberately chosen. All microbes that are human parasites are capable of producing illness and disease (Youmans et al. 1980). Whether they do depends on a number of factors discussed below. When symptoms of illness develop in the host, the infection is termed *disease*. If not associated with illness, the infection is *latent*, and the host is termed a *carrier* (Christie 1974; Wehrle and Haddad 1976). Following infection, the host recovers, dies, or remains a carrier.

When a host successfully repulses a microbe, the microbe must find other hosts or die, and the host is *immune*. Immunology is a complex and extensive topic that begins with external defense mechanisms of the host: Skin, cilia, tears, mucous membranes, pH of the stomach and gastrourinary tract all act to repel potential parasites (Youmans et al. 1980). If, despite defenses, invasion occurs, immunoglobins and immunogens, collectively termed antibodies, continue the warfare biochemically. In general, antibody systems of the host may be either active or passive (Fenner et al. 1974; Wehrle and Haddad 1976).

Active immunity develops from exposure to foreign antigens; passive immunity occurs through maternal-foetal, or maternal-neonatal transfers of antibodies (Burnet and White 1972; Wehrle and Haddad 1976).

Environment is a third major variable that mediates interactions between hosts and parasites. Environment is defined as anything external to a single host and its parasites, including other potential hosts and parasites. Given the range of possible environmental factors, host-parasite interactions can be extensively modified.

Two basic offensive-defensive strategies define interactions between potential hosts and parasites. *Acute* diseases are characterized by abrupt onsets, relatively short durations, and nonrecurrence. Parasites surviving by this strategy depend on continual pools of susceptible individuals because host immunity guarantees nonrecurrence. As a result, acute diseases are frequently termed crowd infections. By contrast, *chronic* infections tend to be long-lived or to recur regularly. Parasitism has little or no effect on immunity, and parasitic survival is not contingent on the number of susceptibles (Cockburn 1963, 1971; Fenner 1971; Fenner et al. 1974).

At the scale of population or species, host-parasite interactions become more complex. In the simplest of host-parasite systems, parasites are specific in their cellular requirements and colonize only a single host species. The host species then can be considered the appropriate environment for reproduction and survival of the parasite. Over time, three evolutionary alternatives may develop: (1) Parasites may be so successful reproductively that both host and parasite species become extinct. (2) Host defenses may neutralize invasive properties of the parasite; in which case, hosts survive, but parasites face extinction. (3) Parasites and hosts develop a commensal relationship that can take one of several forms, depending on antibody systems of the host population and virulence and pathogenicity of the parasitic species.

The final terms requiring definition are *endemic* and *epidemic*. Both describe temporal and spatial aspects of the disease experience in a host species that are determined by a number of factors: adaptive strategy of the parasite including latency and incubation periods, and reproductive requirements, and size and density of the host species.

Endemicity defines a condition in which a host population indefinitely maintains a parasitic species. Because of repeated exposure, immunity is maintained at the level of population. Although individual hosts may experience an infectious episode from the parasite, these are isolated events. The population or species is not at risk for the parasite.

Epidemicity, by contrast, defines a concentration of disease in time and space (Burnet and White 1972). Such events occur because the host population lacks immunity; this condition is, in turn, explained by mutation of the parasite, parasitic invasion of new host species or virgin populations of existing host species, and loss of immune status in the hosts because of demographic factors or mutation of the parasite. Although initial invasions produce the highest levels of morbidity and mortality, reintroduction in previously exposed populations causes some degree of morbidity and mortality.

Finally, although I have drawn dichotomies between concepts of acute-chronic, and endemic-epidemic, there is considerable variability in the application of terms to disease outbreaks. Acute, as well as chronic, diseases can be either endemic or epidemic. Leprosy is a chronic disease for individuals, but occasionally irrupts in a population as an epidemic (Stanhope et al. 1968). Although the course of this illness is longer and slower than that of measles, for instance, it is, nonetheless, an epidemic. Further, some bacteria, such as *Staphylococci*, or *Streptococci* are indigenous to all human populations but cause epidemics when they successfully invade new tissue. *Streptococcus pneumoniae* is part of the normal flora of the human upper respiratory tract. It creates epidemics only when it becomes lodged in human lung tissue.

CLASSIFICATION OF ACUTE AND EPIDEMIC DISEASES

Table 45 presents fourteen diseases that affected Native Americans during the early centuries of European contact. Before discussing either the classification itself or classes of acute infections, biases in the construction of the classification need to be considered.

I restricted the field of the classification to infectious diseases that are acute and can periodically irrupt as epidemics. Although Old World and New World populations certainly differed with respect to chronic or endemic ailments,

Table 45 Classification of Some Acute Infectious Diseases

Mode of Transmission	*Disease Agents*		
	Viral	*Bacterial*	*Protozoal*
Direct Transmission	Class I:	Class II:	
	Chickenpox		
	Influenza	Pneumonia	
	Measles	Scarlet Fever	
	Mumps	Pertussis	
	Rubella		
	Smallpox		
Indirect Transmission	Class III:	Class IV:	Class V:
	Yellow Fever	Anthrax	Malaria
		Bubonic Plague	
		Epidemic Typhus	

identifying the nature of these differences is difficult. Chronic or endemic diseases are frequently masked by the more dramatic epidemic diseases and are rarely the cause of large-scale population mortality. In the United States, for instance, public health officials turned their attention to chronic disabilities including hypertension, coronary heart disease, and arthritis only after the epidemic killers such as plague, smallpox, and yellow fever were controlled. Undoubtedly, chronic infections were introduced to the Americas, but to include these in the classification would not materially alter the description.

Time was another criterion for inclusion or exclusion of specific infections. Because my archaeological tests demonstrated unquestionable catastrophic decline by the seventeenth century, I restricted parasites to those introduced no later than A.D. 1700. Although new diseases such as cholera (Benenson 1976a) and diptheria (Creighton 1894) spread to the New World in later centuries, such additions did not drastically alter earlier patterns.

Finally, diseases must have been either known autochthons of the Old World, or arguments must weigh heavily in favor of such an origin. This requirement had two effects on the discussion: Since I considered only those acute and epidemic infections for which Native Americans lacked immunity, arguments in favor of catastrophic decline were strengthened. In addition, I could eliminate the large, and frequently contentious, literature involving origins. Since my goal was to build a description of the early epidemic environment in North America, these discussions have little relevance.

The most obvious diseases excluded by the criterion of known origin were epidemic, or venereal, syphilis and tuberculosis. Although both diseases have caused high levels of mortality among native populations since European contact (Bushnell 1922; Ferguson 1955; Indian Health Service 1978, 1979a, 1979b), postcontact patterns of illness are inadequate tests for resolving the controversy about origins. Current status of both infections will be briefly reviewed, but for more extensive treatments, I recommend Buikstra 1981; Buikstra and Cook 1981; Bushnell 1922; Cockburn 1963; Crosby 1972; Dubos and Dubos 1952; El-Najjar 1979; Hackett 1963; Hudson 1968; Ortner and Putschar 1981; Powell 1985; Steinbock 1976; Stewart and Spoehr 1952; Wood 1979.

Epidemic Syphilis

As Crosby (1972:123) has stated, "the origin of syphilis is the most controversial subject in all medical historiography." Several factors, including the bias of historical documents, epidemiological patterns, and taxonomic status of the treponemes are causative in this controversy. First, historical records of Europe describe a new and highly virulent disease in the early decades following the voyages of Columbus. The disease raged across Europe for nearly a century, after which it became less prominent and an equilibrium was established between causative agent and host populations (Crosby 1972). The absence of comparable descriptions for the Americas, however, does not mean that the disease originated on this continent. As I have repeatedly stressed, sixteenth century descriptions of Native North American illness are the exception not the rule. Once such descriptions become part of European consciousness, infections similar to venereal syphilis are recorded (Swanton 1969). Thus, the bias of history precludes resolving the question of origins.

Of equal importance in the origin problem is taxonomic confusion. Venereal syphilis is one expression of four diseases, pinta, yaws and nonvenereal syphillis, collectively referred to as the Treponematoses or Treponematosis. *Treponema pallidum*, a bacterium, is the causative organism in venereal syphilis, and the question is whether this form is a distinct species from the other treponemal infections or a strain of one species. Although arguments have gone both ways, the currently accepted approach is unitarian (Crosby 1972). Essentially, what is suggested is that one species, separated into four strains, is responsible for all treponemal infections. Differences in expression are explained by environmental factors, climate, geography, and demography. The incidence of nonveneral syphilis, for instance, is highest in rural populations in temperate and subtropical nonhumid climates. Only epidemic syphilis is free of climate, but it is largely restricted to urban populations.

Although the unitarian approach does not resolve all the problems with epidemic syphilis, it is certainly the most inclusive hypothesis. First, it accounts for the presence of treponemal infections found in both Europe and America prior to European contact. Precolumbian identifications in the New World are drawn from osteological samples (D. Cook 1976; El-Najjar 1979; Powell 1985; Robbins 1978; Williams 1932, 1935, 1936). Old World identifications are largely based on historical documents (Hudson 1968).

Further, the evolution of a new disease that devastated populations in both hemispheres can be explained as a product of genetic mixing or mutation between previously isolated strains. The new strain found environments conducive for reproduction and survival; venereal contact became the mode of transmission. Although initial cycles of infection and death were high, they leveled out with time.

Tuberculosis

Unlike epidemic syphilis, tuberculosis had been part of the disease load of Europeans long before the fifteenth century. Unmistakable evidence derived from Egyptian mummies and early medical writings indicate the presence of the parasite *Mycobacterium tuberculae* in Europe and western Asia no later than 2000 B.C. (Chapman and Eickenhoff 1976; Cockburn 1980; Ortner and Putschar 1981). The question is whether this same genus of bacteria was also present in the New World, causing the same type of illness. Because tubercular-like infections have been found in skeletons (Buikstra 1976, 1981; D. Cook 1976, 1983; Powell 1985) and soft tissue (Allison et al. 1973; Allison et al. 1981) of pre-Columbian native populations, the tentative answer to the question is yes. A yes, however, requires suggestions of why and how the same genus was present in two continents. Two hypotheses have been suggested; both are subject to difficulties.

Currently, Buikstra (1976, 1981) and Cook (1976; 1983) (Buikstra and Cook 1980, 1981) are the major proponents of the position who argue for an autochthonous evolution of tubercular-causing Mycobacterium in North America during the late prehistoric or Mississippi period. Because tuberculosis is density-dependent and because Mississippian populations were large and nucleated, the association is possible. The argument for an independent evolution of tuberculosis during the Mississippi period is strengthened by positive and negative evidence: presence of skeletal, and especially spinal, resorptive lesions of osteological series from the Mississippi period in central Illinois and absence of similar lesions from earlier temporal periods with smaller population sizes and different settlement patterns.

Unfortunately, the argument in favor of an independent evolution of Mycobacterium in the Americas cannot be supported logically. By employing density as causative in the appearance of tuberculosis in pre-Columbian America, Buikstra and Cook seem to be using an argument of convergence: similar environments produce similar adaptive responses. Although convergence is common in nature (Mooney 1977; Orians and Solbrig 1977), it is a morphological response to selection by phylogenetically unrelated organisms. By suggesting that the same genus causes tuberculosis in both continents, Buikstra and Cook are violating a key principle of convergence.

Buikstra seems to be aware of the problem with convergence because she attempts to find a natural, nonhuman reservoir for Mycobacteria in the Americas. Domestic cattle may have been the natural reservoir for tuberculosis in Europe (Cockburn 1963; Pagels et al. 1953). Absence of these herds in precontact America leads Buikstra to suggest that "animals such as llamas, turkeys, dogs, or perhaps bison could have served as the New World reservoir" (1981:13).

The problem here is finding an American analogue that could have been a carrier of a Mycobacteria and could have caused tuberculosis in humans. My research into this topic has been largely negative. There is an avian form of tuberculosis (Chapman and Eikenhoff 1976; Feldman 1963; Sinnecker et al. 1982), but human groups appear to be unaffected by this bacterium. Dogs are highly susceptible to both human and bovine tuberculosis (Feldman 1963) but do not support their own Mycobacterium. Mycobacterium have not been recorded for other animal groups suggested by Buikstra.

To recapitulate, if different genera or perhaps families of microbes caused tuberculosis in both continents, then arguments of convergence can be logically invoked. If the same genus is responsible, then convergence is not possible; and one or more analogous species for the purported reservoir in Europe must be found. Either way, the hypothesis of independence, suggested by Buikstra and Cook, cannot be accepted in its present form.

The alternative to an independent evolution is diffusion from the Old World, and this is essentially what El-Najjar (1979) suggests. The hypothesis is drawn from earlier researchers (Cockburn 1963; Steinbock 1976; Stewart 1960) who argued that *Mycobacteria tuberculae* was part of the disease load of the original Asian migration to the Americas. While arctic and subarctic climates acted as a cold screen (Stewart 1960) against the survival of such tropical parasites as malaria, tuberculosis could have survived these climatic rigors.

In support of this position, El-Najjar (1979) uses certain features of the tuberculosis syndrome. First, tuberculosis is a long-lived, frequently chronic, infection. While it may require crowd conditions to evolve, it can persist in small isolated populations (Black 1975). Since initial founding populations in the Americas were quite small, the analysis does not violate current ideas about either the disease or initial population sizes. Furthermore, since tuberculosis is initially pulmonary, the protected environment of the lungs could have contributed to the survival of the parasite.

This hypothesis is not subject to the logical difficulties of the hypothesis of independent evolution. The only question is whether ancestral forms of tuberculosis were present in Asia at a time commensurate with initial migration into the Americas. Although such a question could be tested, I am not sure what these analyses would show.

Again, the problem is uniformity and analogues. In the hypothesis of an independent evolution, an assumption of comparable disease systems across 500 years is possible because tubercular-like ailments have a temporal depth of at least 2000 years in the Old World. Continuity across 10,000 years is much harder to accept. Importantly, El-Najjar does not make such an assumption. In fact, he is explicit about the continuing adaptations of parasites to changing environmental conditions. Consequently, even if tuberculosis were present in Asiatic populations 12,000 years ago, I am not sure that the evidence, if present, could be recognized.

In summary then, this classification of acute and epidemic diseases was restricted to known, Old World autochthons that spread to the New World between the fifteenth and seventeenth centuries. Because there is such contention regarding the origins of epidemic syphilis and tuberculosis, they were excluded from this consideration of disease. In both cases, reasons for the contentions are logical: evidence from skeletal or soft tissue evidence suggests that infections comparable to the European diseases were present in the Americas prior to Columbus. Problems arise in explaining the presence of these diseases in the Americas. Before employing epidemic syphilis and tuberculosis as causes of postcontact decline, issues of whether the American forms of the diseases represent independent evolutions by convergence or persistence of Old World forms in new environmental settings must be resolved.

Dimensions of the Classification

Causative agents and methods of transmission are the dimensions of this paradigmatic classification of acute diseases (Dunnell 1971). Causative agents are restricted to unicellular or subcellular parasites, viruses, bacteria, and protozoa. Parasites differ with respect to physical and chemical properties. Type and arrangement of genetic material defines viruses. Bacteria, more variable than viruses, share one feature in common: prokaryotic cell structure. Protozoa are nonphotosynthesizing eukaryotes.

Although transmission ultimately depends on contact between agents and susceptible individuals, the number of links in the contact chain between parasites and human populations determines whether the pathway is direct or indirect (Figure 16). Direct transmission is an uncomplicated process. *Homo sapiens* is the only reservoir for the parasite; and consequently, contact between infectious and susceptible individuals is the only factor determining the spread of disease (Figure 16A).

In this classification, indirect transmissions are zoonoses because parasites are transmitted to human hosts through nonhuman species. Typically, the parasite colonizes *Homo sapiens* through an intermediate host(s); and without that host(s), human parasitization does not occur. As a consequence, the

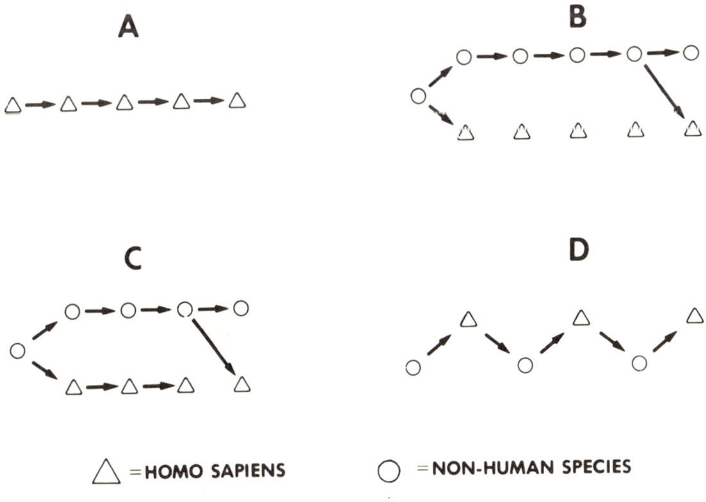

Figure 16. Transmission of Disease Agents

location of potential human host(s) in relation to nonhuman reservoirs and vectors conditions the probability of human infection.

Indirect transmission pathways have three basic structures: (1) the initial reservoir may be the only source of the parasite for *Homo sapiens*. Although *Homo sapiens* can be infected, they are passive recipients of the infection (Figure 16B). (2) Once a person has become infected, he can transmit the pathogen to other susceptible humans (Figure 16C). (3) Transmission alternates between human and nonhuman species, both of which are necessary environments in the life cycles of the parasite. Infection or disease from one individual reaches another individual through the intermediate species (Figure 16D).

CLASS I: DIRECTLY TRANSMITTED VIRUSES Pertinent infectious characteristics of Class I are summarized in Table 46. All agents are highly contagious and are spread while talking, coughing, or sneezing by means of droplets of moisture or mucus. The human respiratory tract is the site of entry of Class I agents, and infections uniformly result in symptoms of illness including coughs, fevers, rashes, and pustules. Virulence and pathogenecity are variable as is the period of communicability. Cold viruses are communicable for no longer than 24 hours; measles and smallpox can be transmitted for as long as two weeks (Dixon 1962; Fenner and White 1976; Gwaltney and Hendley 1976). Consequently, measles and smallpox have a higher probability of reaching more susceptible individuals.

Expected mortality covers the full range of probabilities. In this, as in other tables to be presented, values on expected morbidity and mortality are drawn from western European populations where these infections are endemic and where at least, some of the population is immune. Among nonimmune populations morbidity and mortality estimates would be considerably higher.

Among western Europeans, cold and chickenpox have 0% expected mortality; measles carries up to 25% mortality; smallpox can produce 100% mortality. Further, although initial invasions may not carry a high expected mortality, insults sustained from that infection may allow invasions from other parasites or secondary complications from the initial causative agent (Table 47). Secondary invaders are also autochthons of the Old World. Under appropriate circumstances, secondary infections cause mortality. Complications arising from maternal rubella contracted during the first trimester of pregnancy can be particularly destructive for the fetus, causing such congenital neonatal malformations as cataracts, blindness, microcephaly, and mental retardation (Korones et al. 1965; Swan et al. 1943).

Among Class I agents, *Variola major* holds a unique position. Although the virus is most frequently transmitted through droplet infection, it can survive for a number of years outside human hosts in a dried state (Downie 1967; Upham 1986). As a consequence, *Variola major* can be transmitted through contami-

Table 46 Directly Transmitted Acute Viral Infections

Disease	*Agent*	*Host*	*Means of Transmission*	*Period of Communicability*	*Expected Morbidity*	*Expected Mortality*	*Immunity*
Chickenpox	*Varicella zoster*	*Homo sapiens*	Inhalation	1 or 2 days before rash; 5 days after rash	100%	0	Permanent
Cold	*Rhinovirus*	*Homo sapiens*	Inhalation	Brief; 24 hours	Variable with viral type	0	Varies
Influenza	*Myoxovirus A* and *B*	*Homo sapiens*	Inhalation	1–3 days up to 50%	Variable; but type specific	0	Long term
Measles	*Paramyxovirus*	*Homo sapiens*	Inhalation	7–14 days	100%	10–25%	Permanent
Mumps	*Paramyxovirus*	*Homo sapiens*	Inhalation	More than 7 days	Variable	0	Permanent
German Measles	*Rubella*	*Homo sapiens*	Inhalation	More than 7 days	Variable	Less than 5%	Permanent
Smallpox	*Variola major*	*Homo sapiens*	Inhalation; contamination	9–14 days; several years in dried state	100%	10–100%	Permanent
Smallpox	*Variola minor*	*Homo sapiens*	Inhalation	3–7 days	Variable	1%	Permanent

Sources: American Academy of Pediatrics 1977; Brunell 1976; Dixon 1962; Fenner and White 1976; Gwaltney and Hendley 1976.

Table 47 Secondary Infections following Acute Viral Infections

Primary Disease	*Secondary Disease*	*Expected Agent*	*Mortality*
Chickenpox[a]	Infectious Encephalitis	*Varicella zoster*	?
	Pneumonia	*Streptococcus pneumoniae influenzae* *S. Pyogenes* *Staphylococcus aureus*	?
Influenza[b]	Pneumonia	Same as above	Variable; can be quite high
	Encephalitis	*Myoxovirus*	?
Measles[c]	Encephalitis	*Paramyxovirus*	?
	Pneumonia	Same as above	15%

[a]Brown and Leedom 1976; Brunell 1976; Chin 1976.
[b]Chin 1976; Jordon 1927; Mogabgab 1976.
[c]Brown and Leedom 1976; Chin 1976; Kaschula et al. 1978.

nated articles such as clothing or blankets (Dixon 1962). In the nineteenth century, the U.S. Army sent contaminated blankets to Native Americans, especially Plains groups, to control the Indian problem (Stearn and Stearn 1945).

With two exceptions, recovery from Class I diseases provides the host with parasite-specific immunity. (1) After a brief episode of illness, *Varicella zoster* may take a latent course and appear, after an unspecified period of time, as *Herpes zoster*. Immunity to Varicella is, however, complete (Brunell 1976). Second, Influenza and cold immunities are specific to antigenic type. At least 100 different rhinoviruses result in the common cold. Serum from a recovered individual with Rhinovirus 1 will neutralize subsequent invasions from that virus, but not from viruses 2 through 100 (Burnet and White 1972). Similarly, major epidemics of human influenza are due to mutational changes of extant *Myoxovirus A*. A2 was responsible for the Asian influenza epidemic of 1957; a variant of A2 caused the 1968 pandemic of Hong Kong Influenza (Burnet and White 1972; Schulman 1978; Stuart-Harris 1981).

Immunological patterns coupled with the fact that humans appear to be the only reproductive environment for Class I agents determines whether viruses are endemic or epidemic to particular populations. Although all human groups can be infected by Class I agents, Class I agents, with the exception of smallpox, can persist indefinitely only in large populations. In areas of high population density, children provide the continual pool of individuals necessary for perpetuation of these viruses, and this pattern leads to the colloquial designation of Class I infections as childhood diseases. In small populations the size of the pool defines the life span of the virus. Although the population can be reinfected, the source of that infection is always external. Reintroduction creates a fundamentally different infectious pattern in such populations. All ages not previously exposed are susceptible, and the course of the illness or epidemic is associated with higher morbidity and mortality rates.

A recent dramatic example of this phenomenon is drawn from the literature on nonhuman disease. When mxyomatosis, an endemic disease of Brazilian rabbits (*Sylvilagus brasiliensis*), was first introduced into Australia to control feral populations of rabbits (*Oryctolagus cuniculus*), mortality was in excess of 99%. Seven years later, mortality of rabbit populations had dropped to 25% (Fenner et al. 1974; Fenner and Ratcliffe 1965).

Bartlett (1956, 1957, 1960, 1972) has considered mathematically the relationship between population size and endemicity of the measles virus. After examining measles notifications from cities in England, Wales, and the United States, Bartlett defined a measles epidemic as 1 case per 4000 population. He then estimated the minimum number of susceptible individuals and total population size necessary to prevent fade-outs in the transmission of measles. Comparison of theoretically based curves with direct observations led Bartlett to conclude that a susceptible population of 7000 and total a population of 200,000 to 300,000 constituted the minimum number required for the persistence of measles.

Black (1966) considered measles persistence in isolated or closed communities and suggested a corollary to Bartlett's formulations. After examining measles notifications from 19 island communities for a 15–year period (Table 48), he concluded that fade-outs in transmission could be expected in populations of less than 500,000.

Differences between figures presented by Black and Bartlett were a result of the ways in which human populations distribute themselves spatially. Where people were concentrated, as in urban centers, contact was more regular; and populations of 300,000 could support measles endemically. Where populations of 300,000 were dispersed, contact was less regular, and measles fade-outs occurred. Consequently, the degree of nucleation or total population size constituted the ecological parameters for persistence of measles and, by extension, other directly transmitted acutely infectious viruses.

CLASS II: DIRECTLY TRANSMITTED BACTERIAL INFECTIONS Table 49 summarizes characteristics of Class II infections. Class II agents share several features with Class I. Class II agents tend to locate in the human respiratory tract and to be almost entirely transmitted by droplet infection. Consequently, in large populations, these parasites persist on an endemic basis. In contrast to Class I, Class II agents can be both latent and chronic and are not associated with secondary invasions. Under a variable set of environmental conditions, Class II infections can be highly communicable.

In previously exposed populations, infants of less than one year constitute the

Table 48 Endemicity of Measles among Island Communities[a]

Island	*Population (Thousands)*	*Annual Population Input*[b]	*Number of Months with Measles*
Hawaii	550.0	16,700	100
Fiji	346.0	1,340	64
Iceland	169.0	4,490	61
Samoa	118.0	4,440	28
Soloman	110.0	4,060	32
Fr. Polynesia	75.0	2,690	8
New Caledonia	68.0	2,600	32
Guam	63.0	2,200	80
Tonga	57.0	2,040	12
New Hebrides	52.0	1,910	30
Greenland	28.0	1,190	24
Bermuda	41.0	1,130	51
Faroe	34.0	774	32
Cook	16.0	678	6
Nieu	4.7	225	5
Naura	3.5	167	5
St. Helena	5.0	116	4
Falklands	2.5	43	0

[a]Black 1966.
[b]1956 births less infant mortality.

appropriate environment for *Bordetella pertussis*; and in spite of vaccination, infant pertussis deaths still pose a serious threat in the United States (Brooks and Buchanan 1970; Wilkens and Bass 1976) and elsewhere (Cooper and Fitch 1983). Between 1960 and 1967, infant mortality from pertussis in the United States accounted for 72% (545/626) of all pertussis mortality. For that same period, death rates from pertussis for individuals over five years were less than 3% (Brooks and Buchanan 1970).

Communicability of the bacterial pneumonias depends on a series of environmental variables including previous exposure, health, sanitation, and socioeconomic conditions of the population. As already shown (Table 47), pneumonia is frequently a secondary infection following viral infections which have already impaired an individual's health. Other predisposing factors for pneumonia include chronic lung disease, age, and alcoholism (Brown and Leedom 1976). This tendency toward secondary infection is explained by the fact that pneumococci have low invasive properties and survive only in the human upper respiratory tract. Once microciliary systems and alveolar macrophage clearing

Table 49 Directly Transmitted Acute Bacterial Infections

Disease	*Agent*	*Host*	*Means of Transmission*	*Period of Communicability*	*Expected Morbidity*	*Expected Mortality*	*Immunity*
Whooping Cough (Pertussis)	*Bordetella pertussis*	*Homo sapiens*	Inhalation	4 weeks	100%	Variable; Extremely high for infants	Permanent
Pneumonia	*Streptococcus pneumoniae* *Haemophilis influenzae* *Klebisella pneumoniae* *Staphylococcus aureus* *Pseudomonas aeruginosa*	*Homo sapiens*	Inhalation	Variable	Variable; Dramatic increase during Influenza epidemics	20–25%	Not permanent
Scarlet Fever	*Streptococcus pyogenes*	*Homo sapiens*	Inhalation	Up to 2 weeks long	Variable	0	Permanent to Strain

Sources: American Academy of Pediatrics 1977; Brooks and Buchanan 1970.

actions have been curtailed by viral pathogenicity, pneumococci can reach the lower respiratory tract and produce infection.

Although expected morbidity from scarlet fever tends to be high, it can occur as a latent infection. All periods of communicability tend to be longer than for Class I agents, and mortality is variable. Under most circumstances, scarlet fever is not fatal (Wannamaker et al. 1976). While mortality from pertussis decreases dramatically with age, mortality from pneumonia dramatically increases. In addition, mortality from pneumonia varies with respect to the specific agent, and whether the infection is primary or secondary. When pneumococcal pneumonias occur as primary infections, expected mortality varies from 20 to 25%. When associated with A2 influenza epidemics, the primary causative agent becomes *Staphylococcus aureus*; and expected mortality may increase to more than 50% (Brown and Leedom 1976; Mogabgab 1976). During the 1918 influenza pandemic, 92% of the more than 2 million deaths were due to pneumonia (Jordan 1927; Mogabgab 1976; Schulman 1978).

With two exceptions, recovery from bacterial infections confers permanent immunity. (1) Immunity to pneumonia is specific to causative agent. (2) Because there are some 60 immunologically distinct types of *Streptococcus pyogenes*, immunity is variable. Recovery from scarlet fever confers immunity to a second attack associated with a rash but does not confer immunity to other serologic strains causing sore throats and tonsillitis (Wannamaker et al. 1976).

CLASS III: INDIRECTLY TRANSMITTED VIRAL INFECTIONS Yellow fever is an acute viral disease of primates (Taylor 1951). Although the virus is transmitted from one population of primates to another by one of several mosquito species (Figure 16D), the process of transmission and infection are complex. The virus has no extrahost existence and, consequently, depends on vectors and hosts for survival (Taylor 1951). Because the virus persists in the mosquito for the duration of the latter's life without the vector experiencing illness (Taylor 1951; Whitman 1951), mosquito species are strictly mechanical vectors. When a mosquito inadvertently spreads the virus through biting a primate, the primate becomes the host and illness may ensure. Because reproduction is confined to the host, rapid transmission between infected and susceptible primates ensures the persistence of the virus (Ward 1972; Whitman 1951).

Currently, yellow fever is confined to the African and American tropics (Taylor 1951). Although two classes of the disease (Table 50) are recognized, that is, urban, and forest or sylvan, distinctions are arbitrary. Unlike directly transmitted diseases, differences in the infectious process do not depend on differences among various strains of the virus. In fact, the causative agent is remarkably similar in all human and nonhuman primate infections (Fenner et al. 1974). Differences reflect environmental and dietary preferences of the numerous vectors. *Aedes aegypti* is a domestic species that prefers breeding in

Table 50 Yellow Fever in Africa and Tropical America

Expected Disease	*Agent*	*Vector*	*Host*	*Morbidity*	*Mortality*	*Immunity*
Urban (America)	*Arbovirus*	*Aedes aegypti*	*Homo sapiens*	Variable	0–10%	Permanent
Urban (W. Africa)	*Arbovirus*	*Aedes aegypti*	*Homo sapiens*		(Same as above)	
Urban (Egypt, Sudan)	*Arbovirus*	*Aedes taylori* *Aedes furcifer* *A. vittatus* *A. metallis* *A. aegypti*	*Homo sapiens*		(Same as above)	
Urban (Uganda)	*Arbovirus*	*A. simpsoni*	*Homo sapiens*		(Same as above)	
Forest (South America)	*Arbovirus*	*Haemagogus spegazzini falco* *H. capricornii* *H. splendens*	*Cebidae* *Homo sapiens*		(Same as above)	
Forest (Africa)	*Arbovirus*	*Aedes africani*	*Lemuridae* *Ceropithecidae* *Homo sapiens*		(Same as above)	

Sources: Carter 1931; Strode 1951; Ward 1972.

artificial clay bottom containers and is the primary source of the infection in urban contexts (Carter 1931). Species of *Haemagogus* and species of *Aedes*, other than *A. aegypti*, breed in the holes of trees in climax rain forests (Taylor 1951). The disease is consequently termed forest or sylvan.

Epidemiologists recognize two distinct yellow fever transmission cycles depending on whether *Homo sapiens* is the primary host species.

In the urban cycle (*A. aegypti—H. sapiens—A. aegypti*), humans are the primary host because adult *Aedes* prefer human blood. In the forest or sylvan cycle, nonhuman primates constitute the primary host species. Even in this context, *Homo sapiens* can become infected through accidents of proximity.

In essence, then, yellow fever is a single disease that varies according to distributions of vector and host. An urban focus can become a sylvan focus if an infected individual is the prey of a forest mosquito. The reverse is also true, and the disease can just as easily be transferred from sylvan to urban contexts.

The fluidity of the transmission cycle is well demonstrated by a recent epidemic of yellow fever in Gambia (Monath et al. 1980). The focus of the epidemic was nine rural villages with a combined population of 1531. Where domestic Aedes (*A. aegypti*) was absent, the infection was spread by *A. furcifer* and *A. taylori*, which in the area are sylvactic. During the dry season, the disease was spread by the domestic Aedes where this species was abundant.

Fluidity of transmission and nonurban foci of infections in both Africa and South America have caused the controversy regarding the origin of yellow fever. (For a complete review of the yellow fever controversy see Carter 1931; Findlay 1940, 1941; Goodyear 1978; Jarcho 1964. For the early history of New World epidemics, see Carter 1931; Creighton 1894; Duffy 1953.) Facts that support the argument in favor of tropical America as the place of origin of yellow fever are (1) the earliest recorded epidemic in the New World (1643) predated the earliest recorded African epidemic by 135 years; (2) the disease was not present in Europe prior to the discovery of the New World.

Arguments in support of an African origin are more convincing. They include the following:

1) *Aedes aegypti* is indigenous of Africa, and was transported to the New World on slave ships. (2) More species of mosquitos are vectors of the disease in Africa. (3) Although both African and American primates are equally susceptible to infection, there is greater tolerance to the virus among African monkeys and perhaps native West Africans than among South American monkeys and Native Americans (Scott 1965; Taylor 1951; Whitman 1951). Even if yellow fever was indigenous to South America, absence of a precontact domestic vector and limited flight territories of all mosquitos would have confined the disease to tropical environments.

When populations lack familiarity with the parasite, or where temperature extremes do not facilitate breeding and survival of appropriate mosquito populations, yellow fever follows an epidemic and acute course. Functional temperature limits for *Aedes aegypti* are between 15.6° and 38.9° C (Carter 1931; Whitman 1951). Outside these ranges, vector and parasite must be reintroduced, and reintroductions lead to new cycles of illness.

Under conditions of nonimmunity, morbidity from yellow fever is high if human populations come into contact with mosquito vectors. The disease is short-lived, and symptoms of illness may be mild to fulminating. Degenerative lesions develop in liver, kidney and stomach. Jaundice can be expected along with stomach hemorrhages and persistent vomiting. Mortality varies from 0 to 10% and typically occurs within three or four days of infection. Recovery from the disease confers permanent immunity (Bugher 1951; Carter 1931; Goodyear 1978; Ward 1972).

The postcontact distribution of yellow fever in North America is intelligible in light of the temperature requirements of *Aedes* and patterns of infections. Yellow fever was a disease of ports, extending from Boston to Buenos Aires on the east coast and as far south as Peru on the west coast. Ships carrying infected individuals or vectors continually reintroduced the illness to colonists and Native Americans. From ports of entry, the disease developed endemic foci in areas commensurate with vector and parasite.

CLASS IV: INDIRECTLY TRANSMITTED BACTERIAL INFECTIONS Table 51 summarizes pertinent characteristics of Class IV diseases. Although human populations acquire these diseases accidentally, once a focus has become established, epidemics can result. Human hosts are infected by contact with nonhuman reservoirs or vectors where the agent has previously been a source of infection of varying severity (Figure 16B).

Anthrax is primarily a disease of domestic ungulates in whom the infection may take a chronic, subacute, or acute course. Of all ungulates, cattle appear to be the most susceptible. Human hosts receive the bacillus in one of three ways: (1) contact with infected animals; (2) inhaling viable spores which have become airborne; or (3) ingesting contaminated meat or milk products (Brachman 1976; Sterne 1959; Whiteford 1979).

Wild rodent populations in wooded, desert, or other areas are the true reservoir of the plague bacterium; and in these areas, the disease is both chronic and endemic (Benenson 1976b; McNeill 1976; Meyer 1963). In Europe, the agent, *Yersinia pestis*, is transmitted to domestic rats through an intermediate vector, *Xenopsylla cheopis*, the rat flea. In these populations, the bacterium encounters no resistance, and the course of the disease is acute and epidemic. Proximity of human populations to rats and their fleas creates a tertiary focus of infection. Because human populations have no immunity, the course of the disease is also acute and epidemic. Transmission cycles of plague terminate with human hosts.

Table 51 Indirectly Transmitted Acute Bacterial Infections

Disease	*Expected Agent*	*Expected Reservoir*	*Vector*	*Host*	*Morbidity*	*Mortality*	*Immunity*
Anthrax	*Bacillus anthracis*	Domestic ungulates	N.A.*	Domestic Ungulates *Homo sapiens*	Variable	Variable	Variable
Plague	*Yersinia pestis*	Wild Rodents	*Xenopsylla cheopis* among others	Wild and Domestic Rodents *Homo sapiens*	Variable	25–50%	Permanent
Primary Septecemic Plague	*Yersinia pestis*	Wild Rodents	*Xenopsylla cheopis*	Domestic Rodents *Homo sapiens*	Variable	100%	
Epidemic Typhus	*Rickettsia prowazekii*	*Pediculus humanus*	*Pediculus humanus*	*Homo sapiens*	Variable	10–40%	Long term, but not permanent

Sources: Benenson 1976b; Brachman 1976; Whiteford 1979; Wisseman 1976; Zinsser 1947.
*Not applicable.

Epidemic typhus is an acute illness for both vector and human populations. The causative agent in this cycle is *Rickettsia prowazekii*, which multiplies in the intestinal canal of *Pediculus humanus*, the human body louse. Following exposure and infection, lice die within seven to ten days. The agent is transmitted to the humans when lice bite and defecate on human skin. The irritation created by biting leads to scratching and diffusion of rickettsial agents via the feces through the human body (Wisseman 1976; Zinsser 1947).

Human morbidity from agents of Class IV depends on contact with vectors or reservoirs as well as other factors. Epidemics of anthrax occur more frequently during periods of drought (Brachman 1976); outbreaks of plague correlate with a lack of sanitation (Benenson 1976b); epidemics of typhus frequently occur when human populations are stressed by political, economic or social circumstances (Zinsser 1947). Mortality varies with the particular pathway of the infection and whether secondary complications ensue (Table 52).

Of all infections of anthrax, 95% are cutaneous and result from contact with infected animals; 80% of these cases recover. Symptoms of illness include the formation of black eschars at the site of infection. Although less than 5% of all cases of anthrax arise from inhaling or ingesting the basillus, expected mortality from these cases is 100%. Under such conditions, pneumonia and septecemia with hemorrhaging may occur (Brachman 1976; Whiteford 1979).

Mortality associated with bubonic plague is well known. Although inaccurate, fourteenth-century European plague statistics indicate a minimum population loss of 25%. England alone lost between one-half to two-thirds of its population (Benenson 1976b; Creighton 1894; Tuchman 1978).

In the bubonic form, infection is initially localized; but within six days, bacteria spread to regional lymph nodes where hemorrhagic inflammation, necrosis, and edema result in the formation of bubos. At this point, the infection may be arrested, and 50% of all cases recover. The disease, however, may take a progressive course, becoming disseminated to secondary lymph nodes and then to the bloodstream. If bacteria reach the lungs, a separate clinical expression is recognized (Table 52) that carries 100% mortality. This form of the disease, pneumonic plague, can be transmitted directly. Because the parasite derives initially from a nonhuman reservoir, transmission structure follows that defined

Table 52 Secondary Complications arising from Class IV Diseases

Primary Disease	*Complication or Secondary Invasion*	*Agent*	*Expected Mortality*
Anthrax	Pneumonia	*S. pneumoniae* *Staphylococcus aureus* *H. influenzae*	100%
Bubonic Plague	Pneumonic Plague	*Yersinia pestis*	100%

in Figure 16C. Death occurs within five days (Benenson 1976b; Meyer 1963). If, for some reason, bacteria bypass local lymphatic systems, and spread directly to capillaries, a primary septicemic form develops that also carries an expected mortality of 100%. Within six days, a rise in temperature, hemorrhaging, severe vomiting, and diarrhea occur. Death follows shortly thereafter (Benenson 1976b).

Expected mortality from typhus ranges from 10 to 40%. Following a brief prodromal stage, the disease irrupts with symptoms of headache, vomiting, nausea, insomnia, and high fevers. The body is frequently covered by discrete, pinkish macules, similar to the rash associated with measles. In severe cases, delirium and coma may occur. In fatal cases, death typically occurs from the seventh to the fifteenth day following initial symptoms (Wolbach et al. 1922).

Immunity to Class IV infections is conferred through exposure and illness. Immunity to further infections by *B. anthracis* depends on the source of the infection, but in most cases, it is not permanent. Immunity to second attacks of *Yersinia pestis* is permanent, while that to *Rickettsia prowazekii* is not.

Class V: Indirectly Transmitted Protozoal Infections

There are superficial resemblances between malaria, the only Class V disease, and yellow fever. Because malaria is an infection of primates, questions of a New World origin have been raised (Bruce-Chwatt 1965; Coatney et al. 1971). Like yellow fever, malaria is characterized by an alternating transmission pathway (Figure 16D); and the causative agent is passed to human populations through female anopheline mosquitos (King and Bradley 1941). Because of reproductive requirements of mosquitos, malaria is classified as a subtropical and temperate disease and is confined to 60°N to 40°S latitudes. These latitudes correspond to the northern and southern limits of the 15.6°C mean isothermal lines (Rieckmann and Silverman 1977; Watson and Hewitt 1941). High fevers are clinical symptoms of both illnesses.

Here, similarities between the two diseases cease. The term malaria covers a large group of diseases with variable properties of virulence, pathogenecity, morbidity, and mortality. The causative agent in all malarias is a protozoa, genus Plasmodium, characterized by complicated reproductive cycles. While sexual reproduction is confined to mosquito vectors, asexual reproduction occurs in primates (Coatney and Young 1941; Coatney et al. 1971). Although more than twenty-eight species of Plasmodium cause malarial infections in primates, natural transmission of parasites across major primate taxa is rare (Rieckmann and Silverman 1977).

For the human malarias, three species of Plasmodium and a number of strains have been identified (Table 53). Each species of the parasite is associated with particular infectious attributes that are scaled from mild and chronic (*P. vivax*)

Table 53 Class V Diseases, The Human Malarias of North America

Disease	*Agent*	*Vector*	*Morbidity*	*Mortality*	*Expected Mortality, All Malarias*
Malaria	*P. vivax*	*A. atropus* *A. punctipennis* *A. quadrimaculatus*	Variable	Variable	
	P. malariae	*A. punctipennis* *A. quadrimaculatus*	Variable	Variable	5–25%
	P. falciparum	*A. punctipennis* *A. quadrimaculatus*	Variable	Highest of all types	

Source: Coatney et al. 1971; Simmons 1941.

to acute and fatal (*P. falciparum*). Finally, more than one species of Plasmodium may cause simultaneous infections in susceptible individuals (Hackett 1941).

Human malaria is a blood-borne disease carried within the red blood corpuscles and then disseminated through the body. Parasites tend to locate in the liver, spleen, and bone marrow. Although defense systems of hosts are typically adequate against further incursions of benign parasites, systems are less effective against the virulent and toxin-producing properties of *P. falciparum*. Secondary infections of the brain, kidneys, and lungs may occur (Rieckmann and Silverman 1977).

Clinically, malaria may be either chronic or acute. The causative agent determines the nature of the acute form, characterized by several phases. Periodic bouts of chills, fever, nausea, vomiting, and diarrhea mark the primary attack. After these febrile paroxysms disappear, recrudescence and relapse can occur months later. Relapses, more commonly observed in the form of Vivax malaria, are caused by the intermittent reinvasion of parasites into the blood stream (Coatney et al. 1971; Hackett 1941; Rieckmann and Silverman 1977). Although each recrudescence or relapse helps develop host immunities, immunity is not always permanent (Coatney and Young 1941; Rieckmann and Silverman 1977). The rate at which immunity is acquired is dependent on climate, density of vectors, and stability of the human population. Unlike other acute infections, the sickling of red blood cells provides some West African populations with genetic immunity against certain types of malaria (Boyd and Stratman-Thomas 1933; Butcher et al. 1973).

Expected morbidity varies with respect to the malarial history of the population and transmission rates of mosquitos. As with all acute infections, introduction of a new strain or species into an unexposed population leads to cycles of infection with high levels of morbidity. Mortality ranges from 5 to 25% (Table 53). Although epidemics of malaria in humans can theoretically occur wherever susceptible individuals come in contact with a sufficient number of anopheline transmitters, most epidemics occur as incidence peaks in areas where malaria is endemic (Coatney and Young 1941; Hackett 1941). During the twentieth century, malaria in the United States has been endemic in approximately 70% of all states, with highest levels of incidence in the Southeast, the Mississippi Delta, and the Red River Valley (Craig 1941; Faust 1941).

Changing rates of vector transmission and human immunities determine whether the disease is endemic or epidemic. Rates of transmission change as densities of vectors rise and fall in relation to climate. If anopheline transmitters are few in number or curtailed by climate, epidemics occur. In more tropical climates, denser populations of vectors normally exist, which, in turn, increases rates of transmission. In response, the amplitude of the epidemic decreases, and incidence rates are relatively low. Finally, where populations of anopheline mosquitos are not curtailed by climate, rates of transmission are high and constant. At this point, even endemicity disappears as human populations develop herd immunity (Hackett 1941; Rieckmann and Silverman 1977). Anophelines may continue to feed on humans, but parasitism does not occur. As applied to distribution of malaria in North America, geographic areas characterized by high levels of endemicity generally did not have epidemic outbreaks of malaria.

Although researchers have debated whether malaria originated in Africa or America, current opinion supports an African origin for this disease (Coatney et al. 1971; Dunn 1965; Jarcho 1964). As compared with Africa, few species of Plasmodium infect New World primates (Coatney et al. 1971; Collins and Aikawa 1977). In spite of differences in nomenclature, Plasmodia that infect certain species of New World monkeys are indistinguishable morphologically from certain African strains. As stated by Coatney, the fact that there are virtual duplicates between Old World and New World species of Plasmodium "severely challenges even the most extravagent view of convergent evolution" (1971:5). Whereas some African populations have genetic resistance to some malarias, no such resistance is found among Native Americans. It, thus, appears that malaria was introduced from the Old World and became another source of postcontact mortality among Native Americans. Like other indirectly transmitted diseases, it had a more restricted distribution within the Americas than did directly transmitted diseases.

Conclusions

The consideration of the infectious process of the disease classes demonstrates a number of important points. Despite the variability between and within classes of infection, features common to all diseases carry certain implications for the nature of the epidemic environment during the early centuries of European contact. Exposure and infection for most of the diseases result in permanent or long-term immunity for hosts. Because Native Americans lacked exposure to these parasites, they were virgin territories for the colonization and reproduction of all these parasites. The parasites, in turn, adopted an acute strategy with the result that epidemics must have been common during the early centuries of contact.

As stated by Burnet and White: ". . . any community which is cut off from the rest of the world for periods of a year or more will, on the arrival of visitors, suffer an epidemic of the feverish cold, or influenza type. . . ." (1972:132). In this context morbidity reaches 100%, while mortality stemming directly from the disease as well as from other factors varies. In some instances, there may be no deaths; in other instances, mortality may be 100%. Table 54 summarizes the pattern of reintroduction among populations where acute infections are not endemic.

The diversity of the infections, on the other hand, suggests that Native Americans were at risk for a wide array of diseases. Although any single parasite may have had a minor effect, the combination of new diseases, secondary invasions, and reexposure to previously introduced diseases must have been devastating on the demography and culture of Native Americans. A small, but dramatic, example of this effect was documented by Marchand (1943) for a small band of Tlingit in the Yukon.

Between September 1942 and June 1943, the band experienced six epidemics

Table 54 Attack and Mortality Rates among Isolated Populations

Disease	*Area*	*Year*	*Population Size*	*Attack Rate (per 1000 population)*	*Mortality Rate (per 1000 population)*
Smallpox[a]	Iceland	1707	57,000	?	315
Measles[b]	Faroes	1846	7,863	776	272
Measles[c]	Greenland	1951	4,247	993	18
Measles[d]	Canadian* Arctic	1952	1,800	1000	35
Influenza[e]	Canadian N.W.T.	1949	90	1000	111
Influenza[f]	Alaska*	1959	658	845	4
Influenza[g]	Caroline Islands	1964	Unknown	1000	7
Influenza[h]	Caroline Islands	1966	1,464	1000	294
Cold[i]	Spitzbergen	1933	507	871	0
Yellow Fever[j]	Gambia*	1978	1,531	2.6–4.4	.8

[a]Dixon 1962.
[b]Panum 1940 [1846].
[c]Christensen et al. 1953.
[d]Peart & Nagler 1954.
[e]Nagler et al. 1949.
[f]Phillip et al. 1959.
[g]Brown & Gajdusek 1970.
[h]Brown et al. 1966.
[i]Paul & Freeze 1933.
[j]Monath et al. 1980.
*Medical assistance available.

including measles, malaria, whooping cough, diarrhea, and meningitis. With each epidemic, health of the population deteriorated, allowing for the invasion of other parasites. Although morbidity was high, mortality resulted only from measles, 24 per 1000, and meningitis, 93 per 1000.

In summary then, features common to all diseases and diversity between diseases suggest the same conclusions. Disease introduction must have been a major cause of postcontact aboriginal decline. The consequences were catastrophic, and they fundamentally changed aboriginal populations and cultures quite early. Precontact population of North America must have been very large, numbering at least 12 million or more.

EPIDEMICS AND SPATIAL DIFFUSION

The topic of spatial diffusion of disease is of some importance to the question of catastrophic decline. If disease spreads like rumors (Dietz 1967), then infections could have spread far away from colonial fronts. If this was the case, the first regional records of disease do not necessarily mark the first aboriginal experience of disease. In this section, I will consider several topics: mathematical modes of epidemics, potential diffusion of disease among Native Americans, and an evaluation of Dobyns's sixteenth-century epidemic hypothesis.

Deterministic Models of Directly Transmitted Infections

A number of different disciplines, mathematics, epidemiology, and geography, have developed deterministic and stochastic models of infectious diseases (Bailey 1957, 1975; Serfling 1952). Deterministic modes are based on a fixed number of susceptibles and infectives and are the more appropriate model when considering large populations (Bailey 1957; Haggett 1975); stochastic models, developed from probability, are applicable when attempting to describe the appearance of epidemic peaks in populations where the parasite is endemic (Bartholomew 1973). Although both sorts of models are relevant for the study of disease in the Americas, I will limit this discussion to deterministic models. Such models are simpler to understand and require fewer assumptions about the population. Since this is the first explicit application of these models to postcontact America, simplicity is desirable.

The discussion is further restricted to directly transmitted viruses and bacteria; although some work has been done with zoonoses (Gilg 1973; MacDonald 1950, 1952, 1953; Ross 1911), their complicated transmission cycles and variable expressions make such diseases rather intractable to model.

Even models of direct transmission present analogical difficulties for making specific predictions about diffusion of epidemics in postcontact America. The focus of these models tends to be urban or industrial, largely because such settings have the most epidemiological data. Within the urban setting, the goals of epidemic modeling have been to predict epidemic events and spatial diffusion (Angulo et al. 1983; Haggett 1976; Haggett and Cliff 1979; Murray and Cliff 1977; Pyle 1979), and to simulate outbreaks of epidemics where parasites persist on an endemic basis (Bartlett 1957, 1960).

Because twentieth-century epidemic models are developed from populations fundamentally different from those of sixteenth-century America and because only directly transmitted viruses have been considered extensively, there are no modern analogues for the early postcontact period in America. As a result, this discussion will be quite general, focusing on the principles of diffusion.

Hamer (1906), interested in mathematically describing the periodicity of measles epidemics in England, is credited with developing the initial deterministic formulations for directly transmitted diseases. His geometric approximations were based on several assumptions that have become the baseline for all later deterministic treatments. In a population where contact between individuals is random, the number of new cases that develop from a specified number of infective cases is proportional to (1) the number of existing infective cases, (2) the number of existing susceptible individuals, and (3) a constant determined by factors relating to contact between an infective and susceptible. Soper (1929) modified Hamer's formula; more recently, Bailey (1957) and Bartlett (1956) have further refined the Hamer-Soper model.

Current deterministic models are based on knowledge of microbial transmission and disease characteristics of human populations. In population size n, there are S susceptibles, I infectives and R removals. R occurs through immunity, isolation, or death; thus, $S + I + R = n$. β is the infection rate, and γ is the absolute removal rate. Because removal rates vary according to β and γ, γ is frequently converted to p, the relative removal rate; p is defined as the ratio between β/γ (Bailey 1957; Haggett 1975).

At the scale of a single community, an epidemic results following exposure if the infection rate is greater than or equal to the relative removal rate ($\beta \geq p$). In this case, in time (dt) there will be (SI) new infectives and (γI) removals (Bailey 1957; Haggett 1975). Equations that describe the change in S, I, and R in time (dt) are as follows:

$$\frac{dS}{dt} = -\beta SI$$

(1) $$\frac{dI}{dt} = \beta SI - \gamma I$$

$$\frac{dR}{dt} = \gamma I$$

Graphic resolution of these equations is summarized in Figure 17. Although the shape of any epidemic curve is a function of the total number of susceptibles and infectives, the epidemic maximum always occurs where the curves for susceptibles and infectives intersect. The curve for the recovered individuals is also approaching its maximum.

Equation (1) can be extended to a regional or multi-regional scale by considering other parameters, including migration and accession of new susceptibles through birth, population concentration, or density. The simplest of these formulas attends only δ, defined as the number of persons per unit area (Bailey 1957; Haggett et al. 1977). If the population is infinitely uniform across a two dimensional plane, then an epidemic wave results if population density, δ, exceeds the threshold ($\beta \geq p$). Then, the number of individuals in area dS, surrounding point P, will be either susceptible (δSds), infective (δIds), or removed (δRds). Consequently, $S + I + R = n$. The equations for spatial diffusion given by Bailey (1957) and Haggett et al. (1977), are summarized as follows:

$$\frac{\delta S}{\delta t} = -\beta \delta S \bar{I}$$

(2)
$$\frac{\delta I}{\delta t} = \delta \beta S \bar{I} - I$$

$$\frac{\delta R}{\delta t} = \gamma I$$

where:
$\bar{I}$ = the weighed spatial average of I.

More complicated spatial models consider migration and birth and are reviewed by Bailey (1957) and Haggett (1975).

From a spatial perspective, the course of such a disease is described as a wave. The structure of the wave varies as a function of density of the population and systems of communication (Hagerstrand 1952; Haggett et al. 1977). If the population is evenly distributed across a plane, the epidemic wave shows only minor fluctuations. The terminus of the wave is defined by loss of susceptibles ($\beta < p$).

If, however, the landscape is punctuated by variable population densities, then the amplitude of the wave reflects such differences. As population densities increase, the amplitude of the wave increases. As population densities decrease, the amplitude of the wave decreases. Finally, where populations are discontinuous spatially, or systems of communication are not commensurate with

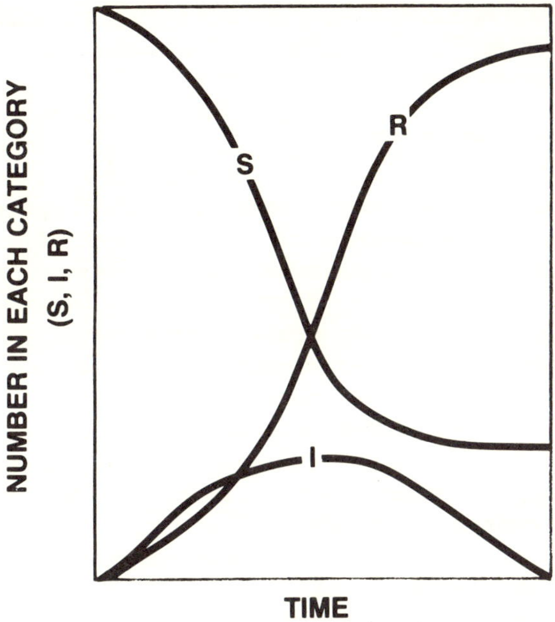

Figure 17. Deterministic Model of an Epidemic in terms of S, I, R

periods of communicability of parasites, fadeouts occur. In this case, the parasite must be introduced to each population cluster.

Velocity of waves is the final aspect of spatial patterning to be considered. A common assumption is that the shorter the period of communicability, the more rapid the spatial dispersion. Haggett (1975) considers this problem in a reexamination of Black's measles data (1966) from insular communities. His equation for velocity is:

$$D_e = \frac{-1}{2\sqrt{S/A}} \qquad (3)$$

where:
D_e = expected spacing of the epidemic
S = size of the susceptible population
A = area of the island in Km^2.

When Haggett applied this equation to Black's island communities, he discovered an inverse relationship between the duration of a measles epidemic and the density of a population. As population density increased, the velocity of the measles wave decreased. Longer epidemic cycles characterized more dispersed populations. The temporal shape of an epidemic curve was altered according to the distribution of the population.

Epidemic Potential among Amerindians

Although archaeologists are a long way from being able to rigorously apply epidemic models to postcontact populations of the Americas, they are important abstractions. Consequently, I will employ the models theoretically and investigate the spatial setting of initial outbreaks and the probability of spatial diffusion.

The significant disease impact occurred at community or regional scales. Because Native Americans lacked immunity, $\beta > p$. Consequently, the earliest introductions produced the most intense episodes of illness within single communities. Time and the relationship between exposure and immunity determined the structure of subsequent cycles of infection. If a sufficient period of time did not elapse before reintroduction of the same parasite, then β would fall below p, and community outbreaks would not occur. The parasite would be repulsed and, without additional susceptibles, the parasite would die out. Spatial diffusion would be curtailed.

Implications from models of spatial diffusion are not quite so straight forward. If all parameters are of equal weight, the earliest epidemics should have produced the most extensive spatial waves. Other factors, however, are not weighted equally. The diffusion potential should vary as a function of (1) the length of the communicability period for each parasite, (2) local and regional population densities around the disease location, (3) the contact mechanisms between communities or regions.

In order to estimate the diffusion potential of directly transmitted parasites, they must be ranked according to some appropriate variable. Periods of communicability are one such measure but are subject to analogical problems: There is no way of knowing whether modern periods of communicability are comparable to those of the past. In the absence of relevant data, I cautiously employ an assumption of continuity. Rankings based on modern periods of communicability may be inappropriate for the past.

Table 55 summarizes rankings of directly transmitted viruses and bacteria. Where periods of communicability could have inhibited the diffusion of viral infections similar to cold and influenza, those of whooping cough or smallpox would have promoted spatial diffusion.

Population density and communication systems are independent variables in relation to diffusion. As shown in Equation (2), the density of the population affects the amplitude of the epidemic wave. Although it is not precisely known how efficiency in communication systems offsets variable densities of populations and, therefore, diffusion potentials, it is likely that the two have an inverse

Table 55 Diffusion Potential of Directly Transmitted Infections

I (*Greater or Equal to 15 Days*)	*II* (*7 to 14 Days*)	*III* (*Less Than or Equal to 6 Days*)
Whooping Cough	Measles	Cold
	Scarlet Fever	Influenza
Smallpox	Chickenpox	
	Mumps	

relationship. As population density decreases and communication systems become more efficient or regular, diffusion potential remains high. In the twentieth century, for instance, jet age transportation turned epidemic influenza into pandemic influenza (Jordan 1927; Stuart-Harris 1981). Conversely, decreases in contact accompanied by increases in population density also lead to high diffusion potentials. Diffusion is unlikely only where there is slow and irregular communication and low population density.

The study of the intersections of the variables causative in the diffusion of parasites has important implications for the epidemic environment of America. First, it is very unlikely that all infections arrived in the Americas during the initial decades of contact. As Snow (1980) has argued, initial crew sizes were too small to harbor most viruses and voyages took longer than a month. Only Rank I, or zoonotic, infections could have survived these conditions. Rank II and III infections were later, perhaps seventeenth century, introductions.

Diffusion potential, once introduced, depended on native population density and transportation mechanisms. Since the Valley of Mexico and the agricultural East supported the greatest population densities at the time of European contact, the entire region could have been one diffusion sphere of infectious disease. Most probably, horses served as efficient mechanisms of diffusion within Mexico; ships spread infections outside of Mexico. After 1598, the horse served a similar function north of Mexico.

The same mechanisms for potential diffusion could not necessarily be maintained across the Great Plains and western United States. Lower population densities, fewer navigable rivers, and greater distances could have created natural barriers against epidemic waves. After the introduction of horses these barriers may have become less significant.

The only reasonable conclusion regarding diffusion of parasites is one that recognizes a time-transgressive pattern. Parasites with longer periods of communicability were introduced earlier and resulted in extensive spatial waves. In some instances, infection may have preceded colonization; in cases like the Valley of Mexico, infection and colonization were simultaneous events. Because aboriginal populations lacked immunity, disease contact caused sharp reductions of native populations. Smaller populations should have curtailed later diffusions, but communication systems between Europe and America, as well as across America, improved. Short-lived parasites gained a foothold, and new epidemic waves resulted.

Assessment of Dobyns's Epidemic Hypothesis

Discussion of deterministic models of acute and directly transmitted diseases has been used as a spring board for suggesting a temporal order of disease introduction and the diffusion potential of pathogens following introduction. These predictions can, in turn, be employed to evaluate Dobyns's sixteenth-century epidemic hypothesis.

As described repeatedly, Dobyns advocates disease diffusion as prior to direct contact. This assumption justifies his reestimation of aboriginal population of North America upwards to 18 million and challenges assumptions of continuity clung to by scholars of the American Historical School. Although my archaeological evaluation of Dobyns's assumptions showed them to be not entirely correct, his arguments need to be considered in an epidemiological framework. Here, two issues are relevant: the contradiction between his estimated precontact population size of Native North Americans and catastrophic decline, and evaluation of sixteenth-century disease introductions. I will consider each in turn.

All available information suggests that large or dense populations are necessary for the evolution and persistence of acute viral and bacterial infections. If Dobyns's estimates of native population size are correct, then why were so few acute infections present in the Americas prior to European contact? In other words, since small populations cannot endemically support most acute infections, the absence of such infections from the Americas seems to support Kroeber's, not Dobyns's, position of population size.

Duplicate forms were absent in the Americas because either they had not evolved in the Old World at the time that founder populations migrated to the Americas or, if fixed as part of the human disease load, they did not survive the climatic rigors of arctic and subarctic winters.

The absence of duplicate forms in the New World does not mean, however, that convergent forms did not evolve here. This, in fact, would be likely if population was as large as Dobyns suggests. Disease transmission and epidemic models in relation to the archaeological record suggest why, with the possible exception of syphilis, there were no New World counterparts for Old World acute diseases.

Survival of acute diseases depends on contact between infected and susceptible individuals. Contact varies according to the density and size of the population. As spatial dispersion decreases, contact and disease diffusion increase. This explains why urban centers constitute the most appropriate environment for persistence of acute viral and bacterial diseases specific to humans. These considerations have direct implications for the evolution of such diseases.

Clearly, viral and bacterial diseases could have appeared numerous times throughout human evolutionary history but they only became part of the human disease load where environmental conditions promoted reproduction of microbes (Cockburn 1963). Such environments occurred when populations became nucleated and developed large sedentary settlements.

In terms of the archaeological record of the Old World, nucleated populations in sedentary settlements began to appear by 5000 B.C (Wenke 1984); by the fifteenth century, they had a consistent distribution across Europe and western Asia. Contact between centers was regularized by communication technologies including horses, wheel drawn carts, and boats.

In the New World, large nucleated and sedentary settlements did not become a consistent feature of the landscape until well after the Christian era (Wenke 1984). Further, urban centers comparable to Old World centers had an irregular distribution, limited to the Valley of Mexico, parts of Peru and the Middle Mississippi Valley. Towns, villages, and hamlets were more frequent; and technologies did not promote regular and rapid contact between settlements. From an evolutionary perspective, it appears that although viral and bacterial diseases could have evolved independently in either the Old or New World, they became fixed only in the Old World. Distribution of population and contact mechanisms in the New World simply did not permit the fixing of crowd infections.

Thus, in addition to population size, factors such as population density and transmission mechanisms are relevant for the evolution and persistence of acute viral and bacterial infections. Using the Old World as the model, it is clear that the American environment was simply not suitable for the persistence of convergent forms, even if they did periodically appear.

This conclusion has relevance for the apparent contradiction between Dobyns's estimates of population size and catastrophic decline from disease. Quite simply, there is no contradiction. Both large and small populations can be at risk for acute pathogens. Large populations, however, have a greater diffusion potential and may be able to sustain pathogens endemically once they are introduced. If the aboriginal population of North America was as large as Dobyns suggests, then introduction implied persistence, not fade-outs of microbes.

Whether Dobyns's sixteenth-century killers (1981, 1983) were actually introduced in that century is the second issue that must be evaluated. The timing of the introductions considered earlier in this chapter forms the basis of this evaluation.

Dobyns uses the 1519–1520 smallpox epidemic in Mexico as the terminus of prehistory for all America. From the point of introduction, the pathogen spread through both continents. Following that pandemic, measles spread into the Southwest from Mexico in 1524 (Crosby 1972; Dobyns 1981). In Florida, acute diseases, carried to that region by ship, were common throughout the sixteenth century. Between 1513 and 1596, Dobyns suggests that twelve parasites diffused into peninsular Florida. Of these, four diseases were zoonoses, typhus, malaria, plague, and an unknown vectored fever; three were due to unidentifiable parasites. The remaining pathogens were directly transmitted viruses or bacteria and included smallpox, typhoid fever, mumps, influenza, and measles.

Nothing in my analysis negates the possibility that smallpox was pandemic in the New World. Not only is smallpox a Rank I virus (Table 55), but it can persist in a dried state (Upham 1986). Since both these factors give it a great diffusion potential, I am in substantial agreement that the smallpox epidemic of 1519 was as significant as Dobyns suggests.

I am, however, in less agreement with the later sixteenth-century diffusions into the Southwest and Florida. Assuming that the past periods of communicability were similar to those of the present, I question whether all of the suggested diseases were present anywhere in the Americas during the sixteenth century. If present, could they have diffused away from their points of introduction?

Since zoonoses depend less on human populations for survival than directly transmitted pathogens and since the specific zoonoses identified by Dobyns can be spread by ship, it is possible that these diseases diffused into sixteenth-century Florida. Diffusion outside of Florida would have been contingent on vector or reservoir dispersion.

With the exception of smallpox, I doubt that any of the other directly transmitted viruses and bacteria were present in sixteenth-century America. Infections, such as measles, mumps, and influenza, seem to require more rapid communication mechanisms or larger population clusters than were present on sixteenth century European ships. If these infections did not survive voyages, they could not have spread to native populations.

While Dobyns's hypothesis may be correct in outline, specific details are erroneous. Major sixteenth-century killers included smallpox, whooping cough, and some zoonoses. Other infections, such as mumps or measles, were probably not even present in the Americas during the sixteenth century. One important conclusion is that fewer diseases than suggested by Dobyns were present and capable of extensive diffusion prior to 1600.

Fewer diseases, however, does not imply a reduction in the magnitude of the initial catastrophe. Since, in the absence of medical assistance, *Variola major* can cause 100% mortality, the presence of other acute killers is quite unnecessary. Cook's research in central Mexico (Borah and Cook 1963; Cook and Borah 1960; Cook and Simpson 1948) suggested that in the first thirteen years of contact native populations experienced a 50% attrition, most of which was due to smallpox. Although environmental parameters of vectors or reservoirs may have restricted the diffusion of zoonoses, plague, which can be directly transmitted, could have been spread by human carriers. In tropical regions, such as Florida and the Gulf Coast, dispersion of anopheline mosquitos insured diffusion of malaria.

CONCLUSIONS

The primary purpose of this chapter was to determine whether disease could have caused the catastrophic decline in population described in Chapter 4. To answer the question, I adopted an actualistic approach, the goal of which was to describe the epidemic environment in the Americas during the early centuries of contact. I developed classes of acute infections and considered these in light of the infectious process.

Once I had described the infectious process of each of the five disease classes, it became apparent that disease was the most important single factor in the demographic catastrophe of Native Americans. Unfortunately, because the description of classes of disease relied on data from modern populations who have some immunity to the diseases, as well as access to medical assistance, it was not possible to estimate the magnitude of loss experienced by Native Americans. Nonetheless, if, in contemporary settings, mortality from acute infectious diseases can be 100%, it is not unreasonable to suggest a minimal population loss of 90% from all introduced diseases.

The second aspect of disease introduction focused on the probability of spatial diffusion of epidemics. Although population clusters could have been wiped out in areas where parasites were introduced, the absence of the potential for diffusion considerably weakens the disease hypothesis.

This question was addressed through exploring deterministic models of disease diffusion and applying properties of those models to virgin soil America. This approach was very fruitful. It suggested that disease introduction did not necessarily imply disease diffusion. The probability of the latter varied according to population density, communication, and periods of communicability of pathogens.

Knowledge of diffusion suggested a temporal order for the introduction of diseases and provided a means of evaluating Dobyns's sixteenth-century epidemic hypothesis. First, there appears to be no conflict between size of aboriginal North American population and the absence of acute pathogens prior to the arrival of Europeans. Environmental conditions were simply unsuitable for the persistence of such pathogens, even if they had independently evolved in the Americas. Although Dobyns may have erred regarding the number of pathogenic microbes present in the sixteenth century, he certainly was correct about the diffusion potential and destructive capacity of those that were present. The sixteenth century must be seen as the watershed of disease contact. Archaeological collapse of populations from the seventeenth century supports the belief that new diseases were introduced and diffusing during that century as well.

Finally, the discussion was helpful for suggesting new directions in historical and epidemiological research. With few exceptions (Cook 1955, 1973a), most historical studies of disease have focused on directly transmitted viruses or bacteria. Although zoonoses are more difficult to identify, they are important to consider. Able to withstand the rigors of initial European voyages, they could have been a major source of postcontact decline during the sixteenth and seventeenth centuries.

Six

Implications and Conclusions

Three issues guided this archaeological study of European contact. I wanted to specify the timing of aboriginal population loss in eastern North America, to determine whether the loss was catastrophic or gradual, and to pinpoint the role of introduced acute infections in that loss. Although these topics have been discussed for nearly 100 years, resolution of the issues has not been possible. Assumptions concerning change of populations made by either the Kroeberians or those of the Cook-Dobyns school have guided the interpretations of incomplete historical records and have lead to continuing controversy. By using the time depth of the archaeological record, I hoped to resolve the specific issues and, thus, contribute to the larger assumptions that have governed the population debate.

The results of this investigation have tended to support the Cook-Dobyns view of European contact at the expense of the Kroeberian one. The onset of aboriginal demographic and systemic change did not begin with regional documentation or sustained presence. Aboriginal population decline tended to precede written documentation and was catastrophic in nature. The timing and nature of the catastrophe logically implicated introduced infectious parasites as causal; the extended discussion of acute infectious diseases explained why and how this could have happened.

This conclusion has lasting implications for anthropology. The assumptions and methods used by the American Historical School for their reconstructions are inappropriate. Because local or regional catastrophic population loss was early and occurred in less than 100 years, survivors were adapting to that loss at the time of initial descriptions. Processes of village fusion and fission, or abandonment of whole regions are evidences of those adaptations.

The historical record of Native Americans, therefore, must be approached from an assumption of change rather than of stability. The applicability of the direct historical approach or any other sort of analogical framework to even the late prehistoric record cannot be presumed. Although traits may have survived across the contact border, survival of traits cannot and should not imply survival of systems.

While generally supporting Dobyns's sequence of contact period events, this analysis demonstrated that the issue is more complex than Dobyns has suggested. The variability is of several types. The timing of the collapse, for instance, varied temporally. Disease was a sixteenth-century phenomenon only in the Lower Mississippi Valley. In central New York and the Middle Missouri, epidemics appeared to impact native populations in the seventeenth century. Furthermore, the pattern of change following the initial epidemic experiences varied considerably. Some groups, like those in the lower valley, disappeared without a trace; others persisted for one or more centuries; a very few, like the Iroquois, have survived into the present.

Such differences raise several questions: Why did the timing of disease contact vary? Why was there differential survival? The demonstration of disease as a sixteenth-century event in the Southeast makes considerable sense. The proximity of the Southeast to the Valley of Mexico and the degree of contact between the two regions and within the Southeast suggested the pathways necessary for an early catastrophic collapse.

Simultaneously, it would be precipitious to negate the possibility of a sixteenth-century collapse in regions that lacked the necessary archaeological evidence. Of great importance here is the differentiation between the record itself and archaeological descriptions of the record. My syntheses of the timing and nature of the collapse were based on regional samples collected for purposes other than the study of the demography of the contact period. As repeatedly shown, these descriptions shaped by other purposes are necessarily biased.

Probability based regional samples of settlements and finer grained chronologies are two necessary means of correcting this serious problem. The first would provide accurate and reliable estimates of settlement counts and of domestic structures through time; the second would facilitate a more accurate determination of the onset of demographic or systemic change. Until we have descriptions of the archaeological record developed according to these guidelines, the question of a sixteenth-century collapse must remain open.

Data of better quality will confirm that the collapse was either a sixteenth-century event or was variable temporally. The confirmation of the former would support another aspect of Dobyns's model; confirmation of the latter would open new avenues of research. As I have indicated, either cultural or natural factors can inhibit the diffusion of parasites. With reasonably large spatial samples, these factors could be specified and measured.

My bias on the question of the timing of disease contact is toward the sixteenth-century. The virgin soil status of Native Americans, the suggested diffusion potential of the earliest microbial imports, and suspected aboriginal population densities in the late fifteenth century converge to make this position probable. Even if this assumption is confirmed by further research, however, the issue of postepidemic change must be assessed systematically. This is a most fruitful area of research for both ethnohistorians and archaeologists. While I cannot consider all the parameters of postepidemic change, it is appropriate to make a few preliminary suggestions.

The potential shape of any survivorship curve is an obviously complex problem that depends on several major classes of variables, including those intrinsic to native systems, predisease adaptations, population size and distribution, as well as magnitude of epidemic loss. Such extrinsic variables as location of native groups relative to European centers, competition between native groups or between European and native populations for resources, and European attitudes toward native populations are also significant. Although evaluating the weight of each variable must be done on a case-by-case basis, several patterns are possible.

In accordance with Morey's Law, Dobyns (1983) has suggested that the largest or densest populations, typically concentrated along river valleys, disappeared earliest. Regardless of size, populations concentrated around European centers may have experienced similar fates, especially if those populations were extraneous to European survival. When selective pressures from disease were coupled with stress factors generated by Europeans who wanted native resources, termination was inevitable.

Those groups that were located farther inland, those that were mobile, or those that were necessary for European survival, were likely to have had different postcontact experiences. In regions like the Middle Missouri, I suspect that the postcontact population curve was bimodal. A preliminary, perhaps sixteenth century, disease experience was followed by at least 100 years of relative peace and health during which time populations adjusted to the catastrophe and recovered demographically. The second and terminal decline began when disease selection was associated with European exploration and settlement and progressive harassment from mounted Plains groups.

Only in two very different situations is long term persistence expected. Because mobile populations intrinsically had less risk of contracting infections, their survivorship curves should be longer. This fact partially explains the school book picture of Native Americans as mounted hunters of the Plains.

In addition, where European survival was contingent on native survival, inadvertent efforts were made to prevent extinction. In central New York, for instance, the British acted as a kind of buffer between the Iroquois and the burgeoning demands of European populations in the Northeast. While the degree of protection provided by the British did not prevent the spread of disease to the Iroquois, it did reduce the total stress on their strategies of survival. The contribution of this reduction in stress to persistence is suggested by the rapid termination of the Iroquois historical record when British support was withdrawn.

This view may also explain the persistence of Puebloans along the Rio Grande. Since contact between the New Mexican colony and Mexico was irregular, survival of Spanish colonists depended on native survival. Rather than competing with native populations, the Spaniards relied on them; and this reliance changed the nature of the competition.

In conclusion, then, a major contribution of this work has been to resolve some very basic questions of Native American population trends during the early centuries of European contact. The independent assessment of archaeology and history showed that demographic and systemic change dominated the Native American record, beginning in the sixteenth century. Although it has not been possible to develop accurate quantitative estimates of population loss or to determine unambiguously the timing of the loss in each instance, this work has shown that the archaeological record can clearly answer these questions, if archaeologist use reliable estimates of site numbers measured over relevant periods of time.

Finally, since I have shown that the Kroeberian assumption of continuity is in error, questions of differential persistence following disease contact become vitally important to ethnohistorians, ethnologists, and archaeologists. I am hopeful that this pilot study will stimulate much needed, cooperative research.

Appendix A Lower Mississippi Valley

TEMPORAL ORDERS

Summary of Temporal Orders

Sixty-eight components are given a temporal assignment in one or more of the three analyses but only sixty-three are listed in Table 56. If the same location was occupied in more than one period, it was treated as two components. This occurred in five cases, Parkin, Clay Hill, Menard, Wallace, and Fatherland. Of the sixty-eight, sixty-six are used in the settlement analyses. Two components, Anna and Emerald, though assigned to the Plaquemine tradition, are excluded because, according to Brain (1978), they were not occupied during the Late Mississippi period.

The occurrence seriations of aboriginal ceramics orders 72% (49/68) of all components; 7% (5/68) have absolute dates; 24% (16/68) are ordered in the analysis of European trade goods. Only 12% (8/68) are ordered by more than one method.

Radiometric Assays

Radiometric dates are of marginal utility in developing the Lower Mississippi Valley chronology. There are very few radiometric determinations for the Late Mississippi period (see Phillips 1970, 2, Table 18 for example), and the reliability of those that do exist is questioned due to biases in the reservoir and the complex histories of many sites. This latter source of bias explains why none of the dates from the same site (Table 57) are averaged. Many radiocarbon samples were from some phase of mound construction; and since mounds were repeatedly modified throughout occupational histories, dates for mounds need not correlate with surface collected samples of pottery.

Table 56 Summary by Component of Temporal Analyses in the Lower Mississippi Valley

Component	*Radiometric Assay*	*Pottery Occurrence Seriation*	*European Trade Goods*
Vernon Paul		X	
Cummings		X	
Castille Landing		X	
Parkin		X	X
Neeley Ferry		X	
Big Eddy		X	
Williamson		X	
Barton Ranch		X	
Welshans Place		X	
Perry		X	
Cramor Place		X	
Hollywood		X	
Woodlyn		X	
Shelby		X	
Upper Nodena	X	X	
Belle Meade		X	
Starkley		X	
Kent Place		X	
Carson Lake		X	
Bradley Place		X	
Bell Place		X	
Clay Hill		X	X
Menard		X	X
Wallace		X	X
Dupree		X	
Vance		X	
Walford		X	
Powell Bayou		X	
Merigold		X	
Salomon		X	
Dockery		X	
Alligator Mounds (B)		X	
Spendthrift		X	
Cason		X	
Old Town		X	

(*continued*)

Table 56 (*Continued*)

Component	*Radiometric Assay*	*Pottery Occurrence Seriation*	*European Trade Goods*
Haynes Bluff		X	
Clarksdale			X
Rice			X
Thoroughbred			X
Greenfield			X
Dead Oak			X
Oliver			X
Satartia			X
Portland			X
Lockgard			X
Magee			
Grace		X	
Failing		X	
Arcola		X	
Silver City		X	
Sherwood		X	
Leland		X	
Winterville		X	
Kinlock		X	
Lake George	X	X	
Campbell		X	
Bay Lake		X	
Refuge		X	
Anna	X		
Emerald	X		
Fatherland	X	X	X
Bayou Goula			X
Trudeau			X

For the lower valley, suites of dates are mandatory for monitoring the occupational history of settlements. Only two sites meet this criterion: Fatherland (Neitzel 1965) and Lake George (Williams and Brain 1983).

In Table 57, radiometric dates from five settlements that presumably date to sometime during the Mississippi period are presented. Upper Nodena is defined as belonging to the Mississippian tradition, Late Mississippi period. Although cultural materials from Lake George cover a great chronological range from *circa* A.D. 500 until the late fifteenth century, Williams and Brain (1983)

Table 57 Lower Mississippi Valley Late Prehistoric and Historic Radiocarbon Dates

Location	*Laboratory Number*	*Provenience*	*Uncorrected Date (A.D.)*	*Dendro Correction (A.D.)*[a]
Upper Nodena[b]	M-385	Unknown	1320 ± 280	1320 ± 251
Lake George[c]	H1206	—	1000 ± 105	1009 ± 90
	H1221	—	1250 ± 110	722 ± 120
	H1229	—	1400–1450 ± 110	470 ± 112
	H1230	—	1250–1300 ± 105	622 ± 107
	H1231	—	1300–1350 ± 110	572 ± 112
	H1232	—	1300 ± 105	1286 ± 109
	H1240	—	1300 ± 110	1286 ± 114
	H1241	—	1075 ± 105	1075 ± 109
	H1242	—	1500 ± 105	1467 ± 111
	H1247	—	1500 ± 105	1467 ± 111
	H1249	—	950 ± 110	961 ± 114
	GX494	—	1315 ± 65	1315 ± 71
	GX495	—	1580 ± 115	1540 ± 121
	GX495	—	1340 ± 115	1339 ± 119
Anna[b]	M-47	Mound 5	1310 ± 250	1311 ± 252
Emerald[b]	M-27	Stage E	1470 ± 100	1461 ± 107
Fatherland[d]	M-1380	Feature 1; Stage 1 (Mound B)	1180 ± 110	195 ± 114
	M-1381	Feature 3; Stage 3 (Mound C)	1225 ± 110	1236 ± 114
	M-1379	Feature 7: Stage 2 (Mound B)	1250 ± 110	1280 ± 114
	M-1382	Feature 30; Mound C	1270 ± 110	1276 ± 114
	M-1378	Feature 7; Mound B	1525 ± 100	1501 ± 107
	M-1376	Feature 101; Mound A	1570 ± 100	1541 ± 107
	M-1383	Feature 44; Mound C	1430 ± 100	1416 ± 107

[a]Damon et al. 1974.
[b]Crane 1956.
[c]William and Brain 1983.
[d]Crane and Griffin 1966.

suggest that the major occupation is confined to the Mississippian tradition. Fatherland is associated with both Plaquemine and Mississippian traditions.

Several dates are thought to be in error, due to contamination of the reservoir or to mixing of deposits. Williams and Brain (1983:346) questioned the accuracy of samples H1206, and H1240. The Fatherland sample from Mound C, M-1383, was taken from nine feet below the surface, but associated pottery appeared to be earlier than the fifteenth century.

Pottery Occurrence Seriations

Forty-nine components are assigned a relative position in one of the five occurrence seriations of pottery. Since more components are ordered by this than by any other temporal method, occurrence seriations are the primary means by which the chronology of the lower valley was developed. Although this work is largely a refinement of Ford's seriations (Phillips, Ford, and Griffin

1951), the refinement is justified: existing chronologies are directed toward answering cultural historical rather than demographic questions.

Even though Phillips's classification of pottery (1970), based on types and varieties, is currently employed by most archaeologists in the lower valley (Brain 1975b; Brain et al. 1974; Brown 1985; Jeter et al. 1979; Morse 1981; Williams and Brain 1983), types defined by Phillips, Ford, and Griffin are used in these seriations.

This decision is based on several considerations. To determine the pattern of change during the contact period requires archaeological samples from an extensive area of space; and Phillips, Ford, and Griffin collected from a much larger area than did Phillips. While it is possible to reassign Phillips's classes to older types, it is impossible to break down older types into Phillips's types and varieties. If Phillips's classes had been used, the archaeological sample would have been restricted to the Yazoo Basin, an area deemed too small to determine the pattern of contact period change. If, as suggested recently by Davis (1981), Phillips's varieties are too fine-grained for developing chronologies, then the logical alternative is to use the next higher scale which are Phillips, Ford, and Griffin's types. Since these types have already been successfully employed in seriations, they have demonstrated a degree of historicity that Phillips's types and varieties have not.

Twenty shell tempered pottery types are characteristic of the Mississippi Period. Table 58 summarizes fifteen of those types employed in these seriations. All components with occurrences of these types are considered in developing temporal orders, regardless of the temporal assignment made by Phillips, Ford, and Griffin. Five of the original types, (Hollywood White Filmed, Carson Red on Buff, Fortune Noded, Walls Engraved, and Hull Engraved) are excluded. Occurrences of the first three types were so infrequent that they caused breaks in the orders. There is some controversy regarding the relationship between Walls and Hull Engraved.

In 1951, Phillips, Ford, and Griffin (1951) suggested that Hull Engraved might be an interior bowl design closely related to Walls Engraved. Phillips (1970) attempted to clarify this problem by making Walls and Hull two varieties of the same type. His opinion was that Hull was a more southern expression than Walls and that decorations of the two were distinct. Nonetheless, in the 1951 publication, the most frequent occurrences of both pottery types was in Memphis, a northern seriation area. Because limits of the existing data precluded resolving this difficulty, both types were excluded. Since frequencies of both were very rare, the exclusion did not change the suggested orders.

To control for the problem of spatial diffusion of style, I divided the region into five smaller areas used by Ford in his seriations (Phillips, Ford, and Griffin 1951) (Figure 18). Although Phillips's phases could have been used for this

Table 58 Pottery Types of the Late Mississippi Period

ARCOLA INCISED
Phillips, Ford, and Griffin 1951:140
Phillips 1070:45 (Barton Incised, var. Arcola)

AVENUE POLYCHROME
Phillips, Ford, and Griffin 1951:134
Phillips 1970:40–41

BARTON INCISED
Phillips, Ford, and Griffin 1951:114–119
Phillips 1970:43–47

BELL PLAIN
Phillips, Ford, and Griffin 1951:122–126
Phillips 1970:58–61

KENT INCISED
Phillips, Ford, and Griffin 1951:126–127
Phillips 1970:46 (Barton Incised, var. Kent)

LELAND INCISED
Phillips, Ford, and Griffin 1951:137–140
Phillips 1970:104–107

NEELEY'S FERRY PLAIN
Phillips, Ford, and Griffin 1951:105–110
Phillips 1970:133 (Mississippi Plain, var. Neeley's Ferry)

NODENA RED ON WHITE
Phillips, Ford, and Griffin 1951:133–134
Phillips 1970:141–143

OLD TOWN RED
Phillips, Ford, and Griffin 1951:129–132
Phillips 1970:144–147

OWENS PUNCTUATED
Phillips, Ford, and Griffin 1951:136–137
Phillips 1970:149–150

PARKIN PUNCTUATED
Phillips, Ford, and Griffin 1951:110–114
Phillips 1970:150–152

RANCH INCISED
Phillips, Ford, and Griffin 1951:119–120
*Phillips 1970:156

RHODES INCISED
Phillips, Ford, and Griffin 1951:127
Phillips 1970:167

VERNON PAUL APPLIQUE
Phillips, Ford, and Griffin 1951:120
Phillips 1970:167

WALLACE INCISED
Phillips, Ford, and Griffin 1951:134–136
Phillips 1970:168

WALLS ENGRAVED
Phillips, Ford, and Griffin 1951:127–129
Phillips 1970:169

*Phillips (1970) recommends discontinuing this description as a pottery type.

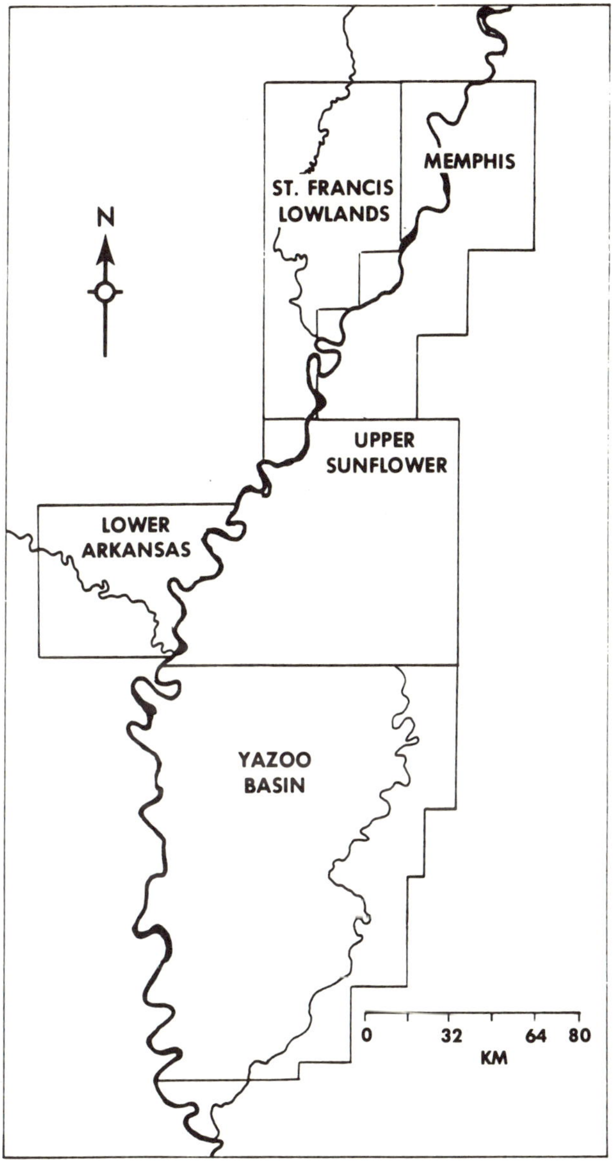

Figure 18. Seriation Areas of the Lower Mississippi Valley

purpose, the spatial division chosen provided a degree of consistency between types and areas used in these seriations. After completing seriations, I noticed that all components from the St. Francis Lowlands were consistent with those identified by Phillips (1970) and Morse (1981) as belonging to the Parkin phase. In this instance, there is agreement between the assignment of components, the spatial boundaries, and the phase designation.

Since the presence or absence of types changes as a function of sample size (Jones et al. 1983), I had to control for differences in size of samples. If type A has a frequency of 5% in a population, for instance, the probability of it being represented in a collection of 100 sherds is considerably less than in a collection of 1000 sherds. As frequencies and sample size decrease or increase, this problem becomes progressively more serious. While in a sample of 5000 sherds, a type with a frequency of 1% is likely to be represented by at least one sherd, in a sample of 50 sherds, a type with a frequency of even 10% may not even be present.

For the ceramic data from the lower valley, sampling errors posed a particularly difficult problem. Ceramic samples collected by both Phillips and Phillips, Ford, and Griffin were judgementally based, and sizes of sample varied greatly. While Phillips's collections from the Yazoo Basin tended to be small, they were of relatively comparable sizes; samples made by Phillips, Ford, and Griffin, even from the same general area, were not comparable in size.

Ford's seriations (Phillips, Ford and Griffin 1951) complicate this problem further. Sample size for each type was not broken down into raw counts but was summarized as percentages and percentages of decorated sherds were low, relative to percentages of plain body sherds.

Although occurrence seriations are the most robust seriation method and can mask differences in samples, sampling errors may still produce spurious conclusions. In short, controlling for differences between samples makes it easier to include samples of various sizes, besides determining whether a particular type is usable in a seriation.

I employed a simple ratio that compared the smallest sample in each area to all others in that same area to determine whether counts in larger samples were a function of the size of the sample. If, in larger samples, type counts were equal to or less than type counts in the smallest sample, presence of that type in the larger sample was regarded as a function of sample size and, therefore, not useful in developing the chronological order.

Table 59 summarizes minimum sample size and range of ceramic counts for each seriation area. Table 60 presents sample size by component and lists those types whose presence in the seriation is due to sampling biases. Once I established sequences, samples less than the minimum could be added. This was possible only in the Yazoo Basin where four components [Haynes Bluff (22-

Table 59 Sample Sizes of Pottery by Seriation Area

Area	*Minimum Sample Size*	*Sample Range*
St. Francis Lowlands	593	593–5848
Memphis	345	345–3034
Lower Arkansas	825	825–1108
Upper Sunflower	405	405–2950
Yazoo Basin	356	356–2777

M-5); Campbell (19-0-9); Sherwood (19-M-3); and Grace (21-M-7)], were added to the order.

Occurrence seriations are presented by area, and appearance and disappearance of pottery types are described in terms of pottery periods (noted by arabic numerals). Although these periods aided in developing the chronological units summarized in the text, they are not equivalent to these units. Pottery periods were strictly an organizational device for describing the stylistic changes in pottery styles. Although I made an effort to place components with trade goods near the top of each sequence, the placement did not guarantee that the direction of the seriation was correct. Most European items were surface finds lacking provenience. Consequently, it is possible that these items did not relate to the same temporal period as the pottery sample.

ST. FRANCIS LOWLANDS SERIATION (TABLE 61) This seriation has ordered nine components. None of the pottery types present in any component were a consequence of sampling. European material has been recovered from 11-N-1 (Parkin) (Klinger 1975–1977; Morse 1981).

Certain shell tempered types, (Neeley's Ferry Plain, Bell Plain, Parkin Punctated, Old Town Red, and Barton Incised), persisted throughout the sequence but were the only types present during Period 1. During Period 2, represented by six occupations, three decorated types were added. Kent Incised appeared first and continued to the end of the sequence. Later, Rhodes Incised and Vernon Paul Applique were added.

The appearance of Avenue Polychrome and Nodena Red on White (single occurrence) marked Period 3. The two types overlapped briefly with decorated types from Period 2. By the end of Period 3, Vernon Paul Applique and Rhodes Incised had disappeared. Seven pottery types (Avenue Polychrome, Barton Incised, Kent Incised, Old Town Red, Parkin Punctated, Bell Plain, Neeley's Ferry Plain) defined Period 4, the terminus of the sequence.

MEMPHIS AREA SERIATION (TABLE 62) Thirteen components were ordered in this sequence. In some assemblages, Kent Incised, Ranch Incised

Table 60 Lower Mississippi Valley Sherd Counts and Unusable Pottery Types by Seriation Area and Component

Area	*Occupation*	*Number*	*Sherd (N)*	*Unusable Types*
St. Francis Lowlands	Vernon Paul	11-N-9	2565	None
	Cummings	11-O-4	715	None
	Castille Landing	13-N-21	2010	None
	Parkin	11-N-1	5848	None
	Neeley Ferry	11-N-4	7215	None
	Big Eddy	12-N-4	728	None
	Williamson	11-N-13	4925	None
	Barton Ranch	11-O-10	4723	None
	Welshans Place	12-N-5	593	None
Memphis	Perry	14-O-4	328	None
	Cramor Place	12-O-5	998	None
	Hollywood	13-O-10	1528	None
	Woodlyn	13-P-11	865	Kent, Ranch, Rhodes
	Shelby	12-P-2	498	None
	Upper Nodena	10-Q-1	3034	None
	Belle Meade	13-O-5	805	Kent, Ranch, Rhodes, Avenue
	Starkley	13-N-16	916	None
	Kent Place	13-N-4	1090	None
	Carson Lake	10-P-1	3508	None
	Bradley Place	11-P-2	479	Old Town, Kent, Avenue
	Bell Place	10-P-2	345	None
	Clay Hill	13-N-7	667	None
Lower Arkansas	Menard	17-K-1	1108	None
	Wallace	17-K-3	1534	None
	Dupree	16-L-6	825	None
Upper Sunflower	Vance	17-N-9	405	None
	Walford	17-N-2	673	None
	Powell Bayou	17-O-9	2254	None
	Merigold	17-N-1	2072	None
	Salomon	15-O-1	1302	None
	Dockery	17-N-11	605	None
	Alligator Mounds (B)	16-N-2b	831	None
	Spendthrift	16-O-2	1045	None
	Cason	17-P-2	2950	None
	Old Town	15-N-3	508	None
Yazoo Basin	Haynes Bluff*	22-M-5	95	
	Magee	20-M-2	1288	Owens
	Grace*	21-M-7	266	
	Failing	19-N-5	371	None
	Arcola	20-M-1	2777	Owens, Nodena, Ranch
	Silver City	20-O-5	625	Nodena
	Sherwood*	19-M-3	239	
	Leland	19-M-1	7981	Old Town
	Winterville	19-L-1	356	None
	Kinlock	19-N-1	884	None
	Lake George	21-N-1	1105	None
	Campbell*	19-O-9	63	
	Bay Lake	19-N-3	1007	None
	Refuge	19-L-6	716	None

*Added after seriations developed.

Table 61 Occurrence Seriation of Pottery from the St. Francis Lowlands

	Types									
Component	*Neeley*	*Bell*	*Parkin*	*Old Town*	*Barton*	*Kent*	*Avenue*	*Vernon Paul*	*Rhodes*	*Nodena*
11-N-4	X	X	X	X	X	X	X			
12-N-4	X	X	X	X	X	X	X		X	
11-N-1	X	X	X	X	X	X	X	X	X	X
13-N-21	X	X	X	X	X	X		X	X	
11-O-4	X	X	X	X	X	X		X		
11-N-13	X	X	X	X	X	X		X		
11-N-9	X	X	X	X	X	X				
11-O-10	X	X	X	X	X	X				
12-N-5	X	X	X	X	X					

Table 62 Occurrence Seriation of Pottery from the Memphis Area

	Types									
Component	*Neeley*	*Bell*	*Parkin*	*Old Town*	*Barton*	*Kent*	*Ranch*	*Rhodes*	*Avenue*	*Vernon Paul*
11-P-2	X	X	X	X[a]	X	X[a]				X[a]
10-P-1/13-N-7	X	X	X	X	X	X			X	
13-N-16/13-N-4	X	X	X	X	X	X	X		X	
10-Q-1	X	X	X	X	X	X	X	X	X	X
13-O-5	X	X	X	X	X	X[a]	X[a]	X[a]	X[a]	X
12-P-2	X	X	X	X	X	X	X	X		X
13-O-10	X	X	X	X	X	X	X	X		
13-P-11	X	X	X	X	X	X[a]	X[a]	X[a]		
12-O-5	X	X	X	X	X	X	X			
14-O-4	X	X	X	X	X	X				
10-P-2	X	X		X	X	X				

[a]Occurrence of types is a function of sample size.

Rhodes Incised, Avenue Polychrome, or Old Town Red are not reliable since their presence is explained as a function of the size of the sample. European trade goods are reported from 13-N-7 (Clay Hill) (Williams 1980). Although Morse (1973) argued that 10-Q-1 (Upper Nodena) was occupied until A.D. 1700, no European material was reported from the site. Morse based his argument on the presence of a late type pendant and a catlinite pipe that Neitzel (1965) considered a trade item in the Natchez area at *circa* A.D. 1600.

Four pottery periods were established for this sequence. During Period 1, represented by a single component, Neeley's Ferry Plain, Bell Plain, Old Town Red, Barton Incised and Kent Incised, were present. In Period 2, also represented by one component, Parkin Punctated is added to the other types; and all six types persisted to the end of the sequence. Period 3 was represented by six components and was marked by the appearance of three incised types, Ranch Incised, Rhodes Incised, and Vernon Paul Applique. Ranch may have persisted longer, but none of these types survived to the end of the sequence. In Period 4 Vernon Paul and Rhodes disappeared but Avenue Polychrome appeared.

Like the St. Francis seriation, polychrome painting was added late in the sequence. As distinct from the St. Francis seriation, Kent Incised persisted throughout the entire sequence.

LOWER ARKANSAS SERIATION (TABLE 63) This sequence has only three components and was too brief to determine stylistic trends in pottery. Two components, 17-K-1 (Menard), 17-K-3 (Wallace) were associated with European trade goods.

UPPER SUNFLOWER SERIATION (TABLE 64) Ten components were given a relative assignment in the Upper Sunflower seriation. No component was associated with European trade material, and the presence of all pottery types was usable in developing the order

Period 1, marked by the presence of Neeley's Ferry Plain, Bell Plain, Parkin Punctated, Old Town Red, Barton Incised, was represented by three components. During Period 2, also represented by three components, Avenue Polychrome was added to the list of the other five types, but it did not persist throughout the sequence. Four types, Owens Punctated, Rhodes Incised, Ranch Incised, and Leland Incised, appeared during Period 3. In Period 4, Avenue Polychrome disappeared with the exception of Rhodes Incised; all types present during Period 3, also disappeared.

YAZOO BASIN SERIATION (TABLE 65) Ten components were ordered. After the seriation was constructed, 22-M-5, 21-M-7, 19-0-9, 19-M-3 were added. Of the fourteen components, only 22-M-5 (Haynes Bluff) was associated with European trade goods. In four assemblages, occurrences of Owens Punc-

Table 63 Occurrence Seriation of Pottery from the Lower Arkansas Area

	Types								
Component	*Neeley*	*Bell*	*Parkin*	*Old Town*	*Barton*	*Avenue*	*Leland*	*Wallace*	*Rhodes*
17-K-1	X	X	X	X	X	X	X	X	
17-K-3	X		X	X	X	X	X	X	X
16-L-6	X		X	X	X	X	X	X	X

Table 64 Occurrence Seriation of Pottery from the Upper Sunflower Area

	Types									
Component	*Neeley*	*Bell*	*Parkin*	*Old Town*	*Barton*	*Avenue*	*Leland*	*Ranch*	*Rhodes*	*Owens*
17-N-11		X	X	X	X				X	
17-O-9	X	X	X	X	X	X	X	X	X	X
17-N-1	X	X	X	X	X	X	X	X	X	X
15-O-1	X	X	X	X	X	X	X	X		
16-O-2/16-N-2b/15-N-3	X	X	X	X	X	X				
17-N-9/17-P-2/17-N-2	X	X	X	X	X					

Table 65 Occurrence Seriation of Pottery from the Yazoo Basin

	Types									
Component	*Neeley*	*Bell*	*Parkin*	*Old Town*	*Leland*	*Barton*	*Arcola*	*Owens*	*Nodena*	*Ranch*
22-M-5	X	X	X		X	X			X	
20-M-2	X	X	X		X	X	X	X[a]		
19-N-5	X	X	X		X	X	X	X		X
20-M-1	X	X	X		X	X		X[a]	X[a]	X[a]
20-O-5	X	X	X	X	X	X	X	X	X[a]	
19-M-3	X	X	X	X	X	X	X		X	
19-L-1	X	X	X	X	X	X	X			
19-M-1	X	X	X	X[a]	X	X	X			
21-M-7/19-N-3/19-N-1/21-N-1/19-O-9	X	X	X		X	X	X			
19-L-6	X	X	X		X					

[a]Occurrence of type is a function of sample size.

tated, Nodena Red on White, Ranch Incised, and Old Town Red were due to sample size.

I established five pottery periods in this seriation. The presence of four types (Neeley's Ferry Plain, Bell Plain, Parkin Punctated, and Leland Incised) defined Period 1. Five components were assigned to Period 2, during which time Barton Incised and Arcola Incised were added as new types. Barton Incised persisted to the end of the sequence. Arcola Incised was not present at 22-M-5, but this absence may have been due to the sample size recovered from Haynes Bluff. The Period 3 marker was Old Town Red, but it did not survive to the end of the sequence. Four components were assigned to Period 3. In Period 4, three new types (Owens Punctated, Nodena Red on White, Ranch Incised) were added, and all three overlapped with Old Town Red. In Period 5, represented by 22-M-5, Ranch Incised and Owens Punctated were absent as was Arcola Incised.

The Yazoo sequence is somewhat different than sequences generated from other areas. Leland Incised is present throughout the sequence; and, as suggested by Phillips (1970), Arcola Incised is unique to the basin. Rhodes Incised, present in all other seriations, is conspicuously absent from the Yazoo; and Owens Punctated occurs at more locations than in any other sequence. In terms of number of occurrences, incising is more prevalent than painting as a decorative technique. The preponderance of these techniques makes considerable sense given the proximity of the Yazoo Basin to areas farther south where incising or engraving decorative techniques predominate.

In summary, comparison of the five seriations facilitated drawing general conclusions regarding the occurrence, persistence, and diffusion of Late Mississippi period types. Some of these conclusions confirmed ideas suggested previously by either Phillips, Ford and Griffin (1951), or Phillips (1970).

Seriations have demonstrated that certain types persisted throughout the entire Mississippi period. These types included plain shell tempered sherds (Neeley's Ferry Plain and Bell Plain), and decorated or painted, shell tempered rim or body sherds (Barton Incised, Parkin Punctated, and Old Town Red). Certain other types that persisted for a shorter period were specific to the Late Mississippi period. These included Kent Incised, Vernon Paul Applique, Avenue Polychrome, Leland Incised, Arcola Incised, Wallace Incised and Owens Punctated.

Based on presence/absence data, types can be assigned a northern or southern affiliation (Table 66). St. Francis Lowlands and Memphis are northern; Yazoo Basin is southern; and Upper Sunflower and Lower Arknsas are transitional between the two. Kent Incised, Vernon Paul Applique, and Avenue Polychrome were specific to the northern part of the region. Leland and Arcola Incised, and Owens Punctated were specific to the Yazoo Basin. In the transi-

Table 66 Tabulation of Pottery Types by Seriation Area

	Types						
Area	*Kent*	*Vernon Paul*	*Avenue*	*Leland*	*Arcola*	*Wallace*	*Owens*
St. Francis Lowlands	X	X	X				
Memphis	X	X	X				
Lower Arkansas			X	X		X	X
Upper Sunflower			X	X		X	
Yazoo Basin				X	X		X

tional area, some northern and southern types and one unique type, Wallace Incised, were found.

If the frequency or occurrence of types within and between areas is used as an indicator, then suggestions regarding the diffusion of types can be made. Painted types, including Avenue Polychrome and Old Town Red, were diffusing south, while Leland Incised and Owens Punctated were diffusing north. If the suggested Upper Sunflower order is correct, then Avenue Polychrome reached this area before Leland and Arcola Incised did.

Finally, these seriations suggest that aboriginal ceramic styles and presumably systems, indeed, terminated prior to the seventeenth century. Of the forty-nine components seriated in this analysis, only five (10%) (Parkin, Clay Hill, Menard, Wallace and Haynes Bluff) were associated with European material. In two cases, recovered European materials were surface finds and may be reflecting later use than the ceramic sample. Only three components, therefore, crossed the border defined by the presence of European trade goods. Since there is no reason to assume that this evidence is incorrect, it appears that assumptions of continuity in to the time of French settlement are inappropriate.

Analysis of European Trade Goods

Seventeen components from the lower valley were associated with European trade goods (Table 67), five of which were given a temporal assignment in one of the pottery seriations. Haynes Bluff was excluded from the analysis of European artifacts. Although it has been assigned to the late seventeenth century (for example, Brain 1975b; Brown 1979; Ford 1936), the specific composition of the European assemblage has not been reported in the literature. The provenience of European objects from the other sixteen settelements was variable. Some objects were recovered from the surface (Clay Hill and Satartia); others were taken from burial contexts (Wallace and Oliver). The remaining ones were a product of either amateur or professional excavation.

European objects were classified into six classes of European function. Table 68 summarizes the classification; and Table 69 tabulates, by component, the

Table 67 Lower Mississippi Valley Components Associated with European Trade Goods

Component	*Source*
Satartia	Brain 1975a
Clarksdale (16-N-26)	Brain 1975a
Oliver (16-N-6)	Brain 1975a
Parkin (11-N-1)	Davis 1966; Klinger 1975–1977; Morse 1981
Clay Hill (13-N-7)	Williams 1980
Haynes Bluff (22-M-5)	Brain 1975b; I. Brown 1979; Ford 1936
Wallace (17-K-3)	Ford 1961; Moore 1908
Menard (17-K-1)	Ford 1961; Phillips, Ford, and Griffin 1951
Portland (22-M-12)	I. Brown 1979
Lockgard (22-M-17)	I. Brown 1979
Fatherland (26-K-2)	Neitzel 1965
Bayou Goula (32-L-1)	Quimby 1957
Trudeau (29-J-2)	Brain 1970, 1980
Greenfield (26-K-92)	I. Brown 1985
Thoroughbred (26-K-74)	I. Brown 1985
Rice (26-K-91)	I. Brown 1985
Dead Oak (26-K-101)	I. Brown 1985

number of classes represented. According to Table 69, the classification separates components into two groups. One group of nine components was represented only by Class 4. The six classes of European function were present in the second group of seven components.

As described below, differences between the two groups of components reflect availability of European products. Since availability increased through time, differences between groups of components are ultimately temporal.

Only two types of ornamental items have been reported from the sixteenth and seventeenth centuries, the period of exploration. The first object is the Clarksdale Bell (see Brain 1975a for a description of the bell.) This particular bell has been recovered from five locations (Satartia, Clarksdale, Oliver, Clay Hill, and Parkin). Other examples of these bells have been found in Florida and Tennessee, and Brain (1975a) correlated their spatial occurence with De Soto's route. The second object, also attributed to De Soto, was a Spanish glass trade bead. One of these beads has been recovered from Parkin (Klinger 1975–77); Morse 1981).

Two other components (Wallace and Menard) were also represented by Class 4, but relate to French, rather than the Spanish, exploration. Ford (1961) excavated Menard to determine whether it was the Arkansas (Quapaw) village of Osotouy where, in 1686, de Tonti established a small fort. Six European

Table 68 Lower Mississippi Valley Functional Classes of European Objects

1. EATING
Bottles
Pottery
Cutlery
2. SUBSISTENCE
Knives
Guns
3. DRESS
Buttons
Needles
Braid
Material
4. ORNAMENTATION
Beads
Bells
Bangles
Bracelets
Pendants
Earrings
Rings
5. CONSTRUCTION
Axes
Chisels
Wedges
Nails
Hammers
6. SMOKING
Pipes

items were recovered from the excavation: four glass trade beads different than the Spanish beads, one metal cross, and one boar's tusk. Ford concluded that Menard was occupied in the late seventeenth century. He used ceramic similarities to place Wallace in the same time interval. Brown (1985) recovered only two glass beads from Dead Oak and Rice.

In summary, nine components, summarized on Table 69 appear to belong to the period of exploration in the lower valley and can be assigned a temporal range from A.D. 1541–1700.

The artifactual inventory of the remaining seven settlements is quite different: more classes of European function are present; and diversity of objects ranges from crockery and glass bottles to iron axes, adzes, hoes, chisels, gun parts, buttons, pipes, and quantities of glass trade beads. These data alone suggest the period of French settlement in the lower valley.

Historical records support this suggestion. Portland and Lockgard were discrete occupations that dated between 1698 and 1706, and 1719 and 1729 respectively (Brown 1979). While Portland was affiliated with Tunica, Lock-

Table 69 Tabulation of European Items by Component and Functional Class

Component	*Classes* 1	2	3	4	5	6
Trudeau (n = 187,000[a])	X	X	X	X	X	X
Bayou Goula[b] (n = ?)	X	X	X	X	X	X
Fatherland[c] (n = 128)	X	X	X	X	X	X
Thoroughbred (n = 51)	X	X	X	X	X	X
Greenfield (n = 130)	X	X	X	X	X	X
Lockgard (n = 81)	X	X	X	X	X	X
Portland (n = 135)	X	X	X	X	X	X
Dead Oak (n = 2)				X		
Rice (n = 19)				X		
Menard (n = 6)				X		
Wallace[b] (n = ?)				X		
Clay Hill (n = 1)				X		
Parkin (n = 2)				X		
Clarksdale (n = 3)				X		
Oliver (n = 2)				X		
Satartia (n = 1)				X		

[a]Without glass beads n ≤ 750.
[b]Counts not given.
[c]Without glass beads which are reported in strings not individually.

gard may have been a hybrid community composed of Yazoo, Koroa, and Ofo. The long prehistoric occupation at Fatherland (see Table 57) continued after European trade goods appear. The town was visited regularly between 1682 and its abandonment in 1730 (Neitzel 1965). According to Quimby (1957), the historic component of Bayou Goula dated between 1699 and 1722. Trudeau was the last settlement of the Tunica, following a long series of relocations. The village was occupied from 1731 until 1764.

Qualitative analyses of European trade goods in association with European documents suggest that European materials from the period of exploration (sixteenth and seventeenth centuries) were fundamentally different in quantity and diversity than those affiliated with the period of European settlement (eighteenth centuries).

In summary, I establish three periods: The last prehistoric period in the lower valley terminated in the midsixteenth century. This was followed by a period of Spanish and French exploration, between 1541 and 1700. The second period of European contact coincided with French settlement between 1701–1764.

SETTLEMENT DATA

Table 70 lists locations employed in the analysis of population change. The n (61) is lower than that appearing in the text (Table 12) because five locations were occupied in more than one period.

Table 70 List of Settlements from the Lower Mississippi Valley

Settlement Number	*Settlement Name*	*County*	*State*	*Source*
12-P-2	Shelby	Shelby	TN	Phillips, Ford, and Griffin 1951
10-Q-1	Upper Nodena	Mississippi	AR	Morse 1973; Phillips, Ford, and Griffin 1951
10-P-1	Carson Lake	Mississippi	AR	Phillips, Ford, and Griffin 1951
10-P-2	Bell Place	Mississippi	AR	Phillips, Ford, and Griffin 1951
11-N-9	Vernon Paul	Cross	AR	Phillips, Ford, and Griffin 1951
11-N-13	Williamson	Cross	AR	Phillips, Ford, and Griffin 1951
11-N-1	Parkin	Cross	AR	Klinger 1975–77; Morse 1981; Phillips, Ford, and Griffin 1951
11-N-4	Neeley Ferry	Cross	AR	Phillips, Ford, and Griffin 1951
12-N-5	Welshans Place	Cross	AR	Phillips, Ford, and Griffin 1951
11-O-4	Cummings	Poinsett	AR	Phillips, Ford, and Griffin 1951
11-O-10	Barton Ranch	Crittendon	AR	Phillips, Ford, and Griffin 1951
11-P-2	Bradley Place	Crittendon	AR	Phillips, Ford, and Griffin 1951
13-O-5	Belle Meade	Crittendon	AR	Phillips, Ford, and Griffin 1951
13-N-21	Castille Landing	St. Francis	AR	Phillips, Ford, and Griffin 1951
12-N-4	Big Eddy	St. Francis	AR	Phillips, Ford, and Griffin 1951
12-O-5	Cramor Place	St. Francis	AR	Phillips, Ford, and Griffin 1951
13-N-16	Starkley	Lee	AR	Phillips, Ford, and Griffin 1951

(*continued*)

Table 70 (*Continued*)

Settlement Number	*Settlement Name*	*County*	*State*	*Source*
13-N-7	Clay Hill	Lee	AR	Phillips, Ford, and Griffin 1951
13-N-4	Kent Place	Lee	AR	Phillips, Ford, and Griffin 1951
15-N-3	Old Town	Phillips	AR	Phillips, Ford, and Griffin 1951
16-L-6	Dupree	Phillips	AR	Phillips, Ford, and Griffin 1951
17-K-3	Wallace	Arkansas	AR	Moore 1908; Phillips, Ford, and Griffin 1951
17-K-1	Menard	Arkansas	AR	Ford 1961; Moore 1908; Phillips, Ford, and Griffin 1951
13-O-10	Hollywood	Tunica	MS	Phillips, Ford, and Griffin 1951
14-O-4	Perry	Tunica	MS	Phillips, Ford, and Griffin 1951
13-P-11	Woodlyn	De Soto	MS	Phillips, Ford, and Griffin 1951
16-O-2	Spendthrift	Coahoma	MS	Phillips, Ford, and Griffin 1951
15-O-1	Salomon	Coahoma	MS	Phillips, Ford, and Griffin 1951
16-N-26	Clarksdale	Coahoma	MS	Brain 1975a
16-N-6	Oliver	Coahoma	MS	Brain 1975a
16-N-2b	Alligator Mounds (B)	Bolivar	MS	Phillips, Ford, and Griffin 1951
17-N-1	Merigold	Bolivar	MS	Phillips, Ford, and Griffin 1951
19-N-1	Kinlock	Sunflower	MS	Phillips, Ford, and Griffin 1951; Phillips 1970
19-N-5	Failing	Sunflower	MS	Phillips, Ford, and Griffin 1951; Phillips 1970
19-N-3	Bay Lake	Sunflower	MS	Phillips, Ford, and Griffin 1951
17-N-2	Walford	Sunflower	MS	Phillips, Ford, and Griffin 1951
17-N-9	Vance	Sunflower	MS	Phillips, Ford, and Griffin 1951
17-N-11	Dockery	Sunflower	MS	Phillips, Ford, and Griffin 1951
17-O-9	Powell Bayou	Sunflower	MS	Phillips, Ford, and Griffin 1951

(*continued*)

Table 70 (*Continued*)

Settlement Number	*Settlement Name*	*County*	*State*	*Source*
17-P-2	Cason	Le Flore	MS	Phillips, Ford, and Griffin 1951
19-O-9	Campbell	Le Flore	MS	Phillips, Ford, and Griffin 1951
20-M-1	Arcola	Washington	MS	Phillips, Ford, and Griffin 1951; Phillips 1970
19-M-3	Sherwood	Washington	MS	Phillips, Ford, and Griffin 1951; Phillips 1970
19-M-1	Leland	Washington	MS	Phillips, Ford, and Griffin 1951; Phillips 1970
20-M-2	Magee	Washington	MS	Phillips, Ford, and Griffin 1951; Phillips 1970
19-L-1	Winterville	Washington	MS	Phillips, Ford, and Griffin 1951; Phillips 1970
19-L-6	Refuge	Washington	MS	Phillips, Ford, and Griffin 1951; Phillips 1970
20-O-5	Silver City	Humphreys	MS	Phillips 1970
21-N-1	Lake George	Yazoo	MS	Phillips, Ford, and Griffin 1951; Phillips 1970
	Satartia	Yazoo	MS	Brain 1975a
21-M-5	Grace	Issaquena	MS	Phillips 1970
22-M-7	Haynes Bluff	Warren	MS	Ford 1936; Phillips 1970
22-M-12	Portland	Warren	MS	I. Brown 1979
22-M-17	Lockgard	Warren	MS	I. Brown 1979
26-K-2	Fatherland	Adams	MS	Neitzel 1965
26-K-92	Greenfield	Adams	MS	I. Brown 1985
26-K-91	Rice	Adams	MS	I. Brown 1985
29-J-2	Trudeau	West Feliciana	LA	Brain 1970, 1980
26-K-74	Thoroughbred	Adams	MS	I. Brown 1985
26-K-101	Dead Oak	Adams	MS	I. Brown 1985
32-L-1	Bayou Goula	Iberville	LA	Quimby 1957

Appendix B Central New York

TEMPORAL ORDERS

Summary of Temporal Orders

I employed eight temporal analyses to order components from central New York (Table 71). Of the twenty-seven components listed in the table, Caughnawaga is the only one to be excluded from these analyses because Grassman (1969) did not include data on artifacts in his lengthy summary of the settlement. Fortunately, Caughnawaga is dated by historical documents, 1667–1693. Twenty-five of the twenty-seven components were employed in archaeological analyses of population change. Tuttle and Nichols were excluded because published descriptions contained no quantitative settlement information.

Radiocarbon Assays

41% (11/27) of all components had at least one radiocarbon date; two components, Maxon Derby and Furnace Brook, had two radiocarbon dates (Table 72). Although the temporal span represented by mean dates ranged from A.D. 1098 until 1590, 46% of all mean dates fell between A.D. 1333 and 1382. The date for Garoga was thought to be in error (Funk 1967; Ritchie 1980; Ritchie and Funk 1973). Based on the size of excavated houses and the presence of European material, Garoga typically is assigned to the early post-European period. If this temporal assessment is correct, then the radiocarbon date is several hundred years too old. The disparity between the date and the context may be explained by changes in the ^{14}C reservoir itself. Alternatively, if Garoga is a multicomponent site, then both temporal assignments could be correct.

Ceramic Seriations

Four seriations that employ stylistic attributes of ceramics are presented. Three of these seriations are based on attributes of pottery vessels, and one is based on the shape of clay pipe bowls.

POTTERY SERIATIONS Occurrence seriation 1 and frequency seriation 1 (Dunnell 1970) used twenty types defined by Ritchie and MacNeish (1949), MacNeish (1952), Lenig (1965), and Pratt (1976). (Table 73 lists types and location of original descriptions.) Types 1 through 7 have in common the attribute of cord impression, while types 8 throuh 20 are all incised.

Twelve components (12/27, 44%) are ordered in the occurrence seriation (Table 74) in which sample size ranges from 43-1011. Temporal direction of the seriation was suggested by radiocarbon dates or European trade goods.

For frequency seriation 1, assemblages less than 100 sherds or those that failed to conform to the method (Dunnell 1970) were excluded. The resulting seriation placed eight components (29%) in chronological sequence. Table 75 presents percentages and raw counts by component; Figure 19 is a bar graph of the percentages. Although, relative to the occurrence sequence, there were many gaps separating components in the frequency seriation, the relative position of those components ordered by both seriations was exactly the same.

In occurrence seriation 2, I used a paradigmatic classification to order a larger number of components and to create a more even distribution of sherds across classes. A total of one hundred-ninety-six classes were created through four dimensions and eighteen modes (Dunnell 1971) (Table 76). Eleven of the possible classes were represented by existing variability, and thirty-five type descriptions were assigned to one of the eleven classes (Table 77).

Since the classification for occurrence seriation 2 synthesized stylistic variability into a fewer number of classes, the seriation did accommodate more components (seventeen or 63%) than either occurrence seriation 1 or frequency seriation 1. In occurrence seriation 2, Garoga was deleted; and two components, Tuttle and Cameron, were added. Several Onondaga County samples, have also been added at the top of the order (Table 78). There were several problems with these samples that raised questions about the reliability of the temporal placement.

Tuck's ceramic analysis (1971) could not be reclassified into existing types. Consequently, older ceramic descriptions from these sites had to be employed; and these listed pottery types by percentage only and excluded information on sample size.

Table 79 compares relative positions of components across the three seriations. With three exceptions, positions were consistent. In occurrence seriation 1, Round Top was assigned a later position than Maxon Derby. In occurrence seriation 2, these components held an equivalent temporal status that was

Table 71 Summary of Temporal Orders from Central New York Tabulated by Component

Component	*Radiocarbon Date*	*Occurrence Seriation #1*	*Frequency Seriation #1*	*Occurrence Seriation #2*	*Occurrence Seriation Ceramic Pipes*	*Occurrence Seriation European Metal*	*Cumulative Frequencies European Trade*	*Glass Trade Beads*
Caughnawaga (A.D. 1667–1693)								
Cameron				X		X	X	X
Beecher						X	X	X
Marshall						X		
Thurston						X	X	X
Diable		X	X	X	X	X	X	X
Bach		X		X		X		
Barnes					X	X		X
Chase				X		X	X	X
Quirk				X		X	X	X
Atwell Fort				X			X	X
Garoga	X	X	X		X		X	X
Burke		X			X			

Table 71 (*Continued*)

Tuttle				X	
Goff		X		X	
Buyea		X	X	X	
Nichols		X	X	X	
Temperance					
Nahrwold #1	X	X	X	X	
Getman	X	X	X	X	
Howlett Hill	X				X
Furnace Brook	X				X
Kelso	X	X	X	X	
Chamberlain	X				X
Sackett	X	X		X	X
Round Top	X	X	X	X	X
Maxon Derby	X	X		X	

Table 72 Some Radiocarbon Dates for Central New York Components

Component	*Lab Number*	*Uncorrected Date (A.D.)*	*Average Date*[a]	*Dendrochronological Correction (A.D.)*[b]
Burke	Y-2375[c]	1590 ± 80		1549 ± 89
Nahrwold #1	Y-1650[c]	1450 ± 100		1435 ± 107
Garoga	Y-1381[c]	1390 ± 100		1382 ± 107
Getman	M-763[e]	1390 ± 150		1382 ± 155
Kelso	Y-1380[c]	1390 ± 100		1382 ± 107
Howlett Hill	Y-1689[c]	1380 ± 60		1373 ± 71
Furnace Brook	Y-1818[c] Y-1817[c]	1370 ± 60 1300 ± 60	1335 ± 42	1333 ± 52
Chamberlain	Y-1819[c]	1290 ± 60		1294 ± 67
Sackett	M-1076[d]	1170 ± 50		1187 ± 33
Maxon Derby	Y-1173[c] M-1077[d]	1100 ± 100 1090 ± 50	1096 ± 83	1098 ± 88
Round Top	Y-1650[c]	1070 ± 60		1098 ± 68

[a]Long and Rippeteau 1974.
[b]Damon et al. 1974.
[c]Stuiver 1969.
[d]Crane and Griffin 1962.
[e]Crane and Griffin 1959.

consistent with dendrochronological corrections of radiocarbon dates for the two sites. (See this Appendix, Table 72.) In occurrence seriation 1 and frequency seriation 1, Diable was later in the sequence than in occurrence seriation 2, where the position was shared with Buyea. Since European trade goods were found at Diable, it is possible that more than one occupation was present at the site. Finally, whereas Chase appeared earlier than Quirk in occurrence seriation 1, they held an equivalent position in occurrence seriation 2 and shared that position with a number of other components. Both Chase and Quirk were associated with European trade goods.

Finally, stylistic trends were observed through the temporal range of the sequence. When established types were used, there was a clear separation between cord impressed or incised rims, collars, or castellations. This separation was one criterion employed for differentiating between the Owasco and Iroquois traditions. Lenig (1965) suggested that cord impression was indigenous to central New York and was replaced by incising *circa* A.D. 1400. With my synthetic classification, the dichotomy between cord impression and incision was not so abrupt. Of the four classes with cord impression as a mode, three terminated before the end of the sequence; but one class (4111) persisted into the historical period.

Collared rims occurred throughout the entire sequence but became increasingly popular close to the terminus. In the synthetic classification, seven

Table 73 Central New York Pottery Types and Sources of Descriptions

1. Carpenter Brook Corded
   Ritchie and MacNeish 1949; p. 108; Figs. 39 b,c; 41 g
2. Levanna Cord on Cord
   Ritchie and MacNeish 1949; p. 110; Fig. 39 g,j
3. Sackett Corded
   Lenig 1965; p. 6; Fig. 1 A,B,C,D
   Includes Owasco Corded Horizontal, Owasco Herringbone, Owasco Platted and Owasco Corded Oblique (Ritchie and MacNeish 1949).
4. Oak Hill Corded
   Lenig 1965; p. 6; Fig. 1 G,H
   Includes Lanor Corded (MacNeish 1952).
5. Kelso Corded
   Lenig 1965; p. 6; Fig. 1 E,F
   Includes Owasco Corded Collar, Bainbridge Collared Incised (Ritchie and MacNeish 1949). Also includes Hummel Corded and Dansville Corded (MacNeish 1952).
6. Canandaiga Plain
   Ritchie and MacNeish 1949; p. 110; Fig. 39 e,f
7. Goodyear Lipped
   Lenig 1965; p. 8; Fig. 1 U
   MacNeish (1952) defined this type as Goodyear Corded.
8. Otstungo Notched
   MacNeish 1952; p. 75; Plate 3:1–3.
9. Rice Diagonal
   MacNeish 1952; p. 74; Plate 29:5–8.
10. Castle Creek Incised Neck
    Ritchie and MacNeish 1949; pp. 114–15; Fig. 40 j,m
11. Deowongo Incised
    Lenig 1965; p. 6; Fig. 1 N,O
12. Garoga Incised
    Lenig 1965; pp. 6–8; Fig. 1 P
    Incudes Cayadutta Incised, Otstungo Incised and Fonda Incised (MacNeish 1952).
13. Wagoner-Syracuse Incised
    Pratt 1976; p. 84
    Includes Wagoner Incised and Syracuse Incised (MacNeish 1952).
14. Durfee Underlined
    MacNeish 1952; p. 60; Plate 25:6–10
15. Onondaga Triangular
    MacNeish 1952; p. 6; Plate 24
16. Chance Incised
    MacNeish 1952; p. 78; Plate 33:4–7
17. Richmond Incised
    MacNeish 1952; p. 66; Plate 31
18. Thurston Incised
    MacNeish 1952; p. 66; Plate 23:1–4
19. Roebuck Low Collar
    MacNeish 1952; p. 61; Plate 25:1–3,5
20. Genoa Frilled
    MacNeish 1952; p. 50; Plate 20

Table 74 Central New York Pottery Occurrence Seriation 1

Component	*Types*																				^{14}C	*Trade*
	1	*2*	*3*	*4*	*5*	*6*	*7*	*8*	*9*	*10*	*11*	*12*	*13*	*14*	*15*	*16*	*17*	*18*	*19*	*20*		
Bach n = 260								X	X			X	X	X	X	X		X	X	X		X
Diable n = 189								X	X			X	X	X	X	X	X	X	X	X		X
Goff n = 226								X	X		X	X	X	X	X	X	X	X				
Garoga n = 1011								X	X		X	X	X			X					1382 ± 107	X
Buyea n = 277								X	X		X	X	X			X						
Getman n = 185				X				X			X	X				X					1382 ± 155	
Nahrwold #1 n = 217			X	X	X			X		X						X					1435 ± 107	
Kelso n = 313			X	X	X		X														1382 ± 107	
Sackett n = 46		X	X		X	X															1187 ± 33	
Round Top n = 491	X	X	X		X																1098 ± 68	
Maxon Derby n = 43	X	X	X																		1098 ± 88	

Table 75 Central New York Pottery Frequency Seriation 1

	Types																	
Component	*1*	*2*	*3*	*4*	*5*	*7*	*8*	*9*	*10*	*11*	*12*	*13*	*14*	*15*	*16*	*17*	*18*	*19*	*20*
Diable							2.1	2.1			27.0	15.9	5.8	36.0	.53	3.2	3.7	.53	3.2
n = 189							4	4			51	30	11	68	1	6	7	1	6
Garoga							3.26	1.78		.39	87.3	5.7			1.48				
n = 1011							33	18		4	883	58			15				
Buyea							12.3	6.9		1.4	57.8	8.3			13.4				
n = 277							34	19		4	160	23			37				
Nichols				.43			4.73	2.73		3.87	46.8	6.16	.29	.43	34.0				.43
n = 696				3			33	19		27	326	43	2	3	237				3
Getman				1.08			4.86			16.75	41.8				35.7				
n = 185				2			9			31	77				66				
Nahrwold #1			2.3	8.3	6.9	.5			76.0	2.8					3.2				
n = 217			5	18	15	1			165	6					7				
Kelso			1.6	3.5	93.9	1.0													
n = 313			5	11	294	3													
Round Top	59.9	30.34	6.1		3.67														
n = 491	294	149	30		18														

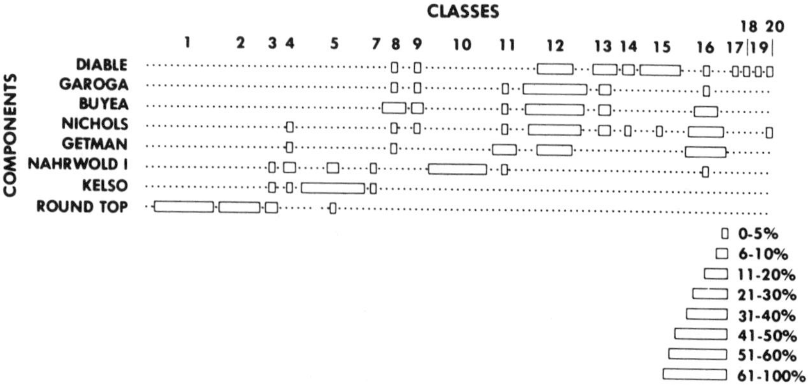

Figure 19. Central New York Pottery Frequency Seriation 1

Table 76 Paradigmatic Classification of Pottery Rim and Lip Attributes for Central New York

Dimension	*Mode*
I. Location of Decoration	1. Rim 2. Lip 3. Rim and Lip 4. Collar 5. Rim and Collar 6. Collar and Lip 7. No Decoration
II. Type of Decoration	1. Cord Impression 2. Incision 3. Impression and Incision 4. Incision and Notching including Gouges 5. Impression and Notching 6. Gouges or Notches 7. No Decoration
III. Collar	1. Present 2. Absent
IV. Castellation	1. Present 2. Absent

classes had collars as a structural feature. Only two of these classes occurred with cord impressions; all others were associated with incision, or incision/gouging. A similar temporal distribution occurred with castellations. Two classes of cord impressions had castellations; three classes with castellations occurred with incising.

The synthetic classification indicated that stylistic diversity, defined by the

Table 77 Assignment of Central New York Pottery Types to Paradigmatic Classes

1122	Carpenter Brook Corded Sackett Corded Owasco Corded Horizontal Owasco Herringbone Owasco Platted Owasco Cord Oblique
2122	Levanna Cord on Cord Canandaiga Plain
2422	Otstungo Notched Rice Diagonal
2522	Goodyear Lipped
3122	Castle Creek Incised
4111	Oak Hill Corded Owasco Corded Collar Bainbridge Collared Incised Hummel Corded Dansville Corded
4211	Chance Incised
4212	Fonda Incised Seed Incised (MacNeish 1952; p. 35; Plate 11:1–5)
4411	Deowongo Incised Durfee Underlined Onondaga Triangular Richmond Incised Roebuck Low Collar Lawson Opposed (MacNeish 1952; p. 13; Plate 1:1–5) Bristol Linear (MacNeish 1952; p. 52; Plate 22:1–2) Genoa Filled
4412	Wagoner-Syracuse Incised Otstungo Incised (MacNeish 1952; p. 77; Plate 31) Cayadutta Incised Cayuga Horizontal (MacNeish 1952; p. 52; Plate 22:3–5) Thurston Incised Ripley Triangular (MacNeish 1952; p. 27; Plate 8:1–4)
5411	Sidey Notched (MacNeish 1952; p. 33; Plate 9:5–8)

largest number of classes represented and the complexity of decoration, occurred during the middle part of the sequence and terminated prior to appearance of European trade goods. In terms of class counts, the earlier stylistic break occurred between Kelso (four classes) and Nahrwold #1 (six classes). Components between Nahrwold #1 and Cameron were represented by at least six classes; following Cameron, class counts decreased to four. Furthermore, number of classes correlated nominally with the complexity of design as seen in classes 4411, 4412, 5411. In these classes, collars tended to be high; well executed and closely space incised designs were confined to the midcollar.

Table 78 Central New York Pottery Occurrence Seriation 2

	Classes										
Component	*1122*	*2122*	*2422*	*2522*	*3122*	*4111*	*4211*	*4212*	*4411*	*4412*	*5411*
Chase*/Quirk*/Atwell Fort*/Temperance House Fort*/Bach (260)/Tuttle (62)/Goff (230)			X					X	X	X	
Cameron (97)			X			X	X	X	X	X	X
Diable (189)/Buyea (303)			X			X	X	X	X	X	
Nichols (696)			X		X	X	X	X	X	X	
Getman (185)			X	X	X	X	X			X	
Nahrwold 1 (217)	X			X	X	X	X			X	
Kelso (320)	X				X	X					
Round Top (491)	X	X				X					
Sackett (46)/Maxon Derby (43)	X	X									

*Sample size not reported.

Table 79 Comparison of Orders Established by Different Pottery Seriations

Occurrence Seriation 1	*Frequency Seriation 1*	*Occurrence Seriation 2*
Bach		Quirk/Chase/Atwell Fort/Temperance House Fort/Bach/Goff/Tuttle
Diable	Diable	
Goff		
Garoga	Garoga	Cameron
Buyea	Buyea	Buyea/Diable
	Nichols	Nichols
Getman	Getman	Getman
Nahrwold 1	Nahrwold 1	Nahrwold 1
Kelso	Kelso	Kelso
Sackett		
Round Top	Round Top	Round Top
Maxon Derby		Maxon Derby/Sackett

Above and below designs were horizontal incisions with gouges or notches. Reed impressions may have extended down from castellations.

Based on this information, I establish three stylistic pottery periods. The earliest period dates roughly from A.D. 1100 to 1400 and is composed of classes 1122, 2122, 3122, 4111. The second period dates to the fifteenth century and lasts until European trade goods appear in central New York. The period is characterized by pottery classes: 2422, 2522, 3122, 4111, 4211, 4212, 4411, 4412, and 5411. The final pottery period coincides with European trade goods and is represented by only four pottery classes: 2422, 4212, 4411, 4412.

CERAMIC PIPE SERIATION The occurrence seriation of ceramic pipes, including whole specimens and fragments, is based on a classification of the shape of the pipe bowl. The bowl of a pipe attaches to the stem and is structurally identified by some type of flare. Eight classes of bowl shape are defined (Table 80), and pipes are placed in the appropriate class based on descriptions or photographs.

Table 81 presents the occurrence seriation of pipe bowls. Sample size ranged from one to fifty-three and the temporal direction was indicated by radiocarbon dates or trade goods. Unlike the pottery seriations, there was considerable disparity between the radiocarbon dates and the relative temporal positions. Nine components (33%) were assigned a relative position in this sequence, and eight of these appeared in one or more of the pottery seriations. Barnes is the only component that did not appear in earlier pottery sequences.

Table 80 Type Descriptions of Shapes of Pipe Bowls

1. Straight Sided Bowl:	No change in dimension of bowl from base to lip.
2. Conical Bowl:	Bowl is constricted at the stem end but flares to the lip. Flare is not as extreme as in the trumpet form (Class 6). Class includes Tuck's (1971) prototrumpet form.
3. Barrel Bowl:	The form is sometimes described as bulbous. The orifice of the bowl is smaller than the midsection.
4. Vasiform Bowl:	Like the barrel form, the bowl has a bulbous section. Above the bulb, the bowl has an extension. Bowl length is longer than the barrel. This form includes Tuck's (1971) puffed sleeve form.
5. Square Bowl:	The bowl is square or rectangular in cross section and shows a slight constriction at the stem end.
6. Trumpet Bowl:	The bowl flares out from the mid section. The bowl and stem intersection are at right angles to each other. The shape resembles a trumpet or a morning glory.
7. Collared Form:	An extra fillet of clay is added to form a collar which begins just below the lip and extends to just above the base of the bowl.
8. Effigy Bowl:	The bowl may be in the shape of a human or nonhuman face.

Table 81 Central New York Occurrence Seriation of Ceramic Pipe Bowls

	Types									
European Component	*1*	*2*	*3*	*4*	*5*	*6*	*7*	*8*	*Trade Goods*	*Dates ¹⁴C (A.D.)*
Garoga (n = 23)/Diable (n = 3)				X				X		1382 ± 107
Barnes (n = 19)						X	X	X	X	
Burke (n = 15)		X				X	X	X		1549 ± 89
Furnace Brook (n = 53)	X	X	X	X	X	X	X			1333 ± 52
Howlett Hill (n = 10)		X	X	X	X					
Round Top (n = 14)/ Chamberlain (n = 1)/ Sackett (n = 2)		X								1098 ± 68 1294 ± 67 1198 ± 88

Classification and Analysis of European Trade Goods

Three temporal analyses are presented: (1) an occurrence seriation of metal objects; (2) cumulative frequencies of European aboriginal assemblages; and (3) frequencies of glass trade beads. The goal of these analyses was to separate sixteenth- from seventeenth-century components.

OCCURRENCE SERIATION OF METAL OBJECTS Metal objects probably first reached populations in New York through diffusion rather than direct interaction. Following European settlement, metal objects were more readily available; and greater availability should be reflected in both the type and the frequency of metal present in aboriginal assemblages. I developed a paradigmatic classification for metal objects to examine the proposed trend (Table 82). After classifying objects, classes were ordered temporally (Table 83).

In the classification, brass/copper was defined as a single mode since published descriptions typically did not differentiate between the two raw materials. 90% (10/11) of all components associated with European trade goods were assigned a relative position. Six of these components were ordered in one or more of the ceramic seriations; three components, Beecher, Marshall and Thurston, were ordered for the first time.

The seriation met the expectations regarding the temporal behavior of metal objects. Sample size increased through time, and scrap preceded shaped objects. Barnes, the earliest component in the sequence, was represented by a single piece of brass/copper scrap. Iron scrap was added next and was followed by shaped brass/copper objects. In assemblages of the most recent components, which Pratt (1976) thought postdated 1613, copper/brass scrap disappeared, but the other classes continued to be represented.

CUMULATIVE FREQUENCY ANALYSIS This analysis examined the number and diversity of classes of European items through time. Cumulative frequency

Table 82 Paradigmatic Classification for Metal from Central New York

	Form	
Type	*Unshaped*	*Shaped*
Brass/Copper	Class 1	Class 3
Iron	Class 2	Class 4

Table 83 Central New York Occurrence Seriation of Metal

	Classes			
Component	*1*	*2*	*3*	*4*
Beecher (n = 30)/Thurston (n = 66)/Marshall*		X	X	X
Bach (n = 9)/Diable (n = 10)/ Cameron (n = 144)		X	X	
Chase (n = 4)	X	X	X	
Quirk (n = 4)	X			
Atwell Fort (n = 6)/Barnes (n = 1)	X			

*Sample size could not be determined. Counts of kettle parts not given by Pratt (1976).

curves were developed from seven classes of European function (Table 84). All objects, exclusive of European trade beads, were assigned to the appropriate class based on published descriptions and photographs.

Although sample size of components treated in this analysis remained exactly the same as in the occurrence seriation of metal objects (90%), one component (Garoga) was added; and another (Bach) was deleted. Table 85 summarizes, by component, percentages and counts for each class.

Differences in curves suggested that there are three distinct temporal intervals (Figure 20). Although four components, Barnes, Garoga, Atwell Fort and Quirk, were assigned to the first interval (Figure 20A), Barnes was excluded from the graph because a cumulative frequency of one is a single point. All components, except Barnes, were characterized by two functional classes: Ornamentation (class 4) and unidentified function or scrap (class 6). There were two components in the second interval, Diable and Chase, both of which were characterized by three classes of European objects (Figure 20B). Both shared

Table 84 Central New York Functional Classification of European Trade Goods

1. Eating	Ceramics Bowls Kettles
2. Subsistence	Harpoons Projectiles of all types Guns Knives Tomahawks
3. Dress	Needles Buttons Cloth Braid
4. Ornamentation	Beads Bangles Rings Earrings Pendants
5. Construction	Adzes Axes Chisels Wedges Nails Awls Picks
6. Function unidentified	Scrap metal
7. Smoking	Pipe stems Pipe bowls

Table 85 Component Percentages and Counts for Classes of European Function

	Classes						
Component	*1*	*2*	*3*	*4*	*5*	*6*	*7*
Thurston (76)	22.4 17	44.7 34	2.6 2	9.2 7	2.6 2	6.6 5	11.8 9
Beecher (34)	14.7 5	35.3 12	5.9 2	5.9 2	32.4 11	5.9 2	
Cameron (143)	18.2 26	13.3 19	2.8 4	52.5 75	11.9 17	1.4 2	
Diable (10)		20.0 2		70.0 7	10.0 1		
Chase (4)				25.0 1	25.0 1	50.0 2	
Quirk (2)				50.0 1		50.0 1	
Atwell (6)				33.0 2		66.0 4	
Garoga (2)				50.0 1		50.0 1	
Barnes (1)						100.0 1	

Class 4 (ornamentation) and Class 5 (construction). Chase had two pieces of scrap (Class 6), and at Diable, one brass spear point and one brass knife blade (Class 2) were recorded.

The most recent interval of time, represented by three components (Cameron, Beecher and Thurston), presumably dated to the seventeenth century (Figure 20C). Six or seven classes of European function were present within these assemblages, representing 100% increase over the previous temporal interval. New classes included: eating (class 1), dress (class 3) and smoking (class 7).

FREQUENCIES OF GLASS TRADE BEADS The popularity of glass beads as a trade item increased after the development of the fur trade; therefore, components thought to date to the seventeenth century should have higher frequencies of glass beads than those that date to the sixteenth century. To determine if this trend was correct, I analyzed aboriginal assemblages used in the cumulative frequency analysis in terms of frequencies of trade beads (Table 86).

The analysis verified the suggested trend. Whereas components placed in the two preseventeenth-century intervals had no glass beads, all three seventeenth-century components had beads in frequencies greater than 50%.

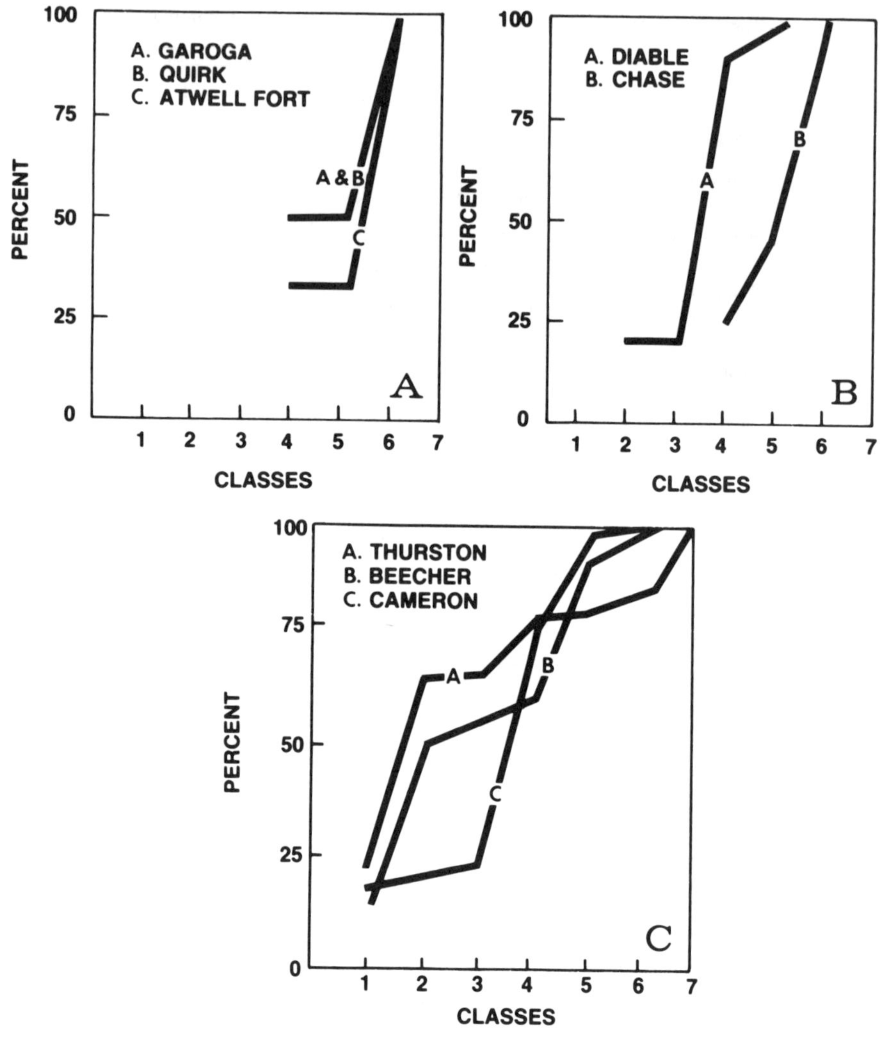

Figure 20. Cumulative Frequencies of European Trade Goods from Central New York

Table 86 Frequencies of Glass Trade Beads in Central New York

Component	*Glass Beads (n)*	*Trade Goods (Total)*	*Percentage (Beads/Total)*
Cameron	505	650	78.0
Beecher	49	83	59.0
Thurston	441	517	87.0
Diable	0		0.0
Chase	0		0.0
Barnes	0		0.0
Garoga	0		0.0
Atwell	0		0.0
Quirk	0		0.0

In summary, the relative positions of components ordered through the temporal analyses of European materials is presented in Table 87. With two minor exceptions, orders are comparable. Whereas Chase appeared earlier than Diable in the occurrence seriation of metal, the two held an equivalent position in the other analyses. Cameron appeared earlier in the occurrence seriation of metal than it did in the other analyses.

Based on analyses of European material, I establish two periods: the earliest dates from the beginning of European trade goods and lasts until the seventeenth century. The second period dates to the seventeenth century.

SETTLEMENT DATA

Twenty-five components were analyzed to determine trends in regional population. Table 88 lists the county location and source of the original description. Table 89 presents measurements of settlement area and roofed area of houses by period and component.

Table 87 Comparison of Component Assignment from Analyses of European Trade Goods

Occurrence Seriation of Metal	*Cumulative Frequencies*	*Glass Trade Beads Frequencies*
Thurston/Beecher/Marshall	Thurston/Beecher/Cameron	Thurston/Beecher/Cameron
Bach/Cameron/Diable	Chase/Diable	Chase/Diable
Chase		
Quirk/Atwell Fort/Barnes	Quirk/Atwell Fort/Garoga/ Barnes	Quirk/Atwell Fort/Barnes/ Garoga

Table 88 Central New York Settlement Summary

Component	*County*	*Settlement Area*	*Excavated Houses*	*Source*
Sackett	Ontario	X	3	Ritchie and Funk 1973
Chamberlain	Onondaga	X	2	Tuck 1971
Furnace Brook	Onondaga	X	4	Tuck 1971
Howlett Hill	Onondaga	X	4	Tuck 1967, 1971
Burke	Onondaga	X	0	Tuck 1971
Barnes	Onondaga	X	0	Tuck 1971
Maxon Derby	Onondaga	X	3	Ritchie and Funk 1973
Quirk	Onondaga	X	0	Tuck 1971
Kelso	Onondaga	X	8	Ritchie 1967; Ritchie and Funk 1973
Temperance	Onondaga-Madison	X	1	Tuck 1971
Chase	Onondaga-Madison	X	0	Tuck 1971
Cameron	Oneida-Madison	X	0	Pratt 1976
Buyea	Madison	X	1	Pratt 1976
Goff	Madison	X	0	Pratt 1976
Diable	Madison	X	0	Pratt 1976
Bach	Madison	X	1	Pratt 1976
Beecher	Madison	X	0	Pratt 1976
Thurston	Madison	X	1	Pratt 1976
Marshall	Madison	X	0	Pratt 1976
Atwell Fort	Madison	X	1	Tuck 1971
Getman	Montgomery	X	5	Ritchie and Funk 1973
Caughnawaga	Montgomery	X	11	Grassman 1969
Round Top	Broome	X	2	Ritchie and Funk 1973
Nahrwold #1	Schoharie	X	2	Ritchie and Funk 1973
Garoga	Fulton	X	8	Ritchie and Funk 1973

Table 89 Measurements of Settlement Areas and Roofed Area of Houses by Component and Period

Period	*Component*	*Settlement Area (Hectares)*	*Houses*	
			House #	*Size (m²)*
I	Sackett	.81	F.1	12.30
			F.2	10.20
			F.7	15.70
	Chamberlain	.71	H.1	177.70
			H.2	106.84
	Furnace Brook	1.01	H.1	174.20
			H.2	259.70
			H.3	419.50
			H.6	100.30
	Howlett Hill	.81	H.1	775.70
			H.3	71.50
			H.2a	183.80
			H.2b	239.30
	Kelso	.81	H.1	56.60
			H.5	49.02
			H.3	261.60
			H.4	228.90
			H.6	23.80
			H.9	262.60
			H.11	77.30
			H.12	29.70
	Round Top	.27	H.1	190.80
			H.2	149.20
	Maxon Derby	.81	H.A	141.70
			H.C	42.70
			H.D	31.60
II	Temperance House Fort	1.82	H.1	209.30
	Nahrwold #1	.81	H.1	63.30
			H.2	98.10
	Burke	1.01		
	Buyea	1.42	H.1	189.00
	Getman	.48	H.1	175.80
			H.2	57.60
			H.3	214.60
			H.4	233.00
			H.5	98.10

(*continued*)

Table 89 (*Continued*)

Period	*Component*	*Settlement Area (Hectares)*	*Houses*	
			House #	*Size (m^2)*
III	Garoga	1.01	H.1	286.14
			H.2	393.90
			H.3	418.10
			H.4	347.50
			H.5	347.50
			H.7	276.90
			H.8	379.10
			H.9	393.90
	Diable	.81		
	Bach	.74	H.1	61.90
	Atwell Fort	1.20	H.1	50.90
	Chase	1.62		
	Quirk	1.01		
	Barnes	2.83		
IV	Caughnawaga	.59	H.1	182.03
			H.2	156.70
			H.3	164.02
			H.4	127.40
			H.5	183.40
			H.6	143.70
			H.8	182.90
			H.9	207.50
			H.10	212.80
			H.11	195.20
			H.12	215.80
	Beecher	1.10		
	Thurston	1.60	H.1	222.00
	Marshall	1.80		
	Cameron	.92		

Appendix C The Middle Missouri

TEMPORAL ORDERS

Summary of Temporal Orders

Thirty-seven components are ordered by at least one of the five temporal analyses (Table 90) used to develop the chronology of the Middle Missouri.

Radiocarbon Assays

Although radiometric, tree ring, and some thermoluminescence dates are available for components in the Middle Missouri, this analysis uses only carbon 14. Dendrochronological dates of components are too few in number (Weakley 1971; Will 1946) to be useful in this analysis; dates by thermoluminescence appeared in press (Ahler and Swenson 1985) too late to be part of this study.

54% (20/37) of all components ordered by one or more temporal methods were associated with at least one radiocarbon date (Table 91). Of these, eighteen (90%) had two or more dates, and four (20%) had four or more dates. The reliability of radiocarbon dates for the Middle Missouri was somewhat better than in the other two test cases since so many components had more than a single date. Nonetheless, severe biases including ambiguities in the determination of dates limit the utility of these data.

Ten components have ^{14}C determinations more recent that A.D. 1400, and several dates are so recent that they can not be calibrated dendrochronologically. Since the magnitude of potential error increases in the recent period, reliability of all these dates is suspect. Nine components (39 ST 9A, 39 ST 9/232B, 32 OL 16, 39 HU 1, 32 OL 14, 39 ST 238, 39 ST 11, 39 LM 232, 39 ST 16) are assigned chronological positions solely on radiometric determinations, and five of the nine have dates more recent than A.D. 1400. Although most of

Table 90 Component Summary of Middle Missouri Ordering Methods

Component		*Radiocarbon Date*	*Pottery Frequency Seriation*	*Metal Occurrence Seriation*	*Cumulative Frequencies*	*Glass Trade Beads Frequencies*
32 ME 5	—Deapolis		X	X	X	X
32 ME 8	—Amahami		X	X	X	X
32 ML 39	—Nightwalker's Butte		X		X	X
32 ME 15	—Rock Village		X		X	X
32 ME 12	—Big Hidatsa				X	X
32 ME 11	—Sakakawea		X	X	X	X
32 ST 14	—Phillips Ranch		X	X	X	X
39 HU 26	—Spotted Bear		X	X	X	X
39 DW 2	—Four Bear			X	X	X
39 ST 15	—Indian Creek			X	X	X
39 ST 6	—Buffalo Pasture		X		X	X
39 LM 215	—Peterson			X	X	X
39 ST 30	—Dodd (Stanley Phase)		X		X	X
39 WW 7	—Swan Creek C/D		X		X	X
39 WW 7	—Swan Creek B		X		X	X
32 OL 16	—Bagnell	X				
39 CO 1	—Demery		X			
39 DW 234	—Molstad	X	X			
32 MO 11	—Huff	X	X			
32 EM 10	—Shermer		X			

Table 90 (*Continued*)

39 ST 9	—La Roche A	X	
39 ST 9/232	—La Roche B	X	
32 SI 19	—South Cannonball	X	
39 HU 6	—Arzberger	X	X
39 HU 1	—Thomas Riggs	X	
39 ST 238	—Durkin	X	
32 OL 14	—Cross Ranch	X	
39 LM 232	—Pretty Head	X	
39 ST 30	—Dodd (Anderson Phase)	X	X
39 LM 208	—Jiggs Thompson	X	X
39 ST 223	—John Ketchen	X	
39 ST 11	—Fay Tolton	X	
32 ME 1	—Clark's Creek	X	
39 ST 9	—La Roche C	X	
39 LM 209	—Langdeau	X	X
32 SI 4	—Paul Brave	X	X
39 ST 16	—Breeden A	X	

Table 91 Middle Missouri Radiocarbon Dates

Component	*Dates (n)*	*Laboratory Number*	*Uncorrected Date (A.D.)*	*Weighted Average*[a] *(A.D.)*	*Dendrochronological Correction*[b] *(A.D.)*
32 ST 9 (A)[d]	2	SI-106	1640 ± 55	1649 ± 37	*
		SI-97	1660 ± 60		
39 ST 9/232 (B)[d]	3	SI-95	1680 ± 50		
		SI-169	1500 ± 120	1604 ± 37	*
		SI-104	1520 ± 60		
39 DW 234[c]	4	I-721	1675 ± 85		
		I-720	1565 ± 95		
		SI-25	1475 ± 100	1586 ± 37	1586 ± 53
		SI-50	1590 ± 50		
32 OL 16[c]	3	WIS-540	1570 ± 55		
		WIS-541	1575 ± 50	1605 ± 31	c.1560
		WIS-542	1690 ± 60		
39 HU 6[f]	2	M-1126	1461 ± 50		
		M-1126a	1531 ± 200	1548 ± 49	1548 ± 62
32 MO 11[c]	9	SI-178		1640 ± 190	
		SI-179	1480 ± 90		
		SI-180	1770 ± 120		
		SI-181	1420 ± 100		
		SI-182	1180 ± 140	1490 ± 45	1458 ± 59
		SI-183	"Modern"		
		SI-446	1560 ± 130		
		SI-447	1450 ± 130		
		SI-448	1350 ± 330		
39 HU 1[c]	2	M-838	1220 ± 100	1482 ± 62	1451 ± 73
		NWV-49	1650 ± 80		
32 OL 14[c]	2	M-2368	1530 ± 100	1445 ± 71	1416 ± 81
		M-2369	1360 ± 100		
39 ST 9C[c]	2	SI-105	1380 ± 55	1381 ± 52	1359 ± 64
		SI-170	1390 ± 150		
39 ST 238[c]	2	WIS-743	1310 ± 55	1303 ± 41	1288 ± 51
		WIS-746	1295 ± 60		
39 LM 232A[c]	1	SI-166	1300 ± 140	—	1285 ± 143
39 LM 208B[c]	2	I-1186	1280 ± 120	1280 ± 85	1267 ± 90
		I-1187	1280 ± 120		
32 ME 1[c]		M-2366	1280 ± 100	1235 ± 74	1227 ± 80
		M-2367	1180 ± 110		
32 SI 19[c]	4	I-4202	1110 ± 90		
		I-4203	1340 ± 95	1224 ± 47	1216 ± 56
		I-4204	1320 ± 95		
		I-4205	1130 ± 100		
39 ST 223[c]	4	SI-378	1260 ± 140		
		SI-477	1140 ± 60	1174 ± 31	1170 ± 44
		WIS-759	1120 ± 60		
		WIS-762	1225 ± 50		

(*continued*)

Table 91 (*Continued*)

Component	*Dates (n)*	*Laboratory Number*	*Uncorrected Date (A.D.)*	*Weighted Average*[a] *(A.D.)*	*Dendrochronological Correction*[b] *(A.D.)*
39 ST 30[c] (Anderson Ph.)	1	M-843	1150 ± 160	—	1148 ± 104
39 LM 209[c]	3	SI-51	1000 ± 65		
		SI-54	1100 ± 55	1080 ± 36	1084 ± 48
		SI-57	1140 ± 70		
32 SI 4[c]	2	M-2364	1030 ± 100	1065 ± 71	1070 ± 77
		M-2365	1100 ± 100		
39 ST 11[c]	4	M-1082	1090 ± 75		
		WIS-722	1065 ± 50	1060 ± 34	1065 ± 46
		WIS-728	1030 ± 60		
		NWV-50	1100 ± 70		
39 ST 16[c]	3	M-608	710 ± 75		
		WIS-513	1220 ± 55	1023 ± 36	1030 ± 48
		WIS-548	990 ± 60		

[a]Long and Rippeteau 1974.
[b]Damon et al. 1974.
[c]Theissen 1977.
[d]Uncorrected dates from Hoffman 1968.
[e]Uncorrected dates from Hoffman 1967.
[f]Uncorrected dates from Wood 1967.
*Too recent for calibration.

the nine components are also associated with pottery samples, classificatory or stratigraphic problems precluded employing samples in seriation analyses. Where possible, traits of each of the nine components have been compared with those of other components dated radiometrically or ordered by relative methods, but the absence of independent evidence for these components casts some doubt on their chronological placement.

Ceramic Classification and Seriations

Although the analysis of stylistic attributes of pottery has played an important chronological role in the Middle Missouri, the classification of pottery is far from consistent.

The type/variety system is the classification most consistently employed (for example, Caldwell and Jensen 1969; Hurt 1954a, 1957; Lehmer 1966; Lehmer and Jones 1968; Wood 1967; Wood and Woolworth 1964), but other classificatory schemes exist (for example, Ahler and Swenson 1985; Deetz 1965; Hoffman 1967, 1968; Spaulding 1956). Even within the type/variety system, there is no archaeological consensus on weighting of attributes. Lehmer (1954b, 1966) and Smith (1951, 1977) placed equal emphasis on rim form and decoration; Hurt (1957), on the other hand, placed greater emphasis on decoration with the result that different shaped rims were placed within the same type. Furthermore, the penchant for naming new styles has resulted in a plethora of types, varieties or sub-varieties, that, in many instances, are component specific, [See for example, Arzberger Diagonal Incised (Spaulding 1956) or Deapolis Collared (Lehmer et al. 1978).] The opposite tendency is also present. Archaeologists have simply transferred existing type/variety names between local areas. In some instances, the transfer is justified stylistically; in other cases, the transfer is not justified, and the same name may refer to quite different stylistic expressions, (for example, Stanley Braced in North and South Dakota).

Because of these problems, I have built a paradigm that synthesizes the variability in existing pottery classifications. The classification utilized nominal characteristics in the form of dimensions and modes (Dunnell 1971) of existing pottery descriptions, photographs and profile drawings (Table 92). The classification is used to order ceramic assemblages by seriations. Although modes of each dimension are designed to be mutually exclusive, the nature of descriptions necessitated that mode (1) of Dimension I and mode (3) of Dimension III have combined attributes.

Once established, eighty-four pottery descriptions were assigned to one of the synthetic classes (Table 93). Scale of placement was variable. In some instances, all varieties of a single type were placed in the same class; in other cases, varieties were placed in different classes; and sometimes, certain sherds of a single variety were placed in different classes.

Using these classes, I ordered 20 (53%) components listed in Table 90 through frequency seriations. To control for the problem of spatial diffusion of style, I divided the Middle Missouri into three smaller areas (Figure 21). Area 1 extended south from the north bank of the Knife River to the South Dakota border; area 2 extended south from the South Dakota border to the north bank of the Cheyenne River. Area 3 extended south from the south bank of the Cheyenne to the mouth of the White River. Direction of seriations is suggested by radiocarbon dates or by the presence of European trade goods.

The frequency seriation from area 1 (Table 94) placed eight components in a relative order; and, according to radiocarbon dates and the presence of Euro-

Table 92 Middle Missouri Paradigmatic Classification of Rim Characteristics

I	Rim Shape	1. Straight to Flared
		2. S-Curve
II	Extra Clay to Rim	1. Brace
		2. Collar
		3. Unmodified
III	Rim Decoration	1. Incision
		2. Cord Impression
		3. Tool Impression and/or Punctates
		4. Finger Impression
		5. No Decoration

Table 93 Assignment of Middle Missouri Pottery Types and Varieties to Paradigmatic Classes

111	La Roche Class 1, var. 2; Hoffman 1967; pp. 39–40; Pls. 11a,b; 12a–c,e
	Le Beau Cord Impressed, var. d; Hurt 1957; p. 39
	Mitchell Incised; Hurt 1954a; Caldwell and Jensen 1969; p. 45
112	Knife River Cord Impressed; Lehmer et al. 1978; pp. 190–195; Figs. 8.1; 8.2; 8.9a–f
	Stanley Cord Impressed; Lehmer 1954b; p. 44; Pl. 13
	Le Beau Cord Impressed, var. a,b,c,e; Hurt 1957; pp. 38–39; Fig. 21, Photo 13; Fig. 26
113	Stanley Tool Impressed; Lehmer 1954b; p. 45; Pl. 14
	Knife River Tool Impressed; Lehmer et al. 1978; pp. 195–196; Fig. 8.3
	Riggs Filleted Rim; Sperry 1968; p. 40; Pls. 6I–L; 7A–B; 9D–E
	La Roche Class 2, var. 1; Hoffman 1968; p. 40; Pls. 12a; 13b,d–h; 14a; 17c
	Iona Indented; Smith and Grange 1957; pp. 98–100; Smith and Johnson 1968; pp. 16–17; Pl. 5a–h
114	Stanley Pinched; Lehmer and Jones 1968; p. 26; Pl. 9e (Originally defined as Stanley Wavy Rim)
	Knife River Pinched; Lehmer et al. 1978; pp. 196–197; Figs. 8.4a–f
115	Stanley Plain; Lehmer 1954b; pp. 45–46
	Knife River Plain; Lehmer et al. 1978; pp. 198–199; Figs. 8.5,8.9
121	Arzberger Crosshatched; Spaulding 1956; pp. 141–145; Pl. 9
	Arzberger Diagonal Incised; Spaulding 1956; pp. 145–148; Pl. 10
	Arzberger Horizontal Incised; Spaulding 1956; pp. 139–141; Pl. 8
	Cadotte Collared, Varieties A,B,C; Smith and Johnson 1968; pp. 15–16; Pl. 4f
	Stuart Horizontal Incised and Stuart Incised Triangle; Hurt 1954a; Caldwell and Jensen 1969; p. 44; Pl. 21a
122	Columbe Collared Cord Impressed; Lehmer and Jones 1968; p. 40; Pl. 7e–k
	Deapolis Collared Rim; Lehmer et al. 1978; pp. 208–211; Figs. 8.4g–i; 8.10a
	Cadotte Collared, Varieties a,b,c,d; Smith and Johnson 1968; pp. 15–16; Pl. 4a,b,e,g
	Columbe Collared Tool Impressed; Lehmer and Jones 1968; p. 29; Pl. 7e–k
	Stuart Collared Tool Impressed; Caldwell and Jensen 1969; p. 44; Pl. 20g–h
124	Cadotte Collared, Variety e; Smith and Johnson 1968; pp. 15–16; Pl. 4a,c
	Columbe Collared Plain; Lehmer and Jones 1968; p. 29; Pl. 7e–k
125	Arzberger Plain; Spaulding 1956; pp. 137–139; Pl. 7
131	Iona Horizontal Incised; Smith and Grange 1957; Smith and Johnson 1968; p. 18; Pl. 41
	Knife River Incised; Lehmer et al. 1978; p. 198
	Hughes Group; Spaulding 1956; pp. 151–164
	La Roche Class 1, Var. 2; Hoffman 1968; p. 40; Pls. 11d–f; 12d,f,h, 16b
	La Roche Class 4; Hoffman 1968; p. 41; Pls. 15c; 17g
	Molstad Group 6, varieties 1,2; Hoffman 1967; pp. 39–41; Pls. 11a,c; 12b; 14c–d,f; 15g; 16a–b; 17a,b,f,g
	Molstad Group 7; Hoffman 1967; pp. 41–42; Pls. 19b–d; 20c
	Nordvold Horizontal Incised; Hurt 1957; pp. 44–45; Fig. 21; Photo 18
	Riggs Incised; Wood and Woolworth 1964; Sperry 1968
	Akaska Stab and Drag, Variety B; Hurt 1954b; pp. 45–46
	Chamberlain Incised Triangle and Chamberlain Horizontal Incised; Hurt 1954a; Caldwell and Jensen 1969; p. 43; Pl. 20a,b
	Grey Cloud Horizontal Incised; Smith and Grange 1957; pp. 102–103; Figs. 4s–u; Pls. 30k–m
	Iona Diagonal Incised; Smith and Grange 1957; Smith and Johnson 1968; p. 18

(*continued*)

Table 93 (*Continued*)

132	Anderson Hi Rim; Lehmer 1954b; p. 46; Pl. 17 Anderson Incised; Caldwell and Jensen 1969; p. 42; Pl. 15f–h Chamberlain Cord Impressed; Hurt 1954a; Caldwell and Jensen 1969; pp. 42–43 Molstad Group 5; Hoffman 1967; pp. 37–38; Pls. 14a,h; 15b,d,e Steamboat Cord Wrapped Rod; Hurt 1957; pp. 43–44; Fig. 23
133	Akaska Tool Impressed; Hurt 1957; pp. 38–39 Le Beau Punctate; Hurt 1957; p. 40; Fig. 21, Photo 19; Fig. 25 Riggs Punctate; Sperry 1968; p. 40; Pl. 6E–H Anderson Tool Impressed; Caldwell and Jensen 1969; p. 42; Pls. 14; 15b–d; 18d Talking Crow Indented; Lehmer and Jones 1968; p. 30 Le Beau Cord Impressed, var. c; Hurt 1957; pp. 38–39
134	Riggs Pinched; Lehmer and Jones 1968; p. 30 Talking Crow Pinched; Lehmer and Jones 1968; p. 30 Le Beau Finger Indented; Hurt 1957; p. 39; Figs. 21:7–10; Fig. 25
135	Talking Crow Indented; Smith 1977; p. 57; Pl. IXi–r Talking Crow Brushed; Smith 1977; p. 57; Pl. IXf–h Talking Crow Straight Rim; Smith 1977; pp. 58–59; Pl. VIII Talking Crow Plain; Lehmer and Jones 1968; p. 30 Riggs Plain; Hurt 1953; Wood and Woolworth 1964; pp. 15–17; Pls. 3 b,d–h; 6e Akaska Plain; Hurt 1957; p. 46 Riggs Decorated Lip; Sperry 1968; pp. 38–39; Pl. 6c–d Anderson Plain; Lehmer 1954b; pp. 48–49; Pl. 17; Caldwell and Jensen 1969; p. 43 Hughes Group; See Class 131 La Roche Class 2, Variety 2; Hoffman 1968; p. 41; Pl. 14b–e,g La Roche Class 5; Hoffman 1968; p. 42; Pls. 15b; 17e,h Le Beau Plain; Hurt 1957; p. 40; Fig. 25 Molstad Group 3; Hoffman 1967; pp. 35–36; Pls. 14a,h; 15b,d,e
221	Arzberger Diagonal Incised; See Class 121 Arzberger Horizontal Incised; See Class 121 Marken Horizontal Incised and Marken Incised Triangle; Caldwell and Jensen 1969; p. 40; Pls. 16i,17c Molstad Group 8; Hoffman 1967; pp. 42–43; Pl. 20b
222	Ft. Rice Cord Impressed; Wood and Woolworth 1964; p. 100; Pls. 11d–h,j–l Marken Cord Impressed Triangle and Marken Cord Impressed Horizontal; Caldwell and Jensen 1969; p. 40; Pl. 16d
225	Marken Plain; Caldwell and Jensen 1969; p. 41
231	Akaska Stab and Drag, Variety A; See Class 131 Foreman Incised Triangle; Hurt 1954a; Caldwell and Jensen 1969; p. 39; Pl. 16b,c Foreman Incised Horizontal and Foreman Incised Crosshatched; Caldwell and Jensen 1969; p. 39 Fort Yates Incised; Wood and Woolworth 1964; Lehmer 1966; pp. 30–31; Pl. 7 Iona S-Rim Incised; Smith and Grange 1957; p. 101; Smith and Johnson 1968; pp. 18–19; Pl. 5i–p La Roche Class 3; Hoffman 1968; p. 41; Pls. 14f,h,i; 16a La Roche Class 6; Hoffman 1968; p. 41; Pls. 15e; 17d,f Le Beau S-Rim Incised; Lehmer et al. 1978; pp. 201–202 Rygh Rainbow Incised; Hurt 1957; p. 42; Fig. 21, Photos 1–2p; Fig. 23, Photos 1–8 Molstad Group 1; Hoffman 1967; pp. 31–34; Pls. 11b,d,e; 12a; 13a; 14a; 17b

(*continued*)

Table 93 (*Continued*)

232	Foreman Horizontal Cord Impressed; Lehmer 1954b; p. 47; Caldwell and Jensen 1969; pp. 38–39; Pls. 15i,j; 16a; 19b Foreman Cord Impressed; Hurt 1954a; Caldwell and Jensen 1969; p. 39; Pl. 16e Fort Yates Cord Impressed; Wood and Woolworth 1964; Lehmer 1966; pp. 30–31; Pl. 7 Le Beau Cord Wrapped Rod; Hurt 1957; Lehmer et al. 1978; pp. 200–201 Le Beau S-Rim Horizontal Cord Impressed; Hurt 1957; p. 41; Fig. 21, Photo 5; Fig. 22, Photos 1–6 La Roche Class 6; See Class 231 Molstad Group 4; Hoffman 1967; pp. 36–37; Pls. 16c,e; 17e
233	Le Beau S-Rim Punctate; Hurt 1957; p. 43
235	Fort Yates Plain; Lehmer 1966; pp. 30–31; Pl. 7 Foreman Plain; Lehmer 1954b; pp. 47–48 Le Beau Plain; Lehmer et al. 1978; p. 203 Molstad Group 2; Hoffman 1967; pp. 34–35; Pl. 15c,f

pean trade goods, the seriation lasted from the eleventh century into the seventeenth century. Of the fourteen classes present, only class 135 is bimodal. Two style periods are evidenced in this seriation.

In the earliest period, unmodified S-Rims that were incised, cord impressed or plain were most popular. During the second pottery period, coincident with European material in North Dakota, these rims all but disappeared and were replaced by braced, straight/flared rims. All decorative modes, except incision, were present on these rims.

As indicated by the radiocarbon date from 39 DW 234, the frequency seriation from area 2 incorporated a relatively short period of time (Table 95). Although the sequence is too short to suggest a definite stylistic pattern, I noted certain similarities and differences with the seriation from area 1.

Although unmodified S-Rims were present in area 2 prior to European trade goods, they persisted after the appearance of European material in frequencies greater than 10%. As distinct from area 1, unmodified straight rim classes were well represented and persisted through the sequence. The greatest similarity between the two seriations occurred in the straight and braced rim classes, where the highest frequencies were obtained after the appearance of European trade goods. All decorative modes were present on these rims. Since, in terms of styles, the area 2 seriation agrees with the pattern found in area 1, it is suggested that two pottery periods may also have been present in area 2.

The frequency seriation from area 3 ordered eight components (Table 96) and, as indicated by radiocarbon dates and the presence of European trade goods, the sequence was as long as that for area 1. Sixteen classes were present in this seriation, two of which (class 112 and 221) were not unimodal. As in the other seriations, two stylistic periods appeared to be present. The earlier period began in the mid eleventh century and lasted until the seventeenth century. The second period began sometime in the seventeenth century.

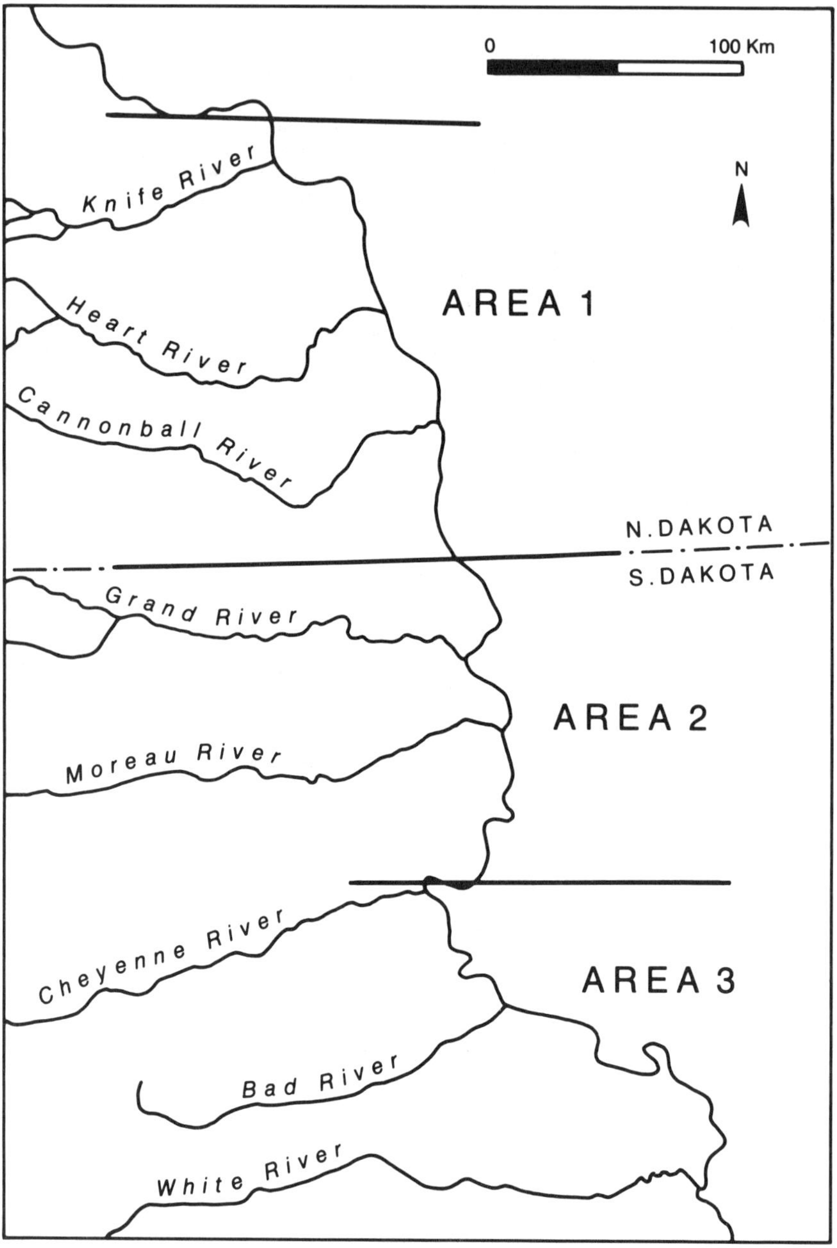

Figure 21. Middle Missouri Seriation Areas

Table 94 Middle Missouri Area 1 Pottery Frequency Seriation

	Classes														
Component	*111*	*112*	*113*	*114*	*115*	*125*	*131*	*132*	*133*	*134*	*135*	*231*	*232*	*235*	*Trade*	^{14}C *Date (A.D.)*
32 ME 5 (329)		30.1 99	2.4 8	0.3 1	54.7 180	10.9 36							1.5 5		X	
32 ME 8 (555)	1.4 8	31.4 174	2.3 13	6.5 36	43.2 240						6.8 37	6.7 36	0.9 5	1.1 6	X	
32 ME 11 (415)	0.5 2	56.6 235	5.8 24	4.3 18	30.6 127	2.2 9									X	
32 ML 39 (394)		49.5 195	12.4 49	8.4 33	23.2 92	4.1 15				0.3 1	0.3 1		2.0 8		X	
32 ME 15 (371)		39.6 147	11.1 41	23.5 87	24.8 92	1.1 4									X	
32 MO 11 (625)			25.1 157		1.1 7						19.6 121	2.2 14	52.2 326			1458 ± 59
32 EM 10 (1541)			31.6 487				0.1 2		20.4 314	0.06 1	10.8 167	4.3 67	28.6 441	4.0 62		
32 SI 4 (489)							12.3 60			5.3 26	48.5 237	16.2 30	27.8 136			1070 ± 77

Table 95 Middle Missouri Area 2 Pottery Frequency Seriation

Component	Classes																Trade	^{14}C Date (A.D.)
	111	*112*	*113*	*114*	*115*	*121*	*131*	*132*	*133*	*134*	*135*	*231*	*232*	*233*	*234*	*235*		
39 WW 7(B)	4.4	9.5	5.9		0.6		1.0	2.6	29.5	16.1	4.3	13.4	11.6	1.0			X	
(492)	22	47	29		3		5	13	145	79	21	66	57	5				
39 WW 7(C/D)	20.4	18.7	10.4	8.2	.75		0.4	1.2	17.3	20.7	9.2	11.1	8.2	.95		0.04	X	
(2008)	41	377	21	165	15		8	25	348	415	184	224	165	19		1		
39 CO 1		0.07	0.4				39.2	0.2			39.1	10.3	6.3	2.8	0.2	1.4		
(1252)		1	5				491	3			489	128	79	35	3	18		
39 DW 234						1.0	67.7	1.1	1.1		11.8	14.4	1.1			1.6		1586 ± 37
(888)						9	602	10	10		105	128	10			14		

Table 96 Middle Missouri Area 3 Pottery Frequency Seriation

Component	Classes 112	113	114	115	121	122	123	125	131	132	133	134	135	221	222	232	Trade	^{14}C Date (A.D.)
39 ST 30	20.2	24.8	47.5	7.3													X	
(Stanley Phase) (395)	80	98	138	29														
39 ST 14	29.9	25.5	16.2	24.5		1.4				.6		.06	1.8				X	
(1497)	447	382	242	367		21				10		1	27					
39 ST 6	25.0	15.9	13.1	37.0		.6	1.2	.16		.16	1.0	1.3	4.5				X	
(1857)	464	295	244	687		7	11	3		3	19	25	83					
39 HU 26	28.6	9.8	5.2	1.5						11.8	9.8		32.9				X	
(788)	226	78	41	12						93	78		260					
39 HU 6					16.3			4.4	14.8		55.4	55.4		10.0				1548 ± 62
(794)					126			35	114		440	440		79				
39 ST 30									8.4	2.9	49.8	38.9						1148 ± 104
(Anderson Phase) (486)									41	14	242	189						
39 LM 208							3.8		5.2	7.6	42.4		24.8	1.4	9.5	5.2		1267 ± 90
(210)							8		11	16	89		52	3	20	11		
39 LM 209							1.3				37.8		27.5	8.9	1.6	2.9		1084 ± 48
(378)							5				143		104	34	6	11		

In the earlier period, S-rims were present. Unlike the other seriations, collared S-rims were present, as well as unmodified S-rims. These latter rims styles disappeared quite early in this sequence. The second characteristic of the earlier period was the presence of straight rims that were either collared or unmodified. The first style was present in very low frequencies; but the latter was extremely popular. Unmodified straight rims were either plain or decorated by incision or tool impression/punctate. Except for class 132, the highest frequencies of unmodified straight rim classes occurred prior to the appearance of European trade goods. Finally, as in the other seriations, all straight and braced rim classes, except that of 111, dominated pottery styles after European trade goods appeared, and, thus, constituted the second style period.

To create a finer resolution of the temporal scale, stylistic trends in each area were simplified (Figure 22). For each area, only those classes present in at least two assemblages with frequencies of 15% or greater were diagrammed. Classes that were not unimodal were also excluded. Based on the patterns, three stylistic periods are suggested, and components were assigned to Periods (Table 97).

During the earliest stylistic period (*circa* A.D. 1100 to 1400), only areas 1 and 3 were inhabited. Lehmer (1971:67) listed eleven components from area 2 that he thought dated to this general temporal interval. Unfortunately, because ceramic data for these components were not available, these components had to be excluded. Area 2 was, therefore, assigned a zero value for this period. In areas 1 and 3, unmodified S-rim styles were increasing in popularity. In area 3, unmodified straight rim styles were present and increased in popularity. These styles were absent from area 1.

The middle period persisted from the fifteenth to the seventeenth century and was present in all three areas. Unmodified S-rims were present only in area 1; and while class 231 was decreasing in popularity, that of class 232 increased.

Table 97 Middle Missouri Component Assignment by Area and Stylistic Period of Pottery

		Components		
Period	*Date (Century)*	*Area 1*	*Area 2*	*Area 3*
Late	17th	ME 5 ME 8 ME 11 ML 39 ME 15	WW 6(B) WW 7(C/D)	ST 30 ST 14 ST 6 HU 26
Middle	15th–17th	MO 11 EM 10	CO 1 DW 234	HU 6
Early	12th–15th	SI 4		ST 30 LM 208 LM 209

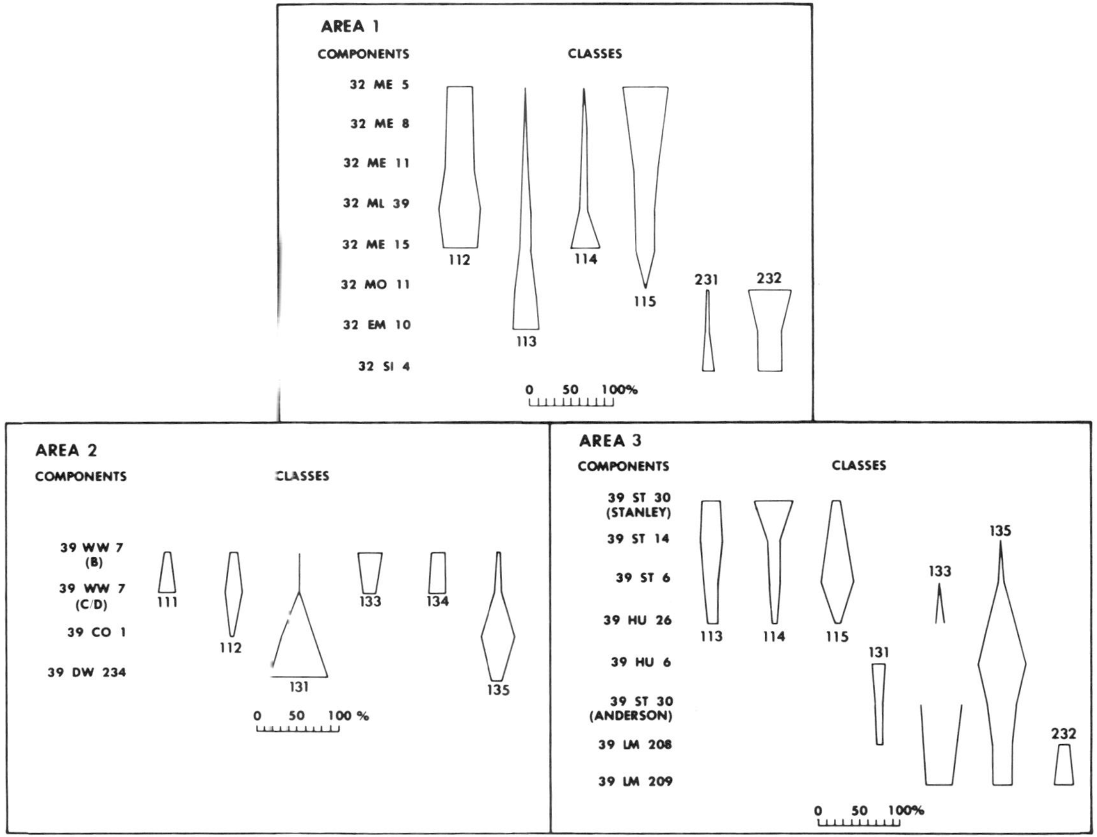

Figure 22. Stylistic Trends in Classes of Pottery from the Middle Missouri

In areas 2 and 3, unmodified straight rims predominated. Finally, in area 1, classes 113 and 115 were present; and both increased in frequency during this period.

In all areas, the latest period was demarcated both by stylistic patterns and by the presence of European trade goods. According to Lehmer's chronology, European trade goods appeared in the Middle Missouri in 1675. Since I am not sure this date is correct, I place the origin of European material sometime during the seventeenth century. The terminal date of the period, which was not indicated by the seriations, is examined in the next section. During this period, braced, straight rim styles predominated. Class 112 was present in areas 1 and 2, while class 111 was present only in area 2. Classes 114, 115 were present in areas 1 and 3.

Classifications and Analyses of European Trade Goods

In the Middle Missouri, the major change in the nature of European material recovered from aboriginal deposits is expected to occur in the late eighteenth or early nineteenth century. This temporal framework is consistent with the establishment of fur trading posts and sustained European presence in the area. I employed three temporal analyses to determine whether or not this assumption was correct. They included: (1) an occurrence seriation of metal objects; (2) cumulative frequencies; (3) frequencies of glass trade beads. Since some components associated with European trade goods were also known from documents, orders developed from archaeological data were compared with historical sources to establish more accurately appropriate temporal intervals. To make this analysis consistent with the frequency seriations, the final summary is presented in terms of the seriation areas previously established.

OCCURRENCE SERIATION OF METAL OBJECTS Metal was probably the earliest type of European material present in the region. Following sustained European presence, both type and frequency of metal objects should have increased. This expectation was tested by developing a classification of metal that included two dimensions and five modes (Table 98). I employed the classification to order aboriginal components through an occurrence seriation (Table 99).

53% (8/15) of Middle Missouri components associated with European trade goods were given a temporal assignment in the seriation. With few exceptions, most of these components were also ordered in one of the frequency seriations. The historical components of 39 ST 30 as well as 39 ST 6 were deleted, and three components not previously ordered (39 LM 215, 39 DW 2, and 39 ST 15) were added.

The order generally meets expectations regarding the temporal occurrence of metal. With the exception of 39 DW 2, sample size increased through time.

Table 98 Classification of Metal for the Middle Missouri

Dimension	Mode
I. Type of Material	1. Copper
	2. Brass
	3. Iron
II. Form	1. Scrap
	2. Definable Shape

Table 99 Occurrence Seriation of Metal from the Middle Missouri

	Classes					
Component	11	12	21	22	31	32
32 ME 5 (997)	X		X	X		X
32 ME 8 (56)	X		X	X	X	X
32 ME 11 (70)/39 ST 14 (25)	X	X	X	X	X	X
39 ST 15 (26)	X	X		X	X	X
39 HU 26 (9)/39 DW 2 (1125)	X	X		X		X
39 LM 215 (2)	X	X				

Copper preceded brass and iron; and all three types of metal persisted to the end of the sequence. Distinctions regarding shaped and unshaped objects were less clear. Copper scrap persisted throughout the sequence, but shaped copper objects did not.

The reverse was true for brass and iron classes. Both brass and iron scrap appeared later than respective types of shaped objects. In addition, while brass scrap persisted to the end of the sequence, iron scrap did not.

The pattern of components in this seriation contained information regarding the abandonment history of the region. South Dakota components dominated the early part of the sequence, while toward the later end of the temporal scale, North Dakota components predominated. The division was sharp enough to support the position argued by Lehmer and others. By the late eighteenth or early nineteenth century, South Dakota was abandoned; aboriginal occupation continued in North Dakota.

CUMULATIVE FREQUENCIES I employed cumulative frequencies to determine temporal trends in the presence of European material in aboriginal components. Eight classes of European function were established (Table 100), and all aboriginal assemblages associated with European material were analyzed. (Glass trade beads, treated in a later section, were excluded.) Table 101 presents raw counts and percentages by component.

Table 100 Middle Missouri Functional Classification for European Materials

1. EATING
Cooking Utensils
Eating Utensils
2. SUBSISTENCE
Cutting Artifacts
Scraping Artifacts
Fishhooks
Knives
Projectiles
Guns
3. DRESS
Thimbles
Buttons
Material
Needles
4. ORNAMENTATION
Beads
Bracelets
Earrings
Pendants
5. CONSTRUCTION
Axes
Chisels
Adzes
Nails
Hammers
Saws
6. SMOKING
Pipes
7. TRANSPORTATION
Bridles
Saddles
8. FUNCTION UNKNOWN
Scrap

Four temporal intervals were suggested by cumulative frequency curves of components (Figure 23). Two components were present in the earliest interval that began in the seventeenth century (Figure 23A). Two classes of European function, ornamentation (4) and unidentified function (8) were present. Five components were placed in the second interval (Figure 23B). Besides the previous classes 4 and 8, subsistence (2), construction (5), and smoking (6) were represented.

Four components were present in the third interval, (Figure 23C) all of which had five classes: 2, 3, 4, 5, 8. Between the second and third interval, the nature of assemblages changed: the frequency of ornamentation decreased while that

Table 101 Component Percentages and Counts by Class of European Function

	Classes							
Component	*1*	*2*	*3*	*4*	*5*	*6*	*7*	*8*
32 ME 5 (840)	4.0	54.5	10.2	11.1	5.6	.6	.4	13.6
	34	458	86	93	47	5	3	114
32 ME 8 (171)	8.2	1.8	4.6	7.6	5.8	1.7		70.2
	14	3	8	13	10	3		120
32 ME 15 (37)	35.1	37.8	2.7	10.8	10.8			2.7
	13	14	1	4	4			1
32 ME 12 (170)	1.1	15.9	14.7	24.7				43.5
	2	27	25	42				74
32 ME 11 (67)		37.3	1.5	7.5	9.0			44.8
		25	15	6				30
32 ML 39 (40)		25.0	2.5	7.5	7.5			57.8
		10	1	3	3			23
39 HU 26 (9)		22.2	11.1	11.1	11.1			44.4
		2	1	1	1			4
39 ST 14 (63)		12.7	3.2	7.9	1.6			74.6
		8	2	5	1			47
39 ST 6 (26)		38.5	3.8	42.3	15.4			
		10	1	11	4			
39 DW 2 (1125)		.3		99.0				.1
		2		1122				1
39 ST 30 (33)				18.0	27.3	6.1		48.5
				6	9	2		16
39 ST 15 (15)				33.3	6.7			60.0
				5	1			9
39 WW 7(C/D) (63)		3.1		93.0				3.1
		2		59				2
39 WW 7(B) (4)				50.0				50.0
				2				2
39 LM 215 (4)				50.0				50.0
				2				2

of subsistence (2) increased. Guns and ammunition became important parts of the subsistence class.

The most recent temporal interval was represented by four components with no less than five functional classes (Figure 23D). Classes 2 through 5 continued to be present; cooking (1) was added for the first time. In addition, smoking items were occasionally present, and at 32 ME 5, transportation items (8) were represented by bridle parts.

Although more components were ordered by this method than by the seriation of metal objects, sequences were quite similar. South Dakota components

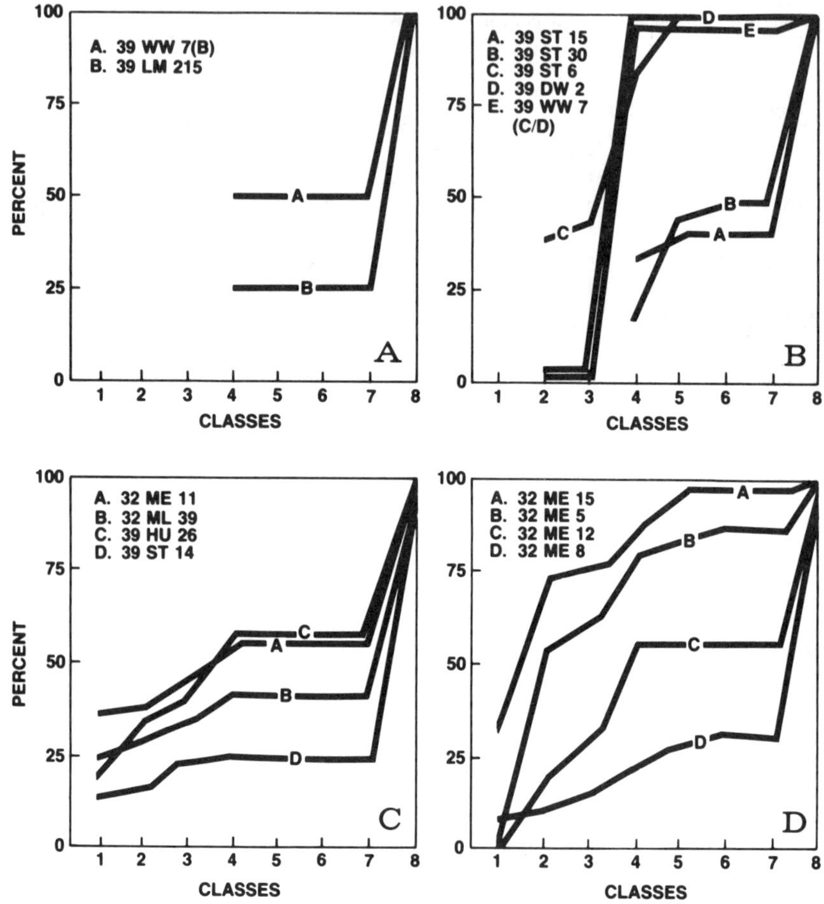

Figure 23. Cumulative Frequencies of European Trade Goods from the Middle Missouri

were represented by fewer classes of European function than North Dakota components; there were no components from South Dakota present in the latest temporal interval. Only components from area 1 were present in the most recent interval.

GLASS TRADE BEADS Table 102 presents frequencies of glass beads as a ratio of all European items. As seen in Table 103, the order developed from frequencies of trade beads was at variance with those developed through the metal seriation and cumulative frequencies. 39 ST 14, 39 HU 26, and 39 DW 2 had earlier temporal assignments in the frequencies of glass beads than in the other

Table 102 Glass Trade Beads by Component

Component	Glass Beads (*n*)	Trade Goods Total (*n*)	Percentage (Beads/Total)
32 ME 5	15,564	16,404	94.9
32 ME 12	2,928	3,098	94.5
32 ME 8	821	995	82.5
32 ME 11	2,365	2,432	97.0
39 ST 6	16	42	38.0
32 ME 15	2	39	5.1
39 ST 30 (Stanley Phase)	8	41	19.5
39 ST 15	2	17	11.5
32 ML 39	0	0	0
39 HU 26	0	0	0
39 ST 14	3	66	4.5
39 DW 2	933	2,058	45.3
39 WW 7(C/D)	1	64	1.5
39 WW 7(B)	0	0	0
39 LM 215	0	0	0

Table 103 Summary of Middle Missouri Components Ordered by Analyses of European Trade Goods

Occurrence Seriation of Metal	*Cumulative Frequencies*	*Glass Trade Bead Frequencies*
32 ME 5/32 ME 8	32 ME 5/32 ME 8/32 ME 15	32 ME 5/32 ME 8/32 ME 11
32 ME 11/39 ST 14	32 ML 39/32 ME 11/39 ST 14/ 39 HU 26	39 ST 6
39 ST 14		
39 HU 26/39 DW 2	39 WW 7(C/D)/39 ST 30/ 39 ST 15/39 ST 6/39 DW 2	39 ST 15/39 ST 30
39 LM 215	39 LM 215/39 WW 7(B)	39 WW 7(B)/39 WW 7(C/D)/ 39 DW 2/39 ST 14/39 HU 26/ 32 ML 39/32 ME 15

two methods. The reverse situation applied to 39 ST 6: it was earlier in the metal and cumulative frequency orders than in the frequencies of trade beads. Since the seriation of metal and the cumulative frequency orders largely agreed with each other, they are accepted as being reasonably accurate temporal measures. Sources of error in the trade bead sequence may be explained by sampling bias and/or irregular diffusion of beads into the Middle Missouri. Given current status of archaeological knowledge, it is not possible to isolate between potential sources of error.

DOCUMENTARY HISTORY Available historical evidence suggests that many North Dakota components ordered archaeologically (32 ME 5, 32 ME 8, 32 ME 11, 32 ME 15, and 32 ML 39) were founded after A.D. 1780 (Ahler et al. 1980; Lehmer et al. 1978; Stewart 1974). Three of these settlements, 32 ME 11, 32 ME 8, and 32 ME 5, persisted until the smallpox epidemic of 1837, while the other two were abandoned following the Lewis and Clark expedition, but before the 1837 smallpox epidemic. Given this information, I suggest that the latest part of both the seriation of metal objects and the analysis of cumulative frequencies date from the late eighteenth through the early nineteenth century.

Secondly, as suggested in the discussion of seriation of metal, South Dakota was abandoned earlier than North Dakota. Between 1738 and 1750, villages between the Grand and White rivers were occupied. By 1804, when Lewis and Clark traveled up the Missouri, resident populations in this same area were gone (Coues 1893; Thwaites, 1904). It would seem, therefore, that the area south of the Grand River dates from the seventeenth to the late eighteenth century.

In summary, archaeological analyses and historical documents, suggest two periods of European trade were present in the Middle Missouri. Component assignment by area and period is summarized on Table 104. The earliest aboriginal period with trade goods dates from the seventeenth and eighteenth centuries, during which time areas 2 and 3 (South Dakota) were occupied. Area 1 may also be occupied. From the late eighteenth century until 1837, the focus of aboriginal occupation was in the Knife-Heart area of North Dakota (area 1). Two components from area 3 also persisted into the later period, but as indicated by the Lewis and Clark journals, they were abandoned before 1804.

Table 104 Assignment of Middle Missouri Components to Period by Area

Period	*Time (Centuries)*	*Areas* 1	2	3
2	18th to early 19th centuries	32 ME 5/32 ME 8/ 32 ME 11/32 ME 12/ 32 ME 15/32 ML 39		39 ST 14/39 HU 26
1	17th to 18th centuries		39 DW 2/ 39 WW 7(B)/ 39 WW 7(C/D)	39 ST 30/39 ST 15/ 39 ST 6/39 LM 215

SETTLEMENT DATA

Table 105 summarizes data on the thirty-seven components employed in the regional analyses of population change. Table 106 lists, by component, measurements of settlement area and roofed area of houses. Table 107 summarizes measurement of settlement area by period and component. Roofed area of settlement pertinent to the calculation of S_{ra} by period is presented in Table 108.

Table 105 Summary of Middle Missouri Settlements

Settlement Number	*Settlement Name*	*County*	*Employed to Calculate S_a*	*Excavated Houses*	*Source*
32 ML 2	Like-A-Fishhook	McLean	X	9	Smith 1972
32 ML 39	Nightwalker's Butte	McLean	X	22	Lehmer et al. 1978
32 ME 1	Clark's Creek	Mercer			Thiessen 1977
32 ME 8	Amahami	Mercer		3	Lehmer et al. 1978
32 ME 5	Deapolis	Mercer			Lehmer et al. 1978
32 ME 11	Sakakawea	Mercer	X	1	Ahler et al. 1980
32 ME 12	Big Hidatsa	Mercer			Ahler and Swenson 1985
32 ME 15	Rock Village	Mercer	X	10	Lehmer et al. 1978
32 OL 14	Cross Ranch	Oliver	X	2	Calabrese 1972
32 OL 16	Bagnell	Oliver		1	Lehmer et al. 1978
32 MO 11	Huff	Morton	X	11	Wood 1967
32 EM 10	Shermer	Emmons	X	3	Sperry 1968
32 SI 4	Paul Brave	Sioux	X	4	Wood and Woolworth 1964
32 SI 19	South Cannonball	Sioux	X	6	Griffin n.d.
39 CO 1	Demery	Corson		4	Woolworth and Wood 1964
39 WW 7(B)	Swan Creek	Walworth			Hurt 1957
39 WW 7(C/D)	Swan Creek	Walworth		2	Hurt 1957
39 DW 234	Molstad	Dewey	X	3	Hoffman 1967
39 DW 2	Four Bear	Dewey	X	1	Hurt et al. 1962
39 ST 16	Breeden A	Stanley		4	Brown 1974
39 ST 30 (Anderson Phase)	Dodd Ranch	Stanley		7	Lehmer 1954b
39 ST 11	Fay Tolton	Stanley	X	2	Wood 1976
39 ST 223	John Ketchen	Stanley	X	3	Johnson 1979
39 ST 238	Durkin	Stanley		3	Johnson 1979
39 ST 9/232(B)	La Roche	Stanley		2	Hoffman 1968
39 ST 9(A)	La Roche	Stanley		7	Hoffman 1968
39 ST 30 (Stanley Phase)	Dodd Ranch	Stanley		9	Lehmer 1954b
39 ST 14	Phillips Ranch	Stanley	X	8	Lehmer 1954b

(*continued*)

Table 105 (*Continued*)

Settlement Number	*Settlement Name*	*County*	*Employed to Calculate* S_a	*Excavated Houses*	*Source*
39 ST 6	Buffalo Pasture	Stanley	X	4	Lehmer and Jones 1968
39 ST 15	Indian Creek	Stanley	X	1	Lehmer and Jones 1968
39 HU 1	Thomas Riggs	Hughes	X	7	Hurt 1953
39 HU 6	Arzberger	Hughes	X	4	Spaulding 1956
39 HU 26	Spotted Bear	Hughes		5	Hurt 1954b
39 LM 215	Peterson	Lyman		1	Caldwell 1966
39 LM 208	Jiggs Thompson	Lyman		2	Caldwell and Jensen 1969
39 LM 209	Langdeau	Lyman	X	5	Caldwell and Jensen 1969
39 LM 232	Pretty Head	Lyman	X	3	Caldwell and Jensen 1969

Table 106 Measurements of Settlement Area and Roofed Area of Houses

Settlement Number	*Settlement Area (Hectares)*	*Houses*	
		Number	*Size (m^2)*
32 ML 2	16.0	3	139.4
		4	228.0
		5	197.3
		7	205.0
		8	245.5
		9(A)	237.0
		10	147.8
		12	237.0
		15	308.3
32 ML 39	0.89	F.1	17.53
		F.7	24.97
		F.16	33.73
		F.18	23.64
		F.19	22.30
		F.31	21.09
		F.35	26.34
		F.36	17.53
		F.37	23.64
		F.38	18.68
		F.42	23.64
		F.46	22.35
		F.47	18.68
		F.48	23.64
		F.49	32.18
		F.55	23.64
		F.60	22.35
		F.4	27.36
		F.27	29.73
		F.29	28.24
		F.66	44.59
		F.75	13.05
32 ME 8		1	161.20
		2	65.67
		3	67.88
32 ME 11	2.1	1	314.20
32 ME 15	1.4	F.69	102.60
		F.53	57.21
		F.60	74.72
		F.8	61.36
		F.19	74.70
		F.10A	74.72
		F.10B	94.30
		F.48	74.70
		F.111	81.90
		F.72	70.10
32 OL 14	5.7	H.3	61.20
		H.7	57.60

(*continued*)

Table 106 (*Continued*)

Settlement Number	*Settlement Area (Hectares)*	*Houses*	
		Number	*Size (m^2)*
32 OL 16		H.1	76.70
32 MO 11	5.2	H.1	90.30
		H.3	57.70
		H.4	100.34
		H.5	103.70
		H.6	118.90
		H.7	125.70
		H.8	118.10
		H.10	112.97
		H.18	156.10
		H.19	173.90
		H.12	86.20
32 EM 10	4.3	H.1	100.34
		H.4	118.90
		H.6	94.50
32 SI 4	1.6	XU1	137.40
		XU2	90.60
		XU3	132.50
		XU8	211.40
32 SI 19	3.7	H.1	85.50
		H.2	91.88
		H.3	105.10
		H.4	73.20
		H.5	75.60
		H.7	83.60
39 CO 1		XU7	53.40
		XU5	35.30
		XU5	89.20
		XU5	42.00
39 WW 7(C/D)		H.1	100.34
		H.2	74.72
39 DW 234	0.37	H.1	148.10
		H.2	160.40
		H.7	336.70
39 DW 2	2.5	H.1	85.60
39 ST 16		XU2	69.90
		XU3	90.60
		XU4	99.90
		XU5	97.50
39 ST 30 (Anderson Phase)		F.17	95.90
		F.29	72.80
		F.34	43.60
		F.61–62	65.70
		F.76	80.10
		F.88	63.20
		F.17	82.90

(*continued*)

Table 106 (*Continued*)

Settlement Number	*Settlement Area (Hectares)*	*Houses*	
		Number	*Size (m²)*
39 ST 11	1.2	H.1	54.40
		H.2	73.30
39 LM 209	2.3	F.4	86.40
		F.7	115.04
		F.10	107.90
		F.11	89.90
		XU5	119.70
39 LM 208		F.2	56.50
		F.4	50.70
39 LM 232	1.8	F.2	95.70
		F.4	184.95
		F.7	99.20
39 ST 223	3.3	XU2	59.95
		F.3	80.30
		XU13	82.30
39 ST 238		XU3	169.10
		XU5	97.60
		XU6	118.80
39 ST 9/232/(B)		H.1 Area A (ST 9)	328.30
		H.1 (ST 232)	469.50
39 ST 9(A)		H.1 Area B	113.90
		H.1 Area E	148.60
		H.1 Area C	94.60
		H.2 Area B	86.90
		H.2 Area E	65.70
		H.3 Area B	80.80
		H.4 Area B	57.80
39 ST 30 (Stanley)		F.1	47.60
		F.7	52.80
		F.8	53.20
		F.11	52.40
		F.15	126.90
		F.35	83.40
		F.73	42.03
		F.106	57.20
		F.107	61.40
39 ST 14	0.69	F.2	69.20
		F.3	48.60
		F.4	95.60
		F.5	64.80
		F.7	79.90
		F.8	76.10
		F.20	73.80
		F.23	111.60
39 ST 6	1.3	H.1	79.50
		H.3B	74.70

(*continued*)

Table 106 (*Continued*)

Settlement Number	*Settlement Area (Hectares)*	*Houses*	
		Number	*Size (m²)*
		H.4	128.70
		H.3A	45.60
39 ST 15	4.8	H.1	49.30
39 HU 1	3.7	H.1A	229.50
		H.1B	193.98
		H.2	134.70
		H.3	95.90
		H.4	106.80
		H.5	69.50
		H.6	166.50
39 HU 6	17.20	H.1	116.70
		H.2	134.90
		H.3	157.70
		H.4	49.20
39 HU 26		H.1	91.60
		H.2	44.60
		H.3	38.60
		H.4	18.04
		H.5	29.20
39 LM 215		H.1	81.90

Table 107 Measurement of Settlement Area by Component and Period

Period	*Settlement Number*	*Area (Hectares)*
V	32 ML 2	16.00
IV	32 ML 39	0.89
	32 ME 11	2.10
	32 ME 15	1.40
	39 ST 14	0.69
III	39 DW 2	2.50
	39 ST 6	1.30
	39 ST 15	4.80
II	39 DW 234	0.37
	39 HU 1	3.70
	39 HU 6	17.20
	32 MO 11	5.20
	32 EM 10	4.30
	32 OL 14	5.70
I	39 LM 209	2.30
	39 LM 232	1.80
	39 ST 223	3.30
	32 SI 4	1.60
	32 SI 19	3.70
	39 ST 11	1.20

Table 108 Measurement of $\overline{S_{ra}}$ by Component and Period

Period	*Settlement Number*	*Excavated Houses*	$\overline{H_{ra}}$ *(m²)*	*Estimate of Total Houses*	$\overline{S_{ra}}$ *(m²)*
IV	32 ME 11	1	314.20	40	12,568.0
	32 ME 15	10	76.60	35	2,681.0
	39 ST 14	8	77.50	21	1,627.5
III	39 DW 2	1	85.60	34	2,910.4
	39 LM 215	1	81.90	56	4,586.4
	39 ST 6	4	81.60	31	2,529.6
II	39 HU 1	7	142.40	20	2,848.0
	39 HU 6	4	114.30	44	5,029.2
	32 EM 10	3	104.58	78	8,157.2
	32 MO 11	11	105.20	102	10,730.4
	39 DW 234	3	215.10	6	1,290.6
	39 CO 1	4	51.04	30	1,531.2
I	32 SI 4	4	142.95	14	2,001.3
	32 SI 19	6	85.50	32	2,736.0
	39 ST 11	2	63.80	33	2,105.4
	39 LM 208	2	53.60	17	911.4
	39 LM 232	3	126.60	16	2,025.6
	39 ST 223	3	75.80	11	833.8

References

Abel, A.

1939 *Tabeau's Narrative of Loisel's Expedition to the Upper Missouri*. University of Oklahoma Press, Norman.

Ackernecht, C. H.

1965 *History and Geography of the Most Important Diseases*. Hafner, New York.

Ahler, S. A.

1978 *A Research Plan for Investigation of the Archeological Resources of the Knife River Indian Villages, National Historic Site*. U. S. National Park Service, Midwest Archeological Center, Lincoln.

1979 *Archeological Field Research in the Knife River Indian Villages, National Historic Site, Summer 1979*. Department of Anthropology and Archeology, University of North Dakota. Submitted to the Midwest Archeological Center. Contract No. CX-6000-6-A061. Grand Forks.

Ahler, S. A., and B. F. Benz

1980 *Analysis of Controlled Surface Artifact Collections from Sakakawea (32 ME 11) and Lower Hidatsa (32 ME 10) Village Sites*. Department of Anthropology and Archeology, University of North Dakota. Submitted to Midwest Archeological Center. Contract No. PX-6115-7-0147. Grand Forks.

Ahler, S. A. and A. A. Swenson

1980 *Analysis of Surface Collections from Poly (32 ME 407), Stanton Ferry (32 ML 6), and Stiefel (32 ME 202) Archeological Sites*. Department of Anthropology and Archeology, University of North Dakota. Submitted to Midwest Archeological Center. Contract No. PX-6115-7-0147. Grand Forks.

1985 *Test Excavations at Big Hidatsa Village (32 ME 12), Knife River Indian Village National Historic Site*. Department of Anthropology, University of North Dakota. Submitted to Midwest Archeological Center. Contract No. CX-6000-6-A061 and CX-6000-1-0045. Grand Forks.

Ahler, S. A., T. Weston, and K. D. McMiller

1980 *Cutbank Profiling and Test Excavations of Sakakawea Village (32 ME 11), Knife River Indian Village, National Historic Site*. Department of Anthropology and

Archeology, University of North Dakota. Sumitted to U.S. National Park Service. Contract No. CX-6000-6-A081. Grand Forks.

Allison, M. J., E. Gerzten, J. Munizaga, C. Santoro, and D. Mendoza

1981 Tuberculosis in Pre-Columbian Andean Populations. In *Prehistoric Tuberculosis in the Americas*, edited by J. E. Buikstra, pp. 49–62. Northwestern University Archeological Program, Scientific Papers 5. Evanston.

Allison, M. J., D. Mendoza, and A. Pezzia

1973 Documentation of a Case of Tuberculosis in Pre-Columbian America. *American Review of Respiratory Disease* 107:985–991.

American Academy of Pediatrics

1977 *Report of the Committee on Infectious Diseases*. 18th ed. American Academy of Pediatrics, Evanston.

Angulo, J. J., C. K. Takiguti, M. E. Sakuma, E. M. Kimura, S. P. Curti, and C. A. Pederneiras

1983 Temporal-Spatial-Social Parameters in the Spread of Contagious Disease. *Ecology of Disease* 2:369–376.

Ashburn, P. M.

1947 *The Ranks of Death*. Coward McCann, New York.

Bailey, N. T. J.

1957 *The Mathematical Theory of Epidemics*. Charles Griffin, London.

1975 *Mathematics of Infectious Diseases and its Applications*. Charles Griffin, London.

Bandelier, A. A.

1890 Final Report of Investigations among the Indians of Southwestern United States, Carried on Mainly in the Years 1880–1885. *Archaeological Institute of North America, Papers, American Series* 3. John Wilson and Sons, Cambridge.

Bartholomew, D. J.

1973 *Stochastic Models for Social Processes*. 2nd ed. John Wiley and Sons, New York.

Bartlett, M. S.

1956 Deterministic and Stochastic Models for Recurrent Epidemics. *Proceedings of the Third Berkeley Symposium on Mathematical Statistics and Probability* 4:81–109.

1957 Measles Periodicity and Community Size. *Journal of the Royal Statistical Society Series A* 120:48–70.

1960 The Critical Community Size for Measles in the United States. *Journal of the Royal Statistical Society Series A* 123:37–40.

1972 Epidemics. In *Statistics: A Guide to the Unknown*, edited by J. M. Tanur, pp. 66–76. Holden-Day, San Francisco.

Barton, B. S.

1799 Observations and Conjectures Concerning Certain Articles which were Taken from Ancient Tumulus, or Grave. *American Philosophical Society Transactions* 4:181–215.

Bartram, J.

1751 *Observations on the Inhabitants, Climate, Soils, Rivers, Productions, Animals and other Matters Worthy of Notice in his Travels from Pennsylvania to Onondaga, Oswego and the Lake Ontario*. J. Whiston and B. White, London.

Beaglehole, J. C. (editor)
1967 *The Journals of Captain James Cook on his Voyages of Discovery. The Voyage of the Resolution and Discovery, 1776–1780*, vol. 3. 2 parts. Hakluyt Society and University Press, Cambridge.

Beauchamp, W. M.
1900 Aboriginal Occupation of New York. *New York State Museum, Bulletin* 7:5–187. Albany.

Beck, C.
1981 Prehistoric Settlement Patterns in the Lower Mississippi Valley during the Late Mississippi Period (A.D. 1200–1600). Paper presented at the 46th Annual Meeting of the Society for American Archaeology, San Diego.

Benenson, A. S.
1976a Cholera. In *Communicable and Infectious Diseases*. 8th ed., edited by F. H. Top Sr., and P. F. Wehrle, pp. 174–183. C. W. Mosby, St. Louis.
1976b Plague. In *Communicable and Infectious Diseases*. 8th ed., edited by F. H. Top Sr. and P. F. Wehrle, pp. 502–507. C.W. Mosby, St. Louis.

Biggar, H. P. (editor)
1911 *The Precursors of Jacques Cartier, 1497–1534. A Collection of Documents Relating to the Early History of the Dominion of Canada*. Government Printing Office, Ottawa.
1924 The Voyages of Jacques Cartier, Published from the Originals with Translations, Notes, and Appendices. *Publications of the Public Archives of Canada* 11. Ottawa.
1925 *The Works of Samuel de Champlain*, vol. 2. Publications of the Champlain Society, Toronto.

Binford, L.
1980 Willow Smoke and Dog's Tails: Hunter-Gatherer Settlement Systems and Archaeological Site Formation. *American Antiquity* 45:4–20.
1982 The Archaeology of Place. *Journal of Anthropological Archaeology* 1:5–31.

Black, F. L.
1966 Measles Endemicity in Insular Populations: Critical Community Size and its Evolutionary Implication. *Journal of Theoretical Biology* 11:207–211.
1975 Infectious Diseases in Primitive Societies. *Science* 187:515–518.

Blanton, R. E.
1972 *Prehispanic Settlement Patterns of the Ixtapalapa Peninsula Region, Mexico*. Pennsylvania State University Occasional Papers in Anthropology 6. University Park.

Bolton, H. E.
1906 *Spanish Exploration in the Southwest, 1542–1706*. Barnes and Noble, New York.
1949 *Coronado on the Turquoise Trail: Knight of Pueblos and Plains*. Coronado Cuarto Centennial Publications, 1540–1940, 1, edited by G. P. Hammond. University of New Mexico Press, Albuquerque.

Borah, W. W.
1976 The Historical Demography of Aboriginal and Colonial America: An Attempt

at Perspective. In *The Native Population of the Americas in 1492*, edited by W. H. Denevan, pp. 13–34. University of Wisconsin Press, Madison.

Borah, W. W., and S. F. Cook
1963 *The Aboriginal Population of Central Mexico on the Eve of Spanish Conquest.* Ibero-Americana 45. Berkeley.

Bourne, E. G.
1904 *Narratives of the Career of Hernando De Soto.* 2 vols. A. S. Barnes, New York.

Bowers, A. W.
1965 Hidatsa Social and Ceremonial Organization. *Bureau of American Ethnology, Bulletin* 194. Washington, D.C.

Boyd, M. F., and W. K. Stratman-Thomas
1933 Studies on Benign Tertian Malaria 4. On the Refractoriness of Negros to Innoculation with *Plasmodium vivax*. *American Journal of Hygiene* 18:485–489.

Brachman, P.S.
1976 Anthrax. In *Communicable and Infectious Diseases*. 8th ed., edited by F. H. Top Sr., and P. F. Wehrle, pp. 137–142. C. W. Mosby, St. Louis.

Bradley, J. W.
1979 *The Onondaga Iroquois: 1500–1655, A Study in Acculturative Change and its Consequences*. Ph.D. dissertation, Syracuse University. University Microfilms, Ann Arbor.

Brain, J. P.
1970 The Tunica Treasure. *Peabody Museum Bulletin* 2. Cambridge.
1971 The Natchez Paradox. *Ethnology* 10:215–222.
1973 Trudeau, an Eighteenth-Century Tunica Village. *Peabody Museum Bulletin* 3. Cambridge.
1975a Artifacts of the Adelantado. *Conference on Historic Site Archaeology Papers, 1973* 5:129–138.
1975b *The Archaeology of the Tunica: Trail on the Yazoo*. Peabody Museum, Harvard University, Cambridge. Ms. in possession of author.
1978 Late Prehistoric Settlement Patterning in the Yazoo Basin and Natchez Bluffs Regions of the Lower Mississippi Valley. In *Mississippian Settlement Patterns*, edited by B. D. Smith, pp. 331–368. Academic Press, New York.
1980 Tunica Treasure. *Peabody Museum of Archaeology and Ethnology Papers* 71. Cambridge.

Brain, J. P., A. Toth, and A. Rodriguez-Buckingham
1974 Ethnohistoric Archaeology and the De Soto *Entrada* into the Lower Mississippi Valley. *Conference on Historic Site Archaeology Papers, 1972* 7:232–289.

Brooks, G. F., and T. M. Buchanan
1970 Pertussis in the United States. *Journal of Infectious Disease* 122(1–2):123–125.

Brose, D. S.
1976 Historical Background. In *The Late Prehistory of the Lake Erie Drainage Basin*, edited by D. S. Brose, pp. 1–24. Cleveland Museum of Natural History, Cleveland.

Browman, D. L.
1981 Isotopic Discrimination and Correction Factors in Radiocarbon Dating. In

Advances in Archaeological Method and Theory, vol. 4, edited by M. B. Schiffer, pp. 241–295. Academic Press, New York.

Brown, B. Mc.

1985 Floor Area and Population: A World-Wide Cross Cultural Study. Ms. submitted to *American Antiquity*.

Brown, I. W.

1975 Excavations at Ft. St. Pierre. *Conference on Historic Site Archaeology Papers, 1974* 9:60–85.

1979 Functional Group Changes and Acculturation: A Case Study of the French and the Indian in the Lower Mississippi Valley. *Midcontinental Journal of Archaeology* 4:147–165.

1982 An Archaeological Study of Culture Contact and Change in the Natchez Bluffs Region. In *La Salle and his Legacy*, edited by P. K. Galloway, pp. 176–193. University Press of Mississippi, Jackson.

1985 *Natchez Indian Archaeology: Culture Change and Stability in the Lower Mississippi Valley*. Mississippi Department of Archives and History, Archaeological Report 15. Jackson.

Brown, I. W., and J. P. Brain

1983 Archaeology of the Natchez Bluffs Region, Mississippi: Hypothesized Cultural and Environmental Factors Influencing Local Population Movements. *Southeastern Archaeological Conference, Bulletin* 20:38–49.

Brown, J. D., and J. M. Leedom

1976 Pneumonia, Bacterial. In *Communicable and Infectious Diseases*. 8th ed., edited by F. H. Top Sr., and P. F. Wehrle, pp. 508–534. C. W. Mosby, St. Louis.

Brown, L. A.

1974 The Archaeology of the Breeden Site. *Plains Anthropologist* 19, *Memoir* 1.

Brown, P., and D. C. Gajdusek

1970 Disease Patterns and Vaccine Response Studies in Isolated Micronesian Populations. *American Journal of Tropical Medicine and Hygiene* 19:170–176.

Brown, P., D. C. Gajdusek, and J. A. Morris

1966 Epidemic A2 Influenza in Isolated Pacific Island Populations without Pre-epidemic Antibodies to Influenza Types A and B, and the Discussion of Still Unexplored Populations. *American Journal of Epidemiology* 83:176–188.

Bruce-Chwatt, L. J.

1965 Paleogenesis and Paleoepidemiology of Primate Malarias. *Bulletin of the World Health Organization* 32: 363–387.

Brunell, P. A.

1976 Chickenpox. In *Communicable and Infectious Diseases*. 8th ed., edited by F. H. Top Sr., and P. F. Wehrle, pp. 165–173. C. W. Mosby, St. Louis.

Bugher, J. C.

1951 Pathology of Yellow Fever. In *Yellow Fever*, edited by G. K. Strode, pp. 141–163. McGraw-Hill, New York.

Buikstra, J. E.

1976 Differential Diagnosis: An Epidemiological Model. *Yearbook of Physical Anthropology* 20:315–328.

1981 Introduction. In *Prehistoric Tuberculosis in the Americas*, edited by J. E. Buikstra, pp. 1–24. Northwestern University Archeological Program, Scientific Papers 5. Evanston.

Buikstra, J. E., and D. C. Cook

1980 Paleopathology: An American Account. *Annual Review of Anthropology* 10: 433–470.

1981 Pre-Columbian Tuberculosis in West-Central Illinois: Prehistoric Disease in Biocultural Perspective. In *Prehistoric Tuberculosis in the Americas*, edited by J. E. Buikstra, pp. 115–140. Northwestern University Archeological Program, Scientific Papers 5. Evanston.

Burnet, Macfarlane Sir, and D. O. White

1972 *Natural History of Infectious Disease*. 4th ed. Cambridge University Press, Cambridge.

Burpee, L. J. (editor)

1927 *Journals and Letters of Pierre Gaultier de Varennes de la Verendrye and his Sons*. Champlain Society Publications 16. Toronto.

Burrage, H. S. D. D. (editor)

1959a The First Relation of Jacques Cartier of St. Maleo, third printing. In *Early English and French Voyages Chiefly from Hakluyt, 1534–1608*, pp. 1–13. Barnes and Noble, New York.

1959b A Short and Brief Narration (Cartier's second voyage), third printing. In *Early English and French Voyages Chiefly from Hakluyt, 1534–1608*, pp. 33–86. Barnes and Noble, New York.

1959c The Third Voyage of Discovery made by Captaine Jaques Cartier, third printing. In *Early English and French Voyages Chiefly from Hakluyt, 1534–1608*, pp. 89–102. Barnes and Noble, New York.

Bushnell, G. E.

1922 *A Study in the Epidemiology of Tuberculosis*. William Wood, New York.

Butcher, G. A., G. H. Mitchell, and S. Cohen

1973 Mechanisms of Host Specificity in Malaria Infections. *Nature* 244:40–42.

Calabrese, F. A.

1972 Cross Ranch: A Study of Variability in a Stable Cultural Tradition. *Plains Anthropologist* 17, *Memoir* 9.

Caldwell, W. W.

1966 *The Black Partisan Site*. River Basin Surveys Publications in Salvage Archaeology 2. Lincoln.

Caldwell, W. W., and R. E. Jensen

1969 *The Grand Detour Phase*. River Basin Surveys Publications in Salvage Archaeology 13. Lincoln.

Carter, H. R.

1931 *Yellow Fever: An Epidemiological and Historical Study of its Place of Origin*, edited by L. A. Carter, and W. H. Frost. Williams and Wilkens, Baltimore.

Casselberry, S. E.

1974 Further Refinement of Formulas for Determining Population from Floor Area. *World Archaeology* 6:117–124.

Chapman, P., and T. Eickenhoff
1976 Tuberculosis. In *Communicable and Infectious Diseases*. 8th ed., edited by F. H. Top Sr., and P. F. Wehrle, pp. 724–753. C. W. Mosby, St. Louis.

Charlevoix, P. F. X. de
1977 *Charlevoix's Louisiana: Selections from the History and the Journal* [1761], edited by Charles E. O'Neill. Louisiana State University Press for Louisiana American Revolution Bicentennial Commission, Baton Rouge.

Chin, T. D. Y.
1976 Encephilitis, Infectious. In *Communicable and Infectious Diseases*. 8th ed., edited by F. H. Top Sr., and P. F. Wehrle, pp. 239–251. C. W. Mosby, St. Louis.

Chittendon, H. M.
1954 *The American Fur Trade of the Far West*, 1 [1902]. Academic Reprints, Stanford.

Chomko, S. A.
1977 Ethnohistory of the Knife-Heart Region, North Dakota. Ms. on file, Department of Anthropology, University of Missouri, Columbia.

Christensen, P. E., H. Schmidt, H. O. Bang, V. Andersen, B. Jordal, and O. Jensen
1953 Measles in Virgin Soil II. The Epidemic Proper. *Acta Medica Scandanavica* 144:430–449.

Christie, A. B.
1974 *Infectious Diseases: Epidemiology and Clinical Practice*. 2nd ed. Churchill Livingstone, Edinburgh.

Clark, R. M.
1975 A Calibration Curve for Radiocarbon Dates. *Antiquity* 49:251–266.

Coatney, G. R., W. A. Collins, W. Hewilson, and P. Contacos
1971 *The Primate Malarias*. U.S. Department of Health, Education and Welfare. National Institute of Health, National Institute of Allergy and Infectious Diseases. Bethesda.

Coatney, G. R., and M. D. Young
1941 The Taxonomy of Malarian Parasites with Notes on Principle American Strains. In *A Symposium on Human Malarias with Special Reference to North America and the Caribbean Region*, edited by F. R. Moulton, pp. 19–24. American Association for the Advancement of Science, Publication 15. Washington, D.C.

Cockburn, A.
1963 *The Evolution and Eradication of Infectious Diseases*. Johns Hopkins Press, Baltimore.
1971 Infectious Diseases in Ancient Populations. *Current Anthropology* 12:45–62.

Cockburn, A. (editor)
1980 *Mummies, Disease, and Ancient Cultures*. Cambridge University Press, New York.

Collins, H. B.
1927 Potsherds from Choctaw Village Sites in Mississippi. *Journal of the Washington Academy of Sciences* 17:259–263.

Collins, W. E., and M. Aikawa

1977 Plasmodia of Nonhuman Primates. In *Parasitic Protozoa*, vol. 3, edited by J. P. Kreier, pp. 467–492. Academic Press, New York.

Cook, D. C.

1976 *Pathologic States and Disease Process in Illinois Woodland Populations: An Epidemiologic Approach*. Ph.D. dissertation, Department of Anthropology, University of Chicago. Chicago.

1983 Paleoepidemiology of the Schild Cemetery: Health Consequences of Regional Integration. Paper presented at 48th Annual Meeting of the Society for American Archaeology, Pittsburgh.

Cook, N. D.

1981 *Demographic Collapse: Indian Peru, 1520–1620*. Cambridge University Press, Cambridge.

Cook, S. F.

1937 *The Extent and Significance of Disease among the Indians of Baja California, 1697–1773*. Ibero-Americana 12. Berkeley.

1940 *Population Trends among California Mission Indians*. Ibero-Americana 17. Berkeley.

1943 *The Conflict between the California Indians and White Civilization I: The Indian versus the Spanish Mission*. Ibero-Americana 21. Berkeley.

1955 The Epidemic of 1830–1833 in California and Oregon. *University of California Publications in American Archaeology and Ethnology* 43:303–36. Berkeley.

1973a The Significance of Disease in the Extinction of the New England Indians. *Human Biology* 45:485–508.

1973b Interracial Warfare and Population Decline among the New England Indians. *Ethnohistory* 25:1–24.

1976 *The Population of the California Indians, 1769–1970*. University of California Press, Berkeley.

1978 Historical Demography. In *California*, edited by R. F. Heizer, pp. 91–98. Handbook of North American Indians, vol. 8, W. G. Sturtevant, general editor. Smithsonian Institution, Washington, D.C.

Cook, S. F., and W. W. Borah

1960 *The Indian Population of Central Mexico: 1531–1610*. Ibero-Americana 44. Berkeley.

1971 *Essays in Population History: Mexico and the Caribbean*, vol. 1. University of California Press, Berkeley.

Cook, S. F., and R. F. Heizer

1965 The Quantitative Approach to the Relationship between Population and Settlement Size. *University of California Archeological Survey Reports* 64. Berkeley.

1968 Relationships among Houses, Settlement Areas, and Population in Aboriginal California. In *Settlement Archaeology*, edited by K. C. Chang, pp. 79–116. National Press Books, Palo Alto.

Cook, S. F., and L. B. Simpson

1948 *The Population of Central Mexico in the Sixteenth Century*. Ibero-Americana 31. Berkeley.

Cook, S. F., and A. E. Treganza
1950 The Quantitative Investigation of Indian Mounds. *University of California Publications in American Archaeology and Ethnology* 40:223–262. Berkeley.

Cooper, D. B.
1965 *Epidemic Disease in Mexico City 1716–1813*. Institute of Latin American Studies, University of Texas, Austin.

Cooper, E., and L. Fitch
1983 Pertussis: Herd Immunity and Vaccination Coverage in St. Lucia. *Lancet* II:1129–1131.

Cordell, L., and S. Upham
1984 Agriculture in the Southwest. In *Culture Resource Management: Stage 1: Site Location Modeling in the Southwestern Region*, pp. 29–44. U.S. Department of Agriculture Forest Service, Southwestern Region, Report 5. Albuquerque.

Coues, E. (editor)
1893 *History of the Expedition of Lewis and Clark; Original Manuscript, Journals and Field Notebooks of the Explorers*. 4 vols. Francis Harper, New York.
1897 *The Manuscript Journals of Alexander Henry and of David Thompson*. 3 vols. Francis Harper, New York.

Cowgill, G. L.
1972 Models, Methods, and Techniques for Seriation. In *Models in Archaeology*, edited by D. L. Clarke, pp. 381–424. Methuen, London.

Craig, C. F.
1941 Cyclical Variation in the Incidence of Malarias. In *A Symposium on Human Malaria with Special Reference to North America and the Caribbean Region*, edited by F. R. Moulton, pp. 131–134. American Association for the Advancement of Science, Publication 15. Washington, D.C.

Crane, H. R.
1956 University of Michigan Radiocarbon Dates I. *Science* 124:664–672.

Crane, H. R., and J. B. Griffin
1959 University of Michigan Radiocarbon Dates IV. *American Journal of Science, Radiocarbon Supplement* 1:173–198.
1962 University of Michigan Radiocarbon Dates VII. *Radiocarbon* 4:183–203.
1966 University of Michigan Radiocarbon Dates XI. *Radiocarbon* 8:256–285.

Creighton, C.
1894 *History of Epidemics in Britain*. 2 vols. Cambridge University Press, Cambridge.

Croix, C. de
1781 Letter to the Governor of New Mexico, September 15. *New Mexico Records Center and Archives* 831. Santa Fe.

Crosby, A.
1972 *The Columbian Exchange: Biocultural Consequences of 1492*. Greenwood Press, Westport.

Crouse, N. M.
1933 The White Man's Discoveries and Explorations. In *History of the State of New York*, vol. 1, edited by A. C. Flick, pp. 137–176. Columbia University Press, New York.

Damon, P. E., C. W. Ferguson, A. Long, and E. I. Wallick
1974 Dendrochronologic Calibration of the Radiocarbon Time Scale. *American Antiquity* 39:350–366.

Darwin, C.
1936 *The Origin of Species* [1859] *and the Descent of Man* [1871]. Modern Library, New York.

Davis, D. D.
1981 Ceramic Classification and Temporal Discrimination: A Consideration of Later Prehistoric Stylistic Change in the Mississippi River Delta. *Midcontinental Journal of Archaeology* 6:55–89.
1984 Protohistoric Cultural Interaction along the Northern Gulf Coast. In *Perspectives on Gulf Coast Prehistory,* edited by D. D. Davis, pp. 216–231. Ripley P. Bullen Monographs in Anthropology and History 5. Florida State Museum, Gainesville.

Davis, H. A.
1966 An Introduction to Parkin Prehistory. The *Arkansas Archeologist* 7:1–40.

Deetz, J.
1965 *The Dynamics of Stylistic Change in Arikara Ceramics*. Illinois Studies in Anthropology 4. Urbana.

Dietz, K.
1967 Epidemics and Rumors: A Survey. *Journal of the Royal Statistical Society Series A* 130:505–528.

Dixon, C. W.
1962 *Smallpox*. J. and A. Churchill, London.

Dixon, R. B.
1913 Some Aspects of North American Archaeology. *American Anthropologist* 15: 549–577.

Dobyns, H.
1963a Indian Extinction in the Middle Santa Cruz Valley, Arizona. *New Mexico Historical Review* 38:163–181.
1963b An Outline of Andean Epidemic History to 1720. *Bulletin of the History of Medicine* 37:493–515.
1966 An Appraisal of Techniques for Estimating Aboriginal American Population with a New Hemispheric Estimate. *Current Anthropology* 7:395–416.
1976 Brief Perspective on a Scholarly Transformation: Widowing the "Virgin" Land. *Ethnohistory* 23:95–104.
1981 *From Fire to Flood: Historic Human Destruction of Sonoran Desert Riverine Oases*. Ballena Press Anthropological Papers 20. Socorro.
1983 *Their Number Become Thinned*. The University of Tennessee Press, Knoxville.

Dodd, C. F.
1982 Ontario Iroquois Tradition Longhouses. *National Museum of Man, Mercury Series, Archaeological Survey of Canada Paper* 124:181–437.

Downie, A. W.
1967 Smallpox. In *Viral and Rickettsial Diseases of Man*. 4th ed., edited by Sir S.

Bedson, A. W. Downie, F. O. MacCollum, and C. H. Stuart-Harris, pp. 84–111. Edward Arnold, London.

Dubos, R.
1971 *Mirage of Health; Utopias, Progress, and Biological Change*. Harper and Row, New York.

Dubos, R., and J. Dubos
1952 *The White Plague; Tuberculosis, Man, and Society*. Little, Brown, Boston.

Duffy, J.
1953 *Epidemics in Colonial America*. Louisiana State University Press, Baton Rouge.

Dunn, F. L.
1965 On the Antiquity of Malaria in the Western Hemisphere. *Human Biology* 37:385–393.

Dunnell, R. C.
1970 Seriation Method and its Evaluation. *American Antiquity* 35:305–319.
1971 *Systematics in Prehistory*. The Free Press, New York.
1980 Evolutionary Theory and Archaeology. In *Advances in Archaeological Method and Theory*, vol. 3, edited by M. B. Schiffer, pp. 35–99. Academic Press, New York.

Elliott, D.
1977 Otsiningo, an Example of an Eighteenth-Century Settlement Pattern. In *Current Perspectives in Northeastern Archaeology: Essays in Honor of William A. Ritchie*. New York State Archaeological Association, Researches and Transactions 17:93–105. Albany.

El-Najjar, M. Y.
1979 Human Treponematosis and Tuberculosis: Evidence from the New World. *American Journal of Physical Anthropology* 51:599–618.

Engelbrecht, W.
1972 The Reflection of Patterned Behavior in Iroquois Pottery Decoration. *Pennsylvania Archaeologist* 42:1–15.

Ewers, J. C.
1955 *The Horse in Blackfoot Culture*. Bureau of American Ethnology, Bulletin 159. Washington, D.C.
1968 *Indian Life on the Upper Missouri*. University of Oklahoma Press, Norman.
1973 The Influence of Epidemics on the Indian Population and Culture of Texas. *Plains Anthropologist* 18:104–115.

Fairbanks, C. H.
1978 The Ethno-Archeology of the Florida Seminole. In *Tacachale: Essays on the Indians of Florida and Southeastern Georgia during the Historic Period*, edited by J. T. Milanich, and S. Proctor, pp. 163–193. The University Presses of Florida, Gainesville.

Faust, E. C.
1941 The Distribution of Malaria in North America, Mexico, Central America and the West Indies. In *A Symposium on Human Malaria with Special Reference to North America and the Caribbean Region*, edited by F. R. Moulton, pp. 8–18.

American Association for the Advancement of Science, Publication 15. Washington D.C.

Feldman, W. K.

1963 Tuberculosis. In *Diseases Transmitted from Animals to Man*. 5th ed., edited by T. G. Hull, pp. 5–81. Charles C. Thomas, Springfield.

Fenner, F.

1971 Infectious Diseases and Social Change. *Medical Journal of Australia* 1:1043–1047; 1099–1201.

Fenner, F., B. J. McAuslan, C. A. Mims, J. Simbrook, and D. O. White

1974 *The Biology of Animal Viruses*, vol. 1. Academic Press, New York.

Fenner, F., and F. N. Ratliffe

1965 *Myxomatosis*. Cambridge University Press, Cambridge.

Fenner, F., and D. O. White

1976 *Medical Virology*. 2nd ed. Academic Press, New York.

Fenton, W. N.

1940 Problems Arising from the Historic Northeastern Position of the Iroquois. In *Essays in Historical Anthropology of North America, Published in Honor of John R. Swanton*. Smithsonian Miscellaneous Collections 100:159–252. Washington, D.C.

1985 Structure, Continuity and Change in the Process of Iroquois Treaty Making. In *The History and Culture of Iroquois Diplomacy*, edited by F. Jennings, pp. 3–36. Syracuse University Press, Syracuse.

Fenton, W. N., and E. Tooker

1978 Mohawk. In *Northeast*, edited by B. G. Trigger, pp. 466–480. Handbook of North American Indians, vol. 15. W. G. Sturtevant, general editor. Smithsonian Institution, Washington, D.C.

Ferguson, R. G.

1955 *Studies in Tuberculosis*. University of Toronto Press, Toronto.

Fernandez, J. B.

1975 *Alvar Nunez Cabesa de Vaca, the Forgotten Chronicler*. Ediciones Universal, Miami.

Findlay, C. E.

1940 *Carlos E. Findlay and Yellow Fever*. Oxford University Press, London.

1941 Present Position of Yellow Fever in Africa. *Transactions of the Royal Society of Tropical Medicine and Hygiene* 35:51–76.

Finlayson, W. R.

1985 *Rescue Excavations at the Draper Site: Introduction and Settlement Patterns*. National Museum of Man, Mercury Series, Archaeological Survey of Canada Paper 130. Ottawa.

Finlayson, W. R., and D. H. Pihl

1980 Some Implications for the Attribute Analysis of Rim Sherds from the Draper Site, Pickering, Ontario. In *Proceedings of the 1979 Iroquois Pottery Conference*, edited by C.F. Hayes III. Rochester Museum and Science Center, Research Records 13:113–131. Rochester.

Fisk, H. N.
1944 *Geological Investigation of the Alluvial Valley of the Lower Mississippi Valley*. U.S. Army Corps of Engineers, Mississippi River Commission, Publication 52. Vicksburg.

Flint, R. F.
1955 Pleistocene Geology of Eastern South Dakota. *U.S. Geological Survey Professional Paper* 262. Washington, D.C.
1957 *Glacial and Pleistocene Geology*. John Wiley and Sons, New York.

Ford, J. A.
1936 *Analysis of Indian Village Site Collections from Louisiana and Mississippi*. Department of Conservation, Louisiana Geological Survey, Anthropological Study 2. New Orleans.
1954 The Type Concept Revisited. *American Anthropologist* 56:42–53.
1961 *Menard Site: The Quapaw Village of Osotouy on the Arkansas River*. American Museum of Natural History, Anthropological Papers 48(2). New York.
1962 *A Quantitative Method for Deriving Cultural Chronology*. Pan American Union, Technical Manual 1.

Ford, J. A., and G. R. Willey
1941 An Interpretation of the Prehistory of the Eastern United States. *American Anthropologist* 43:325–363.

Funk, R. E.
1967 Garoga: A Late Prehistoric Iroquois Village in the Mohawk Valley. In *Iroquois Culture, History, and Prehistory*, edited by E. Tooker, pp. 81–84. University of the State of New York, Albany.

Gerhard, P.
1972 *A Guide to the Historical Geography of New Spain*. Cambridge University Press, Cambridge.

Giardino, M. J.
1984 Documenting Evidence for the Location of Historic Indian Villages in the Mississippi Delta. In *Perspectives on Gulf Coast Prehistory*, edited by D.D. Davis, pp. 232–257. Ripley P. Bullen Monographs in Anthropolgy and History 5. Florida State Museum, Gainesville.

Gibson, J. L.
1973 *Social Systems at Poverty Point: An Analysis of Intersite and Intrasite Variability*. Unpublished Ph.D. dissertation, Department of Anthropology, Southern Methodist University, Dallas.
1980 Speculations on the Origin and Development of Poverty Point Culture. *Louisiana Archaeology* 6:319–348.

Gilg, A. W.
1973 A Study in Agricultural Disease Diffusion. *Institute of British Geographers* 59:77–97.

Giraud, M.
1974 *The History of French Louisiana*, vol. 1. *The Reign of Louis XIV, 1698–1715*, translated by J. C. Lambert. Louisiana State University Press, Baton Rouge.

Goldstein, R. A.
1969 *French-Iroquois Diplomatic and Military Relations 1609–1701*. Mouton, The Hague.

Goodyear, J. D.
1978 The Sugar Connection: A New Perspective on Yellow Fever. *Bulletin of the History of Medicine* 52:5–21.

Gookin, D.
1806 Historical Collections of Indians of New England, 1674. *Collections of the Massachusetts Historical Society, 1st Series* [1792] 1:141–227.

Gould, S. J.
1977 Uniformity and Catastrophe. In *Ever Since Darwin*, edited by S. J. Gould, pp. 147–152. W. W. Norton, New York.

Grassman, T. Fr.
1969 *The Mohawk Indians and their Valley*. Hugo Press, Schenectady.

Graybill, J. R.
1981 *The Eastern Periphery of Fort Ancient (AD 1050–1650): A Diachronic Approach to Settlement Variability*. Unpublished Ph.D. dissertation, Department of Anthropology, University of Washington, Seattle.

Green, W.
1984 Protohistoric Depopulation in the Upper Midwest. Paper presented at the Annual Midwest Archaeological Conference, Evanston.

Griffin, D.
n.d. South Cannonball Village 32 SI 19, North Dakota. Ms. in possession of author. University of Missouri, Columbia.

Griffin, J. B.
1946a Cultural Changes and Continuity in Eastern United States. In *Man in Northeastern North America*, edited by F. Johnson, pp. 37–95. Robert S. Peabody Foundation for Archaeology, Papers 3. Andover.
1946b *The Fort Ancient Aspect, its Cultural and Chronological Position in Mississippi Valley Archaeology*. University of Michigan Press, Ann Arbor.
1952 Culture Periods in the Eastern United States. In *Archaeology of the Eastern United States*, edited by J. B. Griffin, pp. 352–370. University of Chicago Press, Chicago.

Gwaltney, J. M., and J. O. Hendley
1976 Acute Respiratory Infections. In *Communicable and Infectious Diseases*. 8th ed., edited by F. H. Top Sr., and P. F. Wehrle, pp. 91–115. C. W. Mosby, St. Louis.

Haag, W. G.
1985 Federal Aid to Archaeology in the Southeast. *American Antiquity* 50:272–280.

Hackett, C. J.
1963 On the Origin of the Human Treponematoses. *Bulletin of the World Health Organization* 29:1–41.

Hackett, C. W. (editor)
1923–1937 Historical Documents relating to New Mexico, Nueva Viscaya and Approaches Thereto, to 1773. *Adolph A. Bandelier and Fanny R. Bandelier,*

Collections, vols. 1 and 3. Carnegie Institution of Washington 330. Washington, D.C.

Hackett, L. W.

1941 Malaria and Community. In *A Symposium on Human Malaria with Special Reference to North America and the Caribbean Region*, edited by F. R. Moulton, pp. 148–156. American Association for the Advancement of Science, Publication 15. Washington, D.C.

Hagerstrand, T.

1952 The Propogation of Innovation Waves. *Lund Studies in Human Geography* 4:3–23.

Haggett, P.

1975 Simple Epidemics in Human Populations. Some Geographic Aspects of the Hamer-Soper Diffusion Models. In *Processes in Physical and Human Geography*, edited by R. Peel, M. Chishom, and P. Haggett, pp. 372–391. Heinemann Educational Books, London.

1976 Hybridizing Alternative Models of an Epidemic Diffusion Process. *Economic Geography* 52:136–146.

Haggett, P., and A. D. Cliff

1979 Geographic Aspects of Epidemic Diffusion in Closed Communities. In *Statistical Applications in the Spatial Sciences*, edited by N. Wrigley, pp. 5–44. Pion, London.

Haggett, P., A. D. Cliff, and A. Frey

1977 *Locational Analysis in Human Geography*. John Wiley and Sons, New York.

Hamer, W. H.

1906 Epidemic Disease in England—the Evidence of Variability and Persistency of Type. *Lancet* 1:569–574; 655–662; 733–739.

Hariot, T.

1973 A Brief and True Report of the New Found Land of Virginia (1588). In *Virginia Voyages from Hakluyt [1589]*, edited by D. B. Quinn, and A. M. Quinn, pp. 46–76. Oxford University Press, Oxford.

Harris, T. M.

1835 Researches into the Origin of the Indigenes of North and South America. Ms. on file, American Antiquarian Society, Worcester.

Hart, C. W. M.

1943 A Reconstruction of Natchez Social Structure. *American Anthropologist* 45:379–386.

Hassan, F. A.

1981 *Demographic Archaeology*. Academic Press, New York.

Haven, S. F.

1856 *Archaeology of the United States*. Smithsonian Contributions to Knowledge 89 (2). Washington, D.C.

Hayden, B.

1976 Corporate Groups and the Late Ontario Longhouse. *Ontario Archaeology* 28:3–16.

Hayes, C. F. III (general editor)
1983 *Proceedings of the 1982 Glass Bead Conference*. Rochester Museum and Science Center, Records 16. Rochester.
Heizer, R. F.
1941 The Direct Historical Approach in California Archaeology. *American Antiquity* 7:98–122.
Helm, J.
1965 Bilaterality in the Socio-Territorial Organization of the Arctic Drainage Dene. *Ethnology* 4:361–85.
1968 The Nature of Dogrib Socioterritorial Groups. In *Man the Hunter*, edited by R. B. Lee, and I. DeVore, pp. 118–125. Aldine, Chicago.
1980 Female Infanticide, European Diseases and Population Levels among McKenzie Dene. *American Ethnologist* 7:259–285.
Helm J., E. S. Rogers, and J. G. E. Smith
1978 Intercultural Relations and Cultural Change in the Shield and MacKenzie Drainage Borderlands. In *Subarctic*, edited by J. Helm, pp. 146–157. Handbook of North American Indians, vol. 6. W. G. Sturtevant, general editor. Smithsonian Institution, Washington, D.C.
Herskovits, M.
1958 *Acculturation: The Study of Culture Contact* [1938]. Peter Smith, Gloucester.
Hill, J. N.
1970 *Broken K Pueblo: Prehistoric Social Organization in the American Southwest*. University of Arizona, Anthropological Papers 18. Tucson.
Hill, J. N. and R. K. Evans
1972 A Model for Classification and Typology. In *Models in Archaeology*, edited by D. Clarke, pp. 231–273. Methuen, London.
Hoffman, J. J.
1967 *Molstad Village*. River Basin Surveys Publications in Salvage Archaeology 4. Lincoln.
1968 *The La Roche Sites*. River Basin Surveys Publications in Salvage Archaeology 11. Lincoln.
Hoffman, M. P.
1983 Protohistory of the Lower and Central Arkansas River Valley in Arkansas. Paper presented at the Mid-South Archaeological Conference, Memphis.
Hookyas, R.
1963 *Natural Law and Divine Miracle: The Principle of Uniformity in Geology, Biology, and Theology*. Brill, London.
1970 Catastrophism in Geology, its Scientific Character in Relation to Actualism and Uniformitarianism. *Mededlingen der Koninkleke Nederlandse Academie Van Weterschappen AFD. Letterkunde Nieune Reeks-Deel* 33–7:271–316.
House, J.
1984 Kent Phase Investigations in Eastern Arkansas. Paper presented at the 41st Annual Meeting of the Southeastern Archaeological Conference, Pensacola.
Hudson, C.
1976 *The Southeastern Indians*. The University of Tennessee Press, Knoxville.

Hudson, C., M. Smith, D. Hally, R. Polhemus, and C. DePratter
1985 Coosa: A Chiefdom in the Sixteenth-Century Southeastern United States. *American Antiquity* 50:723–737.

Hudson, E. H.
1968 Treponematosis and Human Social Evolution. *American Anthropologist* 67:885–892.

Hunt, G. T.
1967 *The Wars of the Iroquois: A Study in Intertribal Relations*. 3rd printing. The University of Wisconsin Press, Madison.

Hurt, W. R. Jr.
1953 *Report on the Thomas Riggs site, 39 HU 1, Hughes County South Dakota, 1952*. South Dakota Archaeological Commission, Archaeological Studies, Circular 5. Pierre.
1954a Pottery Types of the Over Focus. In Prehistoric Pottery of the Eastern United States edited by J. B. Griffin. Ceramic Laboratory, Museum of Anthropology, University of Michigan. Ann Arbor. Mimeo.
1954b *Report on the Investigation of the Spotted Bear Site, 39 HU 26, and the Cottonwood Site, 39 HU 43, Hughes County, South Dakota, 1953*. The South Dakota Archaeological Commission, Archaeological Studies, Circular 6. Pierre.
1957 *Report on the Investigation of the Swan Creek Site, 39 WW 7, Walworth County, South Dakota, 1954–1956*. South Dakota Archaeological Commission, Archaeological Studies, Circular 7. Pierre.

Hurt, W. R. Jr., W. G. Buckles, E. Fugle, and G. A. Agogino
1962 *Report of the Investigations of the Four Bear Site, 39 DW 2, Dewey County, South Dakota, 1958–1959*. State Museum of South Dakota, Archaeological Studies, Circular 10. Vermillion.

Indian Health Service
1978 *Indian Health Trends and Services*. Department of Health, Education and Welfare, Washington, D.C.
1979a *Selected Vital Statistics for Indian Health Service Areal and Service Units, 1972–1977*. Department of Health, Education and Welfare, Washington, D.C.
1979b *Illness among Indians and Alaska Natives*. Department of Health, Education and Welfare, Washington, D.C.

Innis, H. A.
1956 *The Fur Trade in Canada*. rev. ed. University of Toronto Press, Toronto.

Jablow, J.
1951 *The Cheyenne in Plains Indian Trade Relations*. American Ethnological Society, Monographs 19. Washington, D.C.

Jackes, M. K.
1983 Osteological Evidence for Smallpox: A Possible Case from Seventeenth-Century Ontario. *American Journal of Physical Anthropology* 60:75–81.

Jarcho, S.
1964 Some Observations on Disease in Prehistoric America. *Bulletin of the History of Medicine* 38:1–19.

Jennings, F.
1971 The Constitutional Evolution of the Covenant Chain. *Proceedings of the American Philosophical Society* 115:88–96.
1984 *The Ambiguous Iroquois Empire*. W. W. Norton, New York.
1985 Iroquois Alliances in American History. In *The History and Culture of Iroquois Diplomacy*, edited by F. Jennings, pp. 37–65. Syracuse University Press, Syracuse.

Jennings, J. D.
1985 River Basin Surveys: Origins, Operations, and Results, 1945–1969. *American Antiquity* 50:281–296.

Jeter, M. D., D. B. Kelley, and G. P. Kelley
1979 The Kelley-Grimes Site: A Mississippian Period Burial Mound, Southeast Arkansas, Excavated in 1936. *The Arkansas Archeologist* 20:1–51.

Jochim, M. A.
1976 *Hunter-Gatherer Subsistence and Settlement: A Predictive Model*. Academic Press, New York.
1981 *Strategies of Survival: Cultural Behavior in an Ecological Context*. Academic Press, New York.

Johnson, A. M.
1979 *Extended Middle Missouri Components in the Big Bend Region, South Dakota*. South Dakota Archaeological Society Special Publications 1. University of South Dakota Archaeological Laboratory. Vermillion.

Johnson, G.
1972 A Test of the Utility of Central Place Theory in Archaeology. In *Man, Settlement and Urbanism*, edited by P. J. Ucko, R. Tringham, and G. W. Dimbleby, pp. 769–786. George Duckworth, London.

Jones, G. T., D. K. Grayson, and C. Beck
1983 Artifact Class Richness and Sample Size in Archaeological Surface Assemblages. In *Lulu Linear Punctated: Essays in Honor of George Irving Quimby*, edited by R. C. Dunnell, and D. K. Grayson. Anthropological Papers 72:55–73. Museum of Anthropology, University of Michigan, Ann Arbor.

Jordan, E. O.
1927 *Epidemic Influenza*. American Medical Association, Chicago.

Joutel, H.
1906 *Joutel's Journals of La Salle's Last Voyage, 1684–1687* [1713]. Joseph McDonough, Albany.

Kaschula, R. O. C., C. C. Sinclair-Smith, and P. D. Gajjar
1978 Measles Pneumonia. *South African Medical Journal* 53:1049.

Kellogg, L. (editor)
1917 *Early Narratives of the Northwest, 1634–1699*. Charles Scribner's Sons, New York.

Kidd, K. E., and M. A. Kidd
1970 *A Classification System for Glass Beads for the Use of Field Archaeologists*. Occasional Papers in Archaeology and History 1. National Historic Sites Service, Ottawa.

King, W. V., and G. H. Bradley
1941 General Morphology of Anopheles and Classification of Nearctic Species. In *A Symposium on Human Malaria with Special Reference to North America and the Caribbean Region*, edited by F. R. Moulton, pp. 63–70. American Association for the Advancement of Science, Publication 15. Washington, D.C.

Klein, J., J. C. Lerman, P. E. Damon and E. K. Ralph
1982 Calibration of Radiocarbon Dates: Tables Based on the Consensus Data of the Workshop on Calibrating the Radiocarbon Time Scale. *Radiocarbon* 24:103–150.

Klinger, T.
1975–1977 Parkin Archeology: A Report on the 1966 Field School Test Excavations at the Parkin Site. *The Arkansas Archeologist* 16–18:45–80.

Knight, V. J.
1984 Late Prehistoric Adaptations in the Mobile Bay Region. In *Perspectives on Gulf Coast Prehistory*, edited by D. D. Davis, pp. 198–215. Ripley P. Bullen Monographs in Anthropology and History 5. Florida State Museum, Gainesville.

Korones, S., B. Lorin, E. Ainger, R. Gillis, G. Monif, J. Roane, J. Sever, and F. Fuste
1965 Congenital Rubella Syndrome; a Study of 22 Infants. *American Journal of Disease in Children* 116:434–440.

Krech, S. III
1978 Disease, Starvation, and Northern Athapaskan Social Organization. *American Ethnologist* 5:710–732.
1983 The Influence of Disease and the Fur Trade on Arctic Drainage Dene. *Journal of Anthropological Research* 39:123–146.

Kroeber, A. L.
1925 *Handbook of the Indians of California*. Bureau of American Ethnology, Bulletin 78. Washington, D.C.
1934 Native American Population. *American Anthropologist* 36:1–25.
1939 *Cultural and Natural Areas of Native North America*. University of California Publications in American Archaeology and Ethnology 38. Berkeley.

LeBlanc, S.
1971 An Addition to Naroll's Suggested Floor Area and Settlement Population Relationship. *American Antiquity* 36:210–211.

Leder, L. H. (editor)
1956 The Livingston Indian Records: 1666–1723. *Pennsylvania History* 23:1–240.

Lehmer, D. J.
1952 The Fort Pierre Branch, Central South Dakota. *American Antiquity* 17:329–336.
1954a The Sedentary Horizon on the Northern Plains. *Southwestern Journal of Anthropology* 10:139–159.
1954b Archaeological Investigation in the Oahe Dam Area, South Dakota, 1950–1951. *Bureau of American Ethnology, Bulletin* 158. Washington, D.C.
1966 *The Fire Heart Creek Site*. River Basin Surveys Publications in Salvage Archaeology 1. Lincoln.

1971 *Introduction to Middle Missouri Archaeology*. National Park Service, Anthropological Papers 1. Washington, D.C.

1977 Epidemics among the Indians of the Upper Missouri. *Reprints in Anthropology* 8:105–111. Lincoln.

n.d. Data files. Department of Anthropology, University of Missouri, Columbia.

Lehmer, D. J., and W. W. Caldwell

1966 Horizon and Tradition in the Northern Plains. *American Antiquity* 31:511–516.

Lehmer, D. J., and D. T. Jones

1968 *Arikara Archaeology: The Bad River Phase*. River Basin Surveys Publications in Salvage Archaeology 7. Lincoln.

Lehmer, D. J., W. R. Wood, and C. L. Dill

1978 *The Knife River Phase*. Department of Anthropology and Sociology, Dana College. Submitted to Interagency Archeological Service Center-Denver. Contract No. C3537(68), and Purchase Orders A3514(75), A3521(78). Blair.

Lenig, D.

1965 *The Oak Hill Horizon and its Relation to the Development of Five Nations Iroquois Cultures*. New York State Archaeological Association, Researches and Transactions 15(1). Albany.

1977 Of Dutchmen, Beaver Hats and Iroquois. In *Current Perspectives in Northeastern Archaeology: Essays in Honor of William A. Ritchie*, edited by R. E. Funk, and C. F. Hayes III. New York State Archaeological Association, Researches and Transactions 17:71–84.

Leone, M. P.

1972 Issues in Anthropological Archaeology. In *Contemporary Archaeology*, edited by M. P. Leone, pp. 14–27. Southern Illinois University Press, Carbondale.

Le Page du Pratz, A. S.

1975 *The History of Louisiana* [1758], edited by J. G. Tregle. Reprint, Louisiana State University Press for Louisiana American Revolution Bicentennial Commission, Baton Rouge.

Le Rays, C.

1908 Journal of Charles Le Rays, 1802. *South Dakota Historical Collections* 4:159–169.

Long, A., and B. Rippeteau

1974 Testing Contemporaneity and Averaging Radiocarbon Dates. *American Antiquity* 39:205–215.

Longacre, W. A.

1975 Population Dynamics at Grasshopper Pueblo. In *Population Studies in Archaeology and Biological Anthropology: A Symposium*, edited by A. C. Swedlund, pp. 71–74. Society for American Archaeology, Memoir 30. Washington, D.C.

Lowie, R. H.

1954 *Indians of the Plains*. McGraw-Hill, New York.

MacDonald, G.

1950 The Analysis of Malaria Parasite Rates in Infants. *Tropical Disease Bulletin* 47:915–938.

1952 The Analysis of Equilibrium in Malaria. *Tropical Disease Bulletin* 49:813–829.

1953 The Analysis of Malaria Epidemics. *Tropical Disease Bulletin* 50:871–889.

MacNeish, R. S.
1952 *Iroquois Pottery Types*. National Museum of Canada, Bulletin 124, Anthropological Series 31. Ottawa.
McNeill, W. H.
1976 *Plagues and Peoples: A Natural History of Infectious Diseases*. Anchor Press/ Doubleday, New York.
McWilliams, R. G. (translator and editor)
1981 *Iberville's Gulf Journals*. The University of Alabama Press, University.
Malinowski, B.
1945 *Dynamics of Culture Change*. Yale University Press, New Haven.
Malouf, C.
1963 Crow-Flies-High (32 ML 1), A Historic Hidatsa Village in the Garrison Reservoir Area, North Dakota. *Bureau of American Ethnology, Bulletin* 185:133–166. Washington, D.C.
Marchand, J. F.
1943 Tribal Epidemics in the Yukon. *Journal of the American Medical Association* 123:1019–1020.
Marquardt, W. H.
1978 Advances in Archaeological Seriation. In *Advances in Archaeological Method and Theory*, vol. 1, edited by M. B. Schiffer, pp. 257–314. Academic Press, New York.
Mason, C. I.
1976 Historic Identification and Lake Winnebago Focus Oneota. In *Cultural Change and Continuity: Essays in Honor of James Bennett Griffin*, edited by C. E. Cleland, pp. 335–348. Academic Press, New York.
Meany, E. S. (editor)
1949 *Vancouver's Discovery of Puget Sound*. Binford and Mort, Portland.
Merriam, C. H.
1905 Indian Populations of California. *American Anthropologist* 7:594–606.
Meyer, K. F.
1963 Plague. In *Diseases Transmitted from Animals to Man*. 5th ed., edited by T. G. Hull, pp. 527–587. Charles C. Thomas, Springfield.
Michelson, G.
1977 Iroquois Population Estimates. *Man in the Northeast* 14:3–17.
Milner, G. R.
1980 Epidemic Disease in the Post-Contact Southeast: A Reappraisal. *Midcontinental Journal of Archaeology* 5:39–56.
Mogabgab, W. J.
1976 Influenza. In *Communicable and Infectious Diseases*. 8th ed., edited by F. H. Top Sr. and P. F. Wehrle, pp. 369–378. C. W. Mosby, St. Louis.
Monath, T. P., R. B. Craven, A. Adjukiewicz, M. Germain, D. B. Francy, L. Ferrara, E. M. Samba, H. N'Jie, K. Cham, S. A. Fitzgerald, P. H. Crippen, D. I. Simpson, E. T. Bowen, A. Febiyi, and J-J. Salaun
1980 Yellow Fever in Gambia, 1978–1979: Epidemiologic Aspects with Observations on the Occurrence of Orungo Virus Infections. *American Journal of Tropical Medicine and Hygiene* 29:912–928.

Mooney, H.

1977 *Convergent Evolution in Chile and California*. US/IBP Synthesis Series 5. Dowden, Hutchinson and Ross, Stroudsburg.

Mooney, J.

1910 Population. In *Handbook of American Indians North of Mexico*, edited by F.W. Hodge. Bureau of American Ethnology Bulletin 30 (part 2):28–87. Washington, D.C.

1928 *The Aboriginal Population of America North of Mexico*, edited by J.R. Swanton. Smithsonian Miscellaneous Collections 80(7). Washington, D.C.

Moore, C. B.

1908 Certain Mounds of Arkansas and Mississippi, Parts I, III. *Journal of the Academy of Natural Sciences of Philadelphia, Series 2*, 13:480–600.

Morgan, L. H.

1851 *League of Ho-do-no-sau-nee*. Sage and Brother, Rochester.

Morison, S. E.

1972 *Samuel de Champlain: Father of New France*. Little, Brown, Boston.

Morse, D. F. (editor)

1973 *Nodena: An Account of 75 Years of Archeological Investigation in Southeast Mississippi County, Arkansas*. Arkansas Archeological Survey, Research Series 4. Fayetteville.

Morse, D. F., and P. A. Morse

1983 *Archaeology of the Central Mississippi Valley*. Academic Press, New York.

Morse, P. A.

1981 *Parkin: The 1978–1979 Archeological Investigations of a Cross County, Arkansas Site*. Arkansas Archeological Survey, Research Series 13. Fayetteville.

Murray, G. D., and A. D. Cliff

1977 A Stochastic Model for Measles Epidemics in a Multiregional Setting. *Institute of British Geographers Publication, New Series* 2:158–174.

Nagler, F. P., C. E. Van Rooyen, and J. H. Sturdy

1949 An Influenza Virus Epidemic at Victoria Island, N. W. T., Canada. *Canadian Journal of Public Health* 40:457–465.

Naroll, R.

1962 Floor Area and Settlement Patterns. *American Antiquity* 27:587–589.

Nasatir, A. P.

1952 *Before Lewis and Clark: Documents illustrating the History of the Missouri, 1785–1804*. 2 vols. St. Louis Historical Documents Foundation, St. Louis.

Neitzel, R. S.

1965 *Archaeology of the Fatherland Site, the Grand Village of the Natchez*. American Museum of Natural History, Anthropological Papers 51(1). New York.

Office of Indian Affairs

1829 Letter from Dougherty to William Clark, October 29, 1831. *Microcopy, Reel 883–3*. National Archives. Washington, D.C.

1837 Report from Fulkerson to Clark. *Microcopy, Reel 884–8*. National Archives, Washington, D.C.

1838 Letter from Clark to Harris. *Microcopy, Reel 884–5*. National Archives, Washington, D.C.

1842 Letter from Mitchell to Crawford. *Microcopy, Reel 753–1*. National Archives, Washington, D.C.

Orians, G. H. and O. T. Solbrig

1977 *Convergent Evolution in Warm Deserts*. US/IBP Synthesis Series 3. Dowden, Hutchinson and Ross, Stroudsburg.

Orser, C. E., Jr.

1984 Trade Good Flow in Arikara Villages: Expanding Ray's Middleman Hypothesis. *Plains Anthropologist* 29:1–12.

Ortner, D. and W. G. Putschar

1981 *Identification of Pathological Conditions in Human Skeletal Remains*. Smithsonian Contributions to Anthropology 28. Washington, D.C.

Owsley, D. W. and W. Bass

1979 A Demographic Analysis of Skeletons from the Larson Site (39 WW 2), Walworth County, South Dakota: Vital Statistics. *American Journal of Physical Anthropology* 51:145–154.

Pagels, W., F. A. H. Simmonds, and N. Macdonald

1953 *Pulmonary Tuberculosis: Pathology, Management and Prevention*. 3rd ed. Oxford University Press, London.

Palkovich, A. M.

1981 Demography and Disease Patterns in a Protohistoric Plains Group: A Study of the Mobridge Site (39 WW 1). *Plains Anthropologist* 26 *Memoir* 17:71–84.

Panum, P. L.

1940 *Observations Made during the Epidemic of Measles on the Faroe Islands in the Year 1846*. American Public Health Association, New York.

Parker, A. C.

1907 Excavations in an Erie Village and Burial Site at Ripley, Chautaugua County, New York. *New York State Museum, Bulletin* 117:459–554. Albany.

1916 The Origin of the Iroquois as Suggested by Their Archaeology. *American Anthropologist* 18:479–507.

Parsons, J.

1971 *Prehistoric Settlement Patterns in Texcoco Region, Mexico*. University of Michigan, Museum of Anthropology, Memoirs 3. Ann Arbor.

Paul, J. H., and H. L. Freeze

1933 An Epidemiological and Bacteriological Study of the "Common Cold" in an Isolated Arctic Community (Spitzbergen). *American Journal of Hygiene* 17: 517–535.

Peart, A. F. and F. P. Nagler

1954 Measles in the Canadian Arctic. *Canadian Journal of Public Health* 45:146–156.

Pendergast, J. F., and B. G. Trigger

1972 *Cartier's Hochelaga and the Dawson Site*. McGill-Queens University Press, Montreal.

Perttula, T. K.
1984 The Early Historic Period in the Caddoan Area. Paper presented at the 49th Annual Meeting of the Society for American Archaeology, Portland.

Perttula, T. K., and A. F. Ramenofsky
1981 An Archaeological Model of Caddoan Culture Change: The Historic Period. *Southeastern Archaeological Conference, Bulletin* 24:13–15.

Petsche, J.
1968 *Bibliography of Salvage Archaeology in the United States*. River Basin Survey, Publications in Salvage Archaeology 10. Washington, D.C

Phillip, R. N., W. T. Weeks, and K. Reinghard
1959 Observations on Asia Influenza on Two Alaskan Islands. *Public Health Reports* 74:737–745.

Phillips, P.
1958 Application of the Wheat-Gifford-Wasley Taxonomy to Eastern Ceramics. *American Antiquity* 24:117–125.

1970 *Archaeological Survey in the Lower Yazoo Basin, Mississippi, 1949–1955*. Peabody Museum of Archaeology and Ethnology, Papers 60 (parts I and II). Cambridge.

Phillips, P., J. A. Ford, and J. B. Griffin
1951 *Archaeological Survey in the Lower Mississippi Alluvial Valley, 1940–1947*. Peabody Museum of Archaeology and Ethnology, Papers 25. Cambridge.

Plog, F.
1973 Diachronic Anthropology. In *Research and Theory in Archaeology*, edited by C. L. Redman, pp. 181–198. John Wiley and Sons, New York.

1975 Demographic Studies in Southwestern Prehistory. In *Population Studies in Archaeology and Biological Anthropology: A Symposium*, edited by A. C. Swedlund, pp. 94–103. Society for American Archaeology, Memoir 30. Washington, D.C.

Powell, M. L.
1985 *Health Disease and Social Organization in the Mississippian Community at Moundville*. Unpublished Ph.D. dissertation, Department of Anthropology, Northwestern University, Evanston.

Pratt, P. D.
1976 *Archaeology of the Oneida Iroquois* 1. Minott Printing and Binding, Greenfield, Massachusetts.

Price, J. E.
1978 The Settlement Pattern of the Powers Phase. In *Mississippian Settlement Patterns*, edited by B. D. Smith, pp. 201–231. Academic Press, New York.

Pyle, G.
1979 *Applied Medical Geography*. V. H. Winston and Sons, Washington, D.C.

Quimby, G. I.
1946 Natchez Social Structure as an Instrument of Assimilation. *American Anthropologist* 48:134–137.

1951 *The Medora Site, Western Baton Rouge Parish, Louisiana*. Field Museum of Natural History, Anthropological Series 24(2). Chicago.

1957 *The Bayou Goula Site, Iberville Parish, Louisiana*. Fieldiana: Anthropology 47(2). Chicago.

Ralph, E. K., H. N. Michael, and M. C. Han

1974 Radiocarbon Dates and Reality. *Archaeology of Eastern North America* 2:1–20.

Ramenofsky, A. F.

1982 *Disease and the Archaeology of Population Collapse: Native American Response to European Contact*. Ph.D. dissertation, University of Washington. University Microfilms, Ann Arbor.

1984 Methodological Issues in the Archaeology of European Contact. Paper presented at the 49th Annual Meeting of the Society for American Archaeology, Portland.

1985 The Introduction of European Disease and Aboriginal Population Collapse. *Mississippi Archaeologist* 20:2–18.

Renfrew, C., and R. M. Clark

1974 Problems of the Radiocarbon Calendar and its Calibration. *Archaeometry* 16:5–18.

Rieckmann, K. H., and P. H. Silverman

1977 Plasmodia of Man. In *Parasitic Plasmodia*, vol. 3, edited by J. P. Kreier, pp. 493–527. Academic Press, New York.

Ritchie, W. A.

1944 *The Pre-Iroquoian Occupations of New York State*. Rochester Museum of Arts and Sciences, Memoir 1. Rochester.

1952 The Chance Horizon, an Early Stage of Mohawk Iroquois Cultural Development. *New York State Museum, Circular* 29:3–53. Albany.

1954 *Dutch Hollow, an Early Historic Period Seneca Site in Livingston County, New York*. New York State Archaeological Association, Researches and Transactions 13(1). Albany.

1967 The Kelso Site: Its Significance for the Problem of Iroquois Origin. In *Iroquois Culture, History, and Prehistory*, edited by E. Tooker, pp. 71–73. The University of the State of New York, Albany.

1980 *The Archaeology of New York State*, 2nd rev. ed. [1965]. Harbor Hill Books, Harrison, New York

Ritchie, W. A., and R. E. Funk

1973 *Aboriginal Settlement Patterns in the Northeast*. The University of the State of New York, Memoir 20. Albany.

Ritchie, W. A., and R. S. MacNeish

1949 The Pre-Iroquoian Pottery of New York State. *American Antiquity* 15:97–124.

Robbins, L. M.

1978 Yawslike Disease Processes in a Louisiana Shell Mound. *Medical College of Virginia Quarterly* 14:24–31.

Robinson, D. (editor)

1918 Fort Tecumesh and Fort Pierre Journals and Letter Books (Jacob Halsey [1827–1830]). *South Dakota Historical Collections* 9:69–239.

Rosenblat, A.

1976 The Population of Hispaniola at the Time of Columbus. In *The Native Popula-*

tion of the Americas in 1492, edited by W. H. Denevan, pp. 43–66. University of Wisconsin Press, Madison.

Ross, R. Sir
1911 *The Prevention of Malaria*. 2nd ed. Murray, London.

Sanders, W. T.
1965 The Cultural Ecology of the Teotihuacan Valley. A Preliminary Report of the Results of the Teotihuacan Valley Project. The Pennsylvania State University Department of Sociology and Anthropology, University Park. Mimeo.
1970 The Population of the Teotihuacan Valley, the Basin of Mexico, and the Central Mexican Symbiotic Region in the Sixteenth Century. In *Teotihuacan Valley Project, Final Report. The Natural Environment, Contemporary Occupation and Sixteenth-Century Population of the Valley*, edited by W. T. Sanders, A. Kovar, T. Carlton, and R. Diehl, pp. 388–457. The Pennsylvania State University, Department of Anthropology, Occasional Papers 3. University Park.

Saucier, R. T.
1974 *Quaternary Geology of the Lower Mississippi Valley*. Arkansas Archeological Survey, Research Series 6. Fayetteville.

Sauer, C. O.
1971 *Sixteenth-Century North America: The Land and the People as Seen by Europeans*. University of California Press, Berkeley.

Schacht, R. M.
1981 Estimating Past Population Trends. *Annual Review of Anthropology* 10:119–140.
1984 The Contemporaneity Problem. *American Antiquity* 49:678–695.

Scholes, F.V.
1930 The Supply Service of the New Mexican Missions in the Seventeenth Century. *New Mexico Historical Review* 5:93–115; 186–210; 386–404.

Schoolcraft, H. R.
1853–1857 *Information Respecting the History, Condition and Prospects of Indian Tribes of the United States* (Parts 1–6). Collected and Prepared under Direction of the Bureau of Indian Affairs. Lippencott, Grambo, Philadelphia.

Schroeder, A.
1979 Pueblos Abandoned in Historic Times. In, *Southwest*, edited by A. Ortiz, pp. 236–254. Handbook of North American Indians, vol. 9, W. G. Sturtevant, general editor. Smithsonian Institution. Washington, D.C.

Schulman, J. L.
1978 Epidemiology of Influenza. *American Journal of Clinical Pathology* 70 (Supplement 1): 141–145.

Scott, D.
1965 *Epidemic Diseases in Ghana 1901–1960*. Oxford University Press, London.

Serfling, R. E.
1952 Historical Review of Epidemic Theory. *Human Biology* 24:145–166.

Service, E. R.
1962 *Primitive Social Organization: An Evolutionary Perspective*. Random House, New York.

Shea, J. D. G.

1903 *Discovery and Exploration of the Mississippi Valley: The Original Narratives of Marquette, Allouez, Membre, Hennepin, and Anastase Douay*. 2nd ed. Joseph McDonough, Albany.

Simmons, J. S.

1941 The Transmission of Malaria by Anopheles Mosquitos of North America. In *A Symposium on Human Malaria with Special Reference to North America and the Caribbean Region*, edited by F. R. Moulton, pp. 113–130. American Association for the Advancement of Science, Publication 15. Washington, D.C.

Sinnecker, H., R. Sinnecker, E. Zilske, and D. Koehler

1982 Detection of Influenza A Viruses and Influenza Epidemics in Wild Pelagic Birds by Sentinels and Population Studies. *Zentralblatt fur Bakteriologie Mikrobiologie und Hygiene, Series A*, 253:297–304.

Smith, C. S.

1951 Pottery Types from the Talking Crow Site, Fort Randall Reservoir, South Dakota. *Plains Archaeological Conference Newsletter* 4:32–41.

1977 *The Talking Crow Site*. University of Kansas Publications in Anthropology 9. Lawrence.

Smith, C. S., and R. T. Grange, Jr.

1957 The Spain Site (39 LM 301), a Winter Village in Fort Randall Reservoir, South Dakota. *Bureau of American Ethnology Bulletin* 169:79–128. Washington, D.C.

Smith, C. S., and A. E. Johnson

1968 *The Two Teeth Site*. River Basin Surveys Publications in Salvage Archaeology 8. Lincoln.

Smith, G. H.

1972 *Like-A-Fishhook Village and Fort Berthold, Garrison Reservoir, North Dakota*. National Park Service, Anthropological Papers 2. Washington, D.C.

1980 *The Explorations of the La Verendryes in the Northern Plains 1738–1743*, edited by W. R. Wood. University of Nebraska Press, Lincoln.

Smith, M. T.

1984 *Depopulation and Culture Change in the Early Historic Period Interior Southeast*. Unpublished Ph.D. dissertation, Department of Anthropology. University of Florida, Gainesville.

Snow, D. R.

1980 *Archaeology of New England*. Academic Press, New York.

Snow, D. R. and W. A. Starna

1984 Sixteenth-Century Depopulation: A Preliminary View from the Mohawk Valley. Paper presented at the 49th Annual Meeting of the Society for American Archaeology, Portland.

Soper, H. E.

1929 Interpretations of Periodicity in Disease Prevalence. *Journal of the Royal Statistical Society Series A* 139:468–500.

South, S.

1977 *Method and Theory in Historical Archaeology*. Academic Press, New York.

Spaulding, A.

1956 *The Arzberger Site, Hughes County, South Dakota*. University of Michigan, Museum of Anthropology, Occasional Contributions 16. Ann Arbor.

Sperry, J. E.

1968 The Shermer Site (32 EM 10). *Plains Anthropologist* 13, *Memoir* 9.

Spicer, E. H.

1961 *Perspectives on American Indian Culture Change*. The University of Chicago Press, Chicago.

1962 *Cycles of Conquest: The Impact of Spain, Mexico and the United States on the Indians of the Southwest, 1533–1960*. The University of Arizona Press, Tucson.

Squier, E. G.

1851 Aboriginal Monuments of the State of New York, Comprising the Results of Original Surveys and Explorations. *Smithsonian Contributions to Knowledge* 2(9). Washington, D.C.

Stanhope, J. M., R. J. Stuart, and D. A. Russell

1968 An Outbreak of Leprosy in a Previously Unexposed Population of Eastern New Guinea. *Transactions of the Royal Society of Tropical Medicine and Hygiene* 62:700–711.

Starna, W. A.

1980 Mohawk Iroquois Populations: A Revision. *Ethnohistory* 27:371–382.

Stearn, E. W., and A. E. Stearn

1945 *The Effects of Smallpox on the Destiny of the Amerindian*. Bruce Humphries, Boston.

Steele, J. H.

1979 Introduction. In *Bacterial, Rickettsial and Mycotic Diseases*. Handbook Series in Zoonoses 1, edited by J. H. Steele, pp. 3–13. CRC Press, Boca Raton.

Steinbock, R. T.

1976 *Paleopathological Diagnoses and Interpretations*. Charles C. Thomas, Springfield.

Steponaitis, V. P.

1978 Locational Theory and Complex Chiefdoms: A Mississippian Example. In *Mississippian Settlement Patterns*, edited by B. D. Smith, pp. 417–453. Academic Press, New York.

Sterne, M.

1959 Anthrax. In *Infectious Diseases of Animals: Disease due to Bacteria*, vol. 1., edited by A. W. Stableforth, and I. A. Galloway, pp. 16–52. Academic Press, New York.

Steward, J. H.

1942 The Direct Historical Approach to Archaeology. *American Antiquity* 7:337–343.

1949 The Native Population of South America. In *Handbook of South American Indians*, vol. 5, edited by J. H. Steward. Bureau of American Ethnology, Bulletin 143:655–668. Washington, D.C.

Stewart, F. H.

1974 Mandan and Hidatsa Villages in the Eighteenth and Nineteenth Century. *Plains Anthropologist* 19:287–302.

Stewart, T. D.

1960 A Physical Anthropologist's View of Peopling of the New World. *Southwestern Journal of Anthropology* 16:259–273.

Stewart, T. D., and A. Spoehr

1952 Evidence of the Paleopathology of Yaws. *Bulletin of the History of Medicine* 26:538–553.

Stocking, G. W.

1976 Ideas and Institutions in American Anthropology. Thoughts toward a History of the Interwar Years. In *Selected Papers of the American Anthropologist, 1921–1945*, edited by G.W. Stocking, pp. 1–53. American Anthropological Association. Washington, D.C.

Strode, G. K. (editor)

1951 *Yellow Fever*. McGraw-Hill, New York.

Strong, W. D.

1933 The Plains Culture Area in Light of Archaeology. *American Anthropologist* 35:271–287.

1935 *An Introduction to Nebraska Archaeology*. Smithsonian Miscellaneous Collections 93(10). Washington, D.C.

1940 From History to Prehistory in the Northern Great Plains. In *Essays in Historical Anthropology of North America, in Honor of John R. Swanton*. Smithsonian Miscellaneous Collections 100:353–394. Washington, D.C.

Stuart-Harris, C.

1981 The Epidemiology and Prevention of Influenza. *American Scientist* 69:166–172.

Stuiver, M.

1969 Yale Natural Radiocarbon Measurements IX. *Radiocarbon* 11:545–658.

Swan, C., A. L. Tostewin, B. Moore, H. Mayo, and G. H. Barham-Black

1943 Congenital Defects in Infants following Infectious Disease during Pregnancy. *Medical Journal of Australia* 2:201–210.

Swanton, J. R.

1911 *Indian Tribes of the Lower Mississippi Valley and Adjacent Coast of the Gulf of Mexico*. Bureau of American Ethnology, Bulletin 43. Washington, D.C.

1928 *Aboriginal Cultures of the Southeast*. Forty-second Annual Report of the Bureau of American Ethnology, 1924. Washington, D.C.

1939 *Final Report of the United States De Soto Expedition Commission*. 76th Congress, 1st Session, H.R. 71. Washington, D.C.

1969 *The Indians of the Southeastern United States* [1946]. Greenwood Press, New York.

Taylor, R. M.

1951 Epidemiology. In *Yellow Fever*, edited by G. K. Strode, pp. 426–538. McGraw-Hill, New York.

Tax, S. (editor)

1952 *Heritage of Conquest: The Ethnology of Middle America*. Free Press, Glencoe.

Theissen, T. D.

1977 A Tentative Radiocarbon Chronology for the Middle Missouri Tradition. *Plains Anthropologist* 22 *Memoir* 13: 54–82.

Thomas, C.
1894 *Report on the Mound Explorations of the Bureau of Ethnology*. Twelfth Annual Report of the Bureau of Ethnology, 1890–1891. Washington, D.C.
Thornton, R., and J. Marsh-Thornton
1981 Estimating Prehistoric American Indian Population Size for United States Area: Implications of the Nineteenth Century Population Decline and Nadir. *American Journal of Physical Anthropology* 55:47–54.
Thwaites, R. G.
1904 *Original Journals of Lewis and Clark, 1804–1806*, vols. 1 and 5. Dodd Mead, New York.
Todd, J. E.
1914 Pleistocene History of the Missouri River. *Science* 39:263–274.
Tooker, E.
1978 The League of the Iroquois: Its History, Politics and Ritual. In *Northeast*, edited by B. G. Trigger, pp. 418–41. Handbook of North American Indians, vol. 15, W. G. Sturtevant, general editor. Smithsonian Institution, Washington, D.C.
Trelease, A. W.
1971 *Indian Affairs in Colonial New York: The Seventeenth Century* [1959]. Kennikat Press, New York.
Trigger, B. G.
1962 Trade and Tribal Warfare on the St. Lawrence in the Sixteenth Century. *Ethnohistory* 9:240–256.
1976 *The Children of Aatatensic: A History of the Huron People to 1660*. 2 vols. McGill-Queens University Press, Montreal.
1978 Ethnohistory and Archaeology. *Ontario Archaeology* 30:17–24.
1981a Archaeology and the Ethnographic Present. *Anthropologica* 23:3–17.
1981b Ontario Native Peoples and the Epidemics of 1634–1640. In *Indians, Animals, and the Fur Trade: A Critique of Keepers of the Game*, edited by S. Krech III, pp. 19–38. University of Georgia Press, Athens.
1984 Archaeology at the Crossroads. What's New? *Annual Review of Anthropology* 13:275–330.
1985 *Natives and Newcomers*. McGill-Queen's University Press, Kingston.
Trimble, M. K.
1979 *An Ethnohistorical Interpretation of the Spread of Smallpox in the Northern Plains Utilizing Concepts of Disease Ecology*. National Park Service, Midwest Archeological Center. Lincoln.
Tuchman, B. W.
1978 *A Distant Mirror: The Calamitous 14th Century*. Ballentine, New York.
Tuck, J. A.
1967 The Howlett Hill Site. In *Iroquois Culture, History and Prehistory*, edited by E. Tooker, pp. 75–80. New York State Museum and Science Service, Albany.
1971 *Onondaga Iroquois History: A Study in Settlement Archaeology*. Syracuse University Press, Syracuse.
1974 The Iroquois Confederacy. In *New World Archaeology, Readings from Scientific*

American, edited by E. Zubrow, M. Fritz, and J. Fritz, pp. 190–200. W. H. Freeman, San Francisco.
1985 Unearthing Red Bay's Whaling History. *National Geographic* 168:50–71.

Upham, S.
1982 *Politics and Power: An Economic and Political History of the Western Pueblo.* Academic Press, New York.
1984a Adaptive Diversity and Southwestern Populations at Contact. Paper presented at the 49th Annual Meeting of the Society for American Archaeology, Portland.
1984b Adaptive Diversity and Southwestern Abandonment. *Journal of Anthropological Research* 40:235–256.
1986 Smallpox and Climate in the American Southwest. *American Anthropologist* 88:115–128.

Varner, J., and J. Varner
1951 *The Florida of the Inca.* University of Texas Press, Austin.

Wannamaker, L. W., C. H. Rammelkamp, and F. H. Top, Sr.
1976 Streptococcal Infections. In *Communicable and Infectious Diseases.* 8th ed., edited by F. H. Top Sr., and P. F. Wehrle, pp. 655–671. C. W. Mosby, St. Louis.

Ward, J. A.
1972 *Yellow Fever in Latin America: A Geographical Study.* Center for Latin American Studies, University of Liverpool, Monograph Series 3. Liverpool.

Warrick, G. A.
1983 Reconstructing Ontario Iroquoian Village Organization. *National Museum of Man, Mercury Series, Archaeological Survey of Canada Paper* 124:1–180. Ottawa.

Watson, P. J., R. Redman, and S. LeBlanc
1980 Aspects of Zuni Prehistory: Preliminary Report on Excavations and Survey in the El Morro Valley of New Mexico. *Journal of Field Archaeology* 7:201–218.

Watson, R. B., and R. Hewitt
1941 Topographical and Related Factors in the Epidemiology of Malaria in North America, Central America and the West Indies. In *A Symposium on Human Malaria with Special Reference to North America and the Caribbean Region*, edited by F. R. Moulton, pp. 135–147. American Association for the Advancement of Science, Publication 15. Washington, D.C.

Weakley, W. F.
1971 Tree Ring Dating and Archaeology in South Dakota. *Plains Anthropologist* 16, *Memoir* 8.

Wedel, M. M., and R. J. DeMallie
1980 The Ethnohistorical Approach in Plains Area Studies. In *Anthropology of the Great Plains*, edited by W. R. Wood, and M. Liberty, pp. 129–140. University of Nebraska Press, Lincoln.

Wedel, W. R.
1938 The Direct-Historical Approach in Pawnee Archaeology. *Smithsonian Miscellaneous Collections* 97:1–21. Washington, D.C.

Wehrle, P. F., and Z. Haddad
1976 Infection and Immunity. In *Communicable and Infectious Diseases*. 8th ed., edited by F. H. Top Sr., and P. F. Wehrle, pp. 1–7. C. W. Mosby, St. Louis.

Wenke, R. J.
1984 *Patterns in Prehistory: Man's First Three Million Years*. 2nd ed. Oxford University Press, New York.

White, M. E.
1961 *Iroquois Culture History in the Niagara Frontier Area of New York State*. Anthropological Papers 16, Museum of Anthropology, University of Michigan, Ann Arbor.

Whiteford, H. H.
1979 Anthrax. In *Bacterial, Rickettsial and Mycotic Diseases*. Handbook Series in Zoonoses 1, edited by J. H. Steele, pp. 31–66. CRC Press, Boca Raton.

Whitman, L.
1951 The Arthropod Vectors of Yellow Fever. In *Yellow Fever*, edited by G. K. Strode, pp. 228–298. McGraw-Hill, New York.

Wilkens, J., and J. W. Bass
1976 Pertussis. In *Communicable and Infectious Diseases*. 8th ed., edited by F. H. Top Sr., and P. F. Wehrle, pp. 491–501. C. W. Mosby, St. Louis.

Will, G. F.
1924 *Archaeology of the Missouri Valley*. The American Museum of Natural History, Anthropological Papers 22(6). New York.
1946 *Tree Ring Studies in North Dakota*. Agricultural Experimental Station, North Dakota Agricultural College, Bulletin 338. Fargo.

Will, G. F., and H. J. Spinden
1906 *The Mandans: A Study of their Culture, Archaeology and Language*. Peabody Museum of American Archaeology and Ethnology, Papers 3. Cambridge.

Willey, G. R., and P. Phillips
1958 *Method and Theory in American Archaeology*. University of Chicago Press, Chicago.

Willey, G. R., and J. A. Sabloff
1980 *A History of American Archaeology*. 2nd ed. W. H. Freeman and Co., San Francisco.

Williams, H. U.
1932 The Origin and Antiquity of Syphilis: The Evidence from Diseased Bones. *Archives of Pathology* 13:779–814; 931–983.
1935 The Pathology of Yaws. *Archives of Pathology* 20:596–630.
1936 The Origin of Syphilis from Diseased Bones, a Supplementary Report. *Archives of Dermatology and Syphilis* 33:783–787.

Williams, R.
1863 To John Winthrop [1638]. The Winthrop Papers. *Collections of the Massachusetts Historical Society, 4th Series* 6:229–230.

Williams, S.
1980 Armorel: A Very Late Phase in the Lower Mississippi Valley. *Southeastern Archaeological Conference, Bulletin* 22:105–110.

Williams S. and J. P. Brain
1983 *Excavations at the Lake George Site Yazoo County, Mississippi, 1958–1960.* Peabody Museum of Archaeology and Ethnology Papers 74. Cambridge.

Wisseman, C. L.
1976 Rickettsial Diseases. In *Communicable and Infectious Diseases.* 8th ed., edited by F. H. Top Sr., and P. F. Wehrle, pp. 567–584. C. W. Mosby, St. Louis.

Wissler, C.
1917 *The American Indian.* McMutrie, New York.

Wolbach, S. B., J. L. Todd, and F. Palfrey
1922 *The Etiology and Pathology of Typhus.* League of Red Cross Societies. Harvard University Press, Cambridge.

Wood, C. S.
1975 New Evidence of the Late Introduction of Malaria into the New World. *Current Anthropology* 16:93–104.
1979 *Human Sickness and Health—a Bio-Cultural View.* Mayfield, Palo Alto.

Wood, W. R.
1967 An Interpretation of Mandan Culture History. *Bureau of American Ethnology, Bulletin* 198. Washington, D.C.
1977 David Thompson at the Mandan-Hidatsa Villages, 1797–1798: The Original Journals. *Ethnohistory* 24:329–342.
1978 Notes on the Cartography of the Upper Knife-Heart Region. In *Papers in Plains Prehistory and Ethnohistory*, edited by W. R. Wood. In press, National Park Service, Anthropological Paper 3.
1980 Plains Trade in Prehistoric and Protohistoric Intertribal Relations. In *Anthropology of the Great Plains*, edited by W. R. Wood and M. Liberty, pp. 98–109. University of Nebraska Press, Lincoln.

Wood, W. R. (editor)
1976 *Fay Tolton and the Initial Middle Missouri Variant.* Missouri Archaeology Society, Research Series 3.

Wood, W. R., and A. R. Woolworth
1964 The Paul Brave site (32 SI 4), Oahe Reservoir Area, North Dakota. *Bureau of American Ethnology Bulletin* 189:1–66. Washington, D.C.

Woolworth, A. R., and W. R. Wood
1964 The Demery Site (39 CO 1), Oahe Reservoir Area, South Dakota. *Bureau of American Ethnology Bulletin* 189:67–138. Washington, D.C.

Wray, C. F.
1983 Seneca Glass Trade Beads, *circa* A.D. 1550–1820. In *Proceedings of the 1982 Glass Trade Bead Conference*, edited by C.F. Hayes III, pp. 41–49. Rochester Museum and Science Center Research Records 16. Rochester.

Wray, C. F., and H. L. Schoff
1953 A Preliminary Report on the Seneca Sequence in Western New York, 1150–1687. *Pennsylvania Archaeologist* 23:53–63.

Wright, I. A.
1970 *The Early History of Cuba 1492–1586* [1916]. Octagon Books, New York.

Wylie, A.
1985 The Reaction against Analogy. In *Advances in Archaeological Method and Theory*, vol. 8, edited by M. B. Schiffer, pp. 63–111. Academic Press, New York.
Youmans, G. P., P. Y. Paterson and H. M. Sommers
1980 *The Biologic and Clinical Basis of Infectious Disease*. 2nd ed. W. B. Saunders, Philadelphia.
Zinsser, H.
1947 *Rats, Lice and History*. Atlantic Monthly Press. Little, Brown, New York.

Index

Vectors of Death was
designed by Barbara
Werden. The type was
set by Keystone
Typesetting Company
on the Linotron 202, in
9½/12 Plantin. It was
printed on 50#
Booktext Natural at
BookCrafters, Inc., who
also printed the jackets
and bound the book.